THE INTERNATIONAL PHARMACOPOEIA

THIRD EDITION

VOLUME 2

QUALITY SPECIFICATIONS

THE INTERNATIONAL PHARMACOPOEIA

THIRD EDITION

PHARMACOPOEA INTERNATIONALIS

EDITIO TERTIA

Volume 2

Quality Specifications

WORLD HEALTH ORGANIZATION

GENEVA

1981

ISBN 92 4 154151 2

The designations employed and the presentation of the material in this publication do not imply the expression of any opinion whatsoever on the part of the Secretariat of the World Health Organization concerning the legal status of any country, territory, city or area or of its authorities, or concerning the delimitation of its frontiers or boundaries.

The mention of specific companies or of certain manufacturers' products does not imply that they are endorsed or recommended by the World Health Organization in preference to others of a similar nature that are not mentioned. Errors and omissions excepted, the names of proprietary products are distinguished by initial capital letters.

PRINTED IN SWITZERLAND

80/4839 — Presses Centrales — 9000

CONTENTS

MONOGRAPHS
(Latin names)

6   CONTENTS

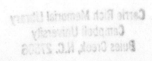

PREFACE

The *International Pharmocopoeia* is published by the World Health Organization by virtue of resolution WHA3.10[1] of the Third World Health Assembly. Information on the publication of the first and second editions of the *International Pharmacopoeia* and on the preparatory work for the third edition will be found in the preface to volume 1 of the third edition[2]. The WHO Expert Committee on Specifications for Pharmaceutical Preparations in its 27th report[3] further reviewed the organization of the work on the revision of the *International Pharmacopoeia* and drew up the tentative production schedule for the third edition, which will published in several volumes. As recommended by the Committee, volume 1 of the third edition contains the description of general methods of analysis, while the succeeding volumes will contain the monographs, i.e., quality specifications for individual drugs, primarily those most widely used in general health care.

The process of establishing and revising the quality specifications included in volume 2 of the third edition was carried out during the period 1977–79 with the help of members of the WHO Expert Advisory Panel on the International Pharmacopoeia and Pharmaceutical Preparations and other specialists. In July 1980, the draft text of volume 2 was sent for final comments to all WHO Member States, to members of the WHO Expert Advisory Panel on the International Pharmacopoeia and Pharmaceutical Preparations, and to other specialists.

The following specialists participated both in person and by correspondence in the preparation of volume 2, and commented on the final draft: Professor H.Y. Aboul-Enein, Riyad University, Riyad, Saudi Arabia; Professor E.A. Babayan, Ministry of Health, Moscow, USSR; Dr D. Banes, The United States Pharmacopeia, Rockville, MD, USA; Mr J.R. Buriánek, State Institute for the Control of Drugs, Prague, Czechoslovakia; Dr T. Canbäck, Swedish Phamacopoeia Commission, Stockholm, Sweden; Mrs E. Castrén, National Control Laboratory for Medicine, Helsinki, Finland; Dr L. Chafetz, Warner-Lambert Research Institute, Morris Plains, NJ, USA; Dr R. Chanda, State Drugs Testing and Research Laboratory, Bhubaneswar, Orissa, India; Professor E. Cingolani, Permanent Commission of the Italian Pharmacopoeia, Higher Institute of Health, Rome, Italy; Dr D. Cook, Drug Research Laboratories, Ottawa, Ontario, Canada; Dr R. Danielak, Institute for Drug Research and Control, Warsaw, Poland; Dr L.F. Dodson, National Biological Standards Laboratory, Canberra, Australia; Dr P. Emafo, Pharmaceutical Services Directorate, Federal Ministry of Health, Lagos, Nigeria; Dr K. Florey, The Squibb Institute for Medical Research, New Brunswick, NJ, USA; Dr H. Gebler, Pharmacists' Board of Lower Saxony,

---

[1] *WHO Handbook of Resolutions and Decisions,* vol. I, 1973, p. 127.

[2] WORLD HEALTH ORGANIZATION, *The International Pharmacopoeia,* third edition, Geneva, vol. 1, 1979.

[3] WHO Technical Report Series, No. 645, 1980.

Hanover, Federal Republic of Germany; Dr A.R. Gennaro, The Philadelphia College of Pharmacy and Science, Philadelphia, PA, USA; Dr T. George, Ciba-Geigy Research Centre, Goregaon, Bombay, India; Dr S.S. Gothoskar, Directorate General of Health Services, New Delhi, India; Dr L.T. Grady, The United States Pharmacopeia, Rockville, MD, USA; Mr J. Gralewicz, Quality Control Department, Polfa-Tarchomin, Warsaw, Poland; Dr T. Inoue, National Institute of Hygienic Sciences, Tokyo, Japan; Professor P. Ionesco-Stoian, Academy of Medical Sciences, Bucharest, Romania; Miss S. Johansson, WHO Collaborating Centre for Chemical Reference Substances, Solna, Sweden; Mr C.A. Johnson, British Pharmacopoeia Commission, London, England; Mrs Preeya Kashemsant, Drug Analysis Division, Ministry of Public Health, Bangkok, Thailand; Dr Kohlmeyer, Bayer AG, Wuppertal, Federal Republic of Germany; Professor L. Krówczyński, Nicolas Copernicus Medical Academy, Kraków, Poland; Dr C.S. Kumkumian, Bureau of Drugs, Food and Drug Administration, Rockville, MD, USA; Professor J. Laszlovszky, National Institute of Pharmacy, Budapest, Hungary; Dr J.W. Lightbown, National Institute for Biological Standards and Control, London, England; Dr K.L. Loening, Chemical Abstracts Service, Columbus, OH, USA; Professor M.D. Maškovskij, Pharmacopoeia Commission of the USSR, Ministry of Health, Moscow, USSR; Professor R. Moreau, Faculty of Pharmaceutical Science and Biology, René Descartes University, Paris, France; Dr E. Nieminen, National Control Laboratory for Medicine, Helsinki, Finland; Dr A.N. Obojmakova, Pharmacopoeia Committee of the USSR, Moscow, USSR; Mr B. Öhrner, WHO Collaborating Centre for Chemical Reference Substances, Solna, Sweden; Dr S. Okamoto, National Institute of Health, Tokyo, Japan; Dr T.O. Oke, Continental Pharmaceuticals Ltd., Yaba, Lagos State, Nigeria; Dr P.R. Pabrai, Central Indian Pharmacopoeia Laboratory, Ghaziabad, Uttar Pradesh, India; Dr V. Parrák, State Institute for the Control of Drugs, Bratislava, Czechoslovakia; Dr M. Pesez, Roussel Uclaf SA, Romainville, France; Professor J. Richter, Institute of Pharmacology and Therapeutics of the GDR, Berlin, German Democratic Republic; Dr S.K. Roy, Central Drugs Laboratory, Ministry of Health, Calcutta, India; Professor R.B. Salama, University of Khartoum, Sudan; Dr K. Satiadarma, Bandung Institute of Technology, Bandung, Indonesia; Dr G. Schwartzman, Association of Official Analytical Chemists, Arlington, VA, USA; Professor St. Skramovský, Czechoslovak Pharmacopoeia Commission, Prague, Czechoslovakia; Professor S.D. Sokolov, All-Union Chemico-Pharmaceutical Research Institute, Moscow, USSR; Dr I. Suzuki, National Institute of Hygienic Sciences, Tokyo, Japan; Mr Tu Guoshi, National Institution for the Control of Pharmaceutical and Biological Products, Beijing, China; Professor H. Vanderhaeghe, Rega Pharmaceutical Institute, Leuven, Belgium; Mr O. Wallén, Port Ripaille, Thonon-les-Bains, France; Dr B.A. Wills, Department of Health and Social Security, London, England; Dr W.W. Wright, The United States Pharmacopeia, Rockville, MD, USA.

Furthermore, comments were obtained from the Finnish Pharmacopoeia Commission; from the Ministries of Health of Austria and the Netherlands; and also from the Drug Research Laboratories, Ottawa, Ontario, Canada, and the National Institute for the Control of Drugs, Hanoi, Viet Nam. The World Health Organization takes this opportunity to express its gratitude to all those persons and institutions.

Dr D. Cook served as Chairman at the 27th meeting of the WHO Expert Committee on Specifications for Pharmaceutical Preparations. The function of Secretary to the Committee was assumed by Dr W. Wieniawski, Chief Pharmaceutical Officer, assisted by Miss M. Schmid, Technical Assistant.

Volume 2 contains quality specifications for 126 individual pharmaceutical substances. For some of these substances no international quality specifications have previously been issued. Specifications that were included in the second edition of the *International Pharmacopoeia* have been subjected to thorough revision.

For substances used in more than one form (e.g., anhydrous and hydrated, or non-injectable and sterile) the requirements for the relevant forms have been put together in a single monograph, but separate tests have been provided, as required, for each specific form.

The methods of analysis used in the monographs included in volume 2 are described in volume 1 of the third edition. The general notices that are given in the present volume should also be taken together with the relevant general notices issued in volume 1. A similar comment applies to the notes on patents, trademarks, and the use of trade names included in volume 1.

The international chemical reference substances referred to in the monographs may be obtained from the WHO Collaborating Centre for Chemical Reference Substances, Box 3045, 171 03 Solna, 3, Sweden.

Infrared reference spectra are mentioned in a number of monographs. A separate publication containing reproductions of such spectra will be issued at a later date.

In accordance with the World Health Assembly resolution WHA3.10 mentioned above, the *International Pharmacopoeia* constitutes a collection of recommended methods and specifications that are not intended to have a legal status as such in any country, unless expressly introduced for that purpose by appropriate legislation, but are offered to serve as reference so that national requirements can be established on a similar basis in any country. Any Member State of the World Health Organization may include all or part of these provisions in its national requirements.

GENERAL NOTICES

Monograph nomenclature

Unless otherwise indicated, the monograph title is a singular Latin form of the recommended or proposed *International Nonproprietary Name (INN)*.

All names with certain traditional exceptions are treated as second declension neuter substantives (e.g., Ethosuximidum).

With salts, the method of nomenclature adopted is the traditional one of placing the name of the acid component in the nominative case (either second declension neuter or third declension masculine) and the other component in the genitive case (e.g., Codeini phosphas). With compounds that are not derived from true acids, both components of the title are placed in the nominative case, treating the main component as a neuter substantive and using an adjectival form of the complementary component in agreement with this substantive (e.g., Cloxacillinum with "Natricus" as the adjectival form of Natrium, thus Cloxacillinum natricum).

The English name of the pharmacopoeial substance is given below the Latin title of each monograph, and the English equivalents of the Latin titles are used throughout the monograph texts of the *International Pharmacopoeia*.

In exceptional cases where a second name is also in general use, it is given as "Other name".

Chemical formulas

When the chemical composition of a pharmacopoeial substance is known or generally accepted, the molecular chemical formula and the relative molecular mass are given at the beginning of the monograph for purposes of information. For organic substances, the graphic formula, when known or generally accepted, is also given. The chemical formulas and relative molecular masses given at the beginning of the monographs are those of the chemically pure substances and are not to be regarded as an indication of the purity of the pharmacopoeial drug. Elsewhere, in statements of specifications of purity and strength, and in descriptions of processes of assay, it is evident from the context that the formulas denote the pure chemical substances.

Chemical names

The chemical names are given in accordance with the rules published by the International Union of Pure and Applied Chemistry (IUPAC). In many cases, when equally acceptable alternative names may be construed under these rules, more than one systematic name is given. Such alternative names are given especially when changes in the interpretation of IUPAC rules occuring in recent years have led to substantial modifications of the chemical names used for the substance. To facilitate further the recognition of the substance, the registry number established by the Chemical Abstracts Service of the American Chemical Society (CAS No.) is also given.

Identity tests

The identity tests are provided for the verification of identity of the substance described in the monograph and a judgement by the analyst is needed as to the extent of testing required, taking into account the available instrumentation.

It is generally recognized that the infrared spectrum provides the best method of identification because of the uniqueness of a well-developed finger print region of the spectrum for a given drug substance.

Wherever possible infrared spectrum characteristics are used as the primary test of identification. Usually this can stand by itself without any additional test. Further identification tests provided in an individual monograph, taken together, are intended to provide verification of identity, should the use of an infrared spectrophotometer be precluded.

It should further be noted that whenever a melting temperature is provided under the heading "Identity tests", only an approximate value is given, since no exact reproduction of the quoted temperature is necessary.

Impurities

The requirements of the monographs are not framed to provide against all possible impurities. It is not to be presumed, for example, that an unusual impurity is to be tolerated, even if it is not precluded by the prescribed tests, should rational considerations and good manufacturing practice require that it be absent. The tests selected have been designed to detect or determine the impurities to which attention is more particularly needed, to fix the limits of those that are tolerated to a given extent, and to indicate convenient methods of ensuring a practical absence of certain others for which no tolerance is approved. In some purity tests limits are indicated additionally in brackets in percentage terms. Such limits are given for information only.

Water

When water is referred to in the tests, distilled or demineralized water of adequate purity is to be used.

Clarity of solution

The determination of the clarity of solution is done as described in volume 1 under "Colour of liquids", but using a black background. The source of light must be such that opalescence standard TS2 can be readily distinguished from water.

A solution is clear if its opalescence is not more pronounced than that of opalescence standard TS2.

Colourless solution

A solution is considered colourless if, when compared as described in volume 1 under "Colour of liquids", it is not more intensely coloured than any of the standard colour solutions Bn0, Yw0, Gn0, or Rd0, the matching being made with the standard colour solution of most appropriate hue.

Indicators for visual determination of pH values

Indicators and indicator papers used in the tests and assays for the determination of the pH value or of its change by visual inspection of colour can be replaced by other indicators that exhibit a colour change at the same pH range.

Water-bath

When a water-bath is referred to in the text, a bath with boiling water (about 100 °C) is to be used unless a specific water temperature is given.

Examination in ultraviolet light

When examination in ultraviolet light (254 nm or 365 nm) is referred to in the text, an ultraviolet lamp having a maximum output at about 254 nm, or at about 365 nm, respectively, is to be used.

Loss on drying

The desiccants mentioned in the loss on drying test may be replaced by other substances of equivalent desiccant capacity.

Containers

The following term describing additional requirements for the permeability of containers is added to those given in volume 1.

Hermetically closed container. It must protect the contents from extraneous matter and from loss of the substance and be impervious to air or any other gas under the ordinary or customary conditions of handling, shipment, or storage.

Stability information

For those substances that are easily degraded in adverse storage conditions such as occur in tropical climates, a warning is given indicating that the substance is degraded on exposure to a humid atmosphere and that the decomposition is faster at more elevated temperatures. In such cases a special mention is added as additional information.

For substances that are stable even in unfavourable conditions of temperature and humidity but are adversely affected on exposure to light, a statement is included in the information on storage conditions indicating the need of protecting such substances from light.

Category

The statements given under this heading are intended *only as information* on the principal pharmacological actions and therapeutic uses of the concerned substances. It should not be assumed that the substance has no other action or use and the statements are in no way intended to be binding.

MONOGRAPHS

ACETAZOLAMIDUM

Acetazolamide

Molecular formula. $C_4H_6N_4O_3S_2$

Relative molecular mass. 222.2

Graphic formula.

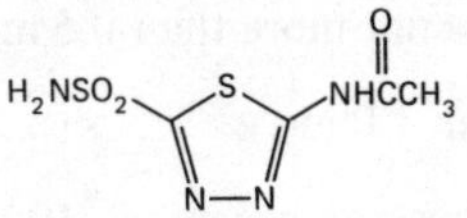

Chemical name. *N*-(5-Sulfamoyl-1,3,4-thiadiazol-2-yl)acetamide; *N*-[5-(amino-sulfonyl)-1,3,4-thiadiazol-2-yl]acetamide; 5-acetamido-1,3,4-thiadiazole-2-sulfonamide; CAS Reg. No. 59-66-5.

Description. A white, or almost white, crystalline powder; odourless.

Solubility. Very slightly soluble in water; slightly soluble in ethanol (~750 g/l) TS; practically insoluble in ether R and chloroform R.

Category. Carbonic anhydrase inhibitor.

Storage. Acetazolamide should be kept in a well-closed container.

REQUIREMENTS

General requirement. Acetazolamide contains not less than 99.0% and not more than 101.0% of $C_4H_6N_4O_3S_2$, calculated with reference to the dried substance.

Identity tests

A. Carry out the examination as described under "Spectrophotometry in the infrared region" (vol. 1, p. 40). The infrared absorption spectrum is concordant with the spectrum obtained from acetazolamide RS or with the *reference spectrum* of acetazolamide.

B. Dissolve 25 mg in 5 ml of water, add 0.15 ml of sodium hydroxide (1 mol/l) VS and 0.1 ml of copper(II) sulfate (80 g/l) TS; a bluish green colour or precipitate is formed.

C.   Triturate 0.5 g with a mixture of 5 ml of water and 1 ml of sodium hydroxide (1 mol/l) VS, add 0.2 g of zinc R powder and 0.5 ml of hydrochloric acid (~420 g/l) TS; hydrogen sulfide is evolved and may be detected by its odour (proceed with caution), or by the use of filter paper soaked in lead acetate (80 g/l) TS which turns black on exposure.

Heavy metals.   Use 1.0 g for the preparation of the test solution as described under "Limit test for heavy metals", Procedure 3 (vol. 1, p. 118); determine the heavy metal content according to Method A (vol. 1, p. 119); not more than 20 μg/g.

Sulfates.   Dissolve 1.0 g in 40 ml of water, warm to 70 °C for 5 minutes, cool and filter.   Proceed with the filtrate as described under "Limit test for sulfates" (vol. 1, p. 116); the sulfate content is not more than 0.5 mg/g.

Sulfated ash.   Not more than 1.0 mg/g.

Loss on drying.   Dry to constant weight at 105 °C; it loses not more than 5.0 mg/g.

pH value.   Shake 1 g with 50 ml of water for 5 minutes; pH of the suspension, 4.0–6.0.

Related substances.   Carry out the test as described under "Thin-layer chromatography" (vol. 1, p. 83), using silica gel R2 as the coating substance and a mixture of 30 volumes of dioxan R, 30 volumes of 2-propanol R, 20 volumes of ammonia (~35 g/l) TS, 10 volumes of toluene R, and 10 volumes of xylene R as the mobile phase.   Apply separately to the plate 20 μl of each of 2 solutions in ethanol (~750 g/l) TS containing (A) 5.0 mg of the test substance per ml and (B) 0.050 mg of the test substance per ml.   After removing the plate from the chromatographic chamber, allow it to dry in air, and examine the chromatogram in ultraviolet light (254 nm).   Any spot obtained with solution A, other than the principal spot, is not more intense than that obtained with solution B.

Assay.   Dissolve about 0.45 g, accurately weighed, in 90 ml of dimethylformamide R and titrate with tetrabutylammonium hydroxide (0.1 mol/l) VS determining the endpoint potentiometrically as described under "Non-aqueous titration", Method B (vol. 1, p. 132). Each ml of tetrabutylammonium hydroxide (0.1 mol/l) VS is equivalent to 22.22 mg of $C_4H_6N_4O_3S_2$.

ACIDUM ACETYLSALICYLICUM

Acetylsalicylic acid

Molecular formula. $C_9H_8O_4$

Relative molecular mass. 180.2

Graphic formula.

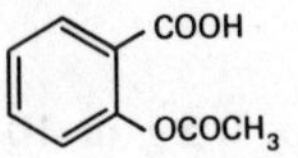

Chemical name. 2-(Acetyloxy)benzoic acid; 2-acetoxybenzoic acid; CAS Reg. No. 50-78-2.

Description. Colourless crystals or a white, crystalline powder; odourless or almost odourless.

Solubility. Soluble in about 300 parts of water; freely soluble in ethanol ($\sim$750 g/l) TS; soluble in ether R and chloroform R.

Category. Analgesic; antipyretic.

Storage. Acetylsalicylic acid should be kept in a tightly closed container, protected from light.

Additional information. Even in the absence of light, Acetylsalicylic acid is gradually degraded on exposure to a humid atmosphere, the decomposition being faster at higher temperatures.

REQUIREMENTS

General requirement. Acetylsalicylic acid contains not less than 99.0% and not more than 100.5% of $C_9H_8O_4$, calculated with reference to the dried substance.

Identity tests

A. Heat 0.05 g in 2 ml of water for several minutes, cool, and add 1–2 drops of ferric chloride (25 g/l) TS; a violet-red colour is produced, which does not change on the addition of ethanol ($\sim$750 g/l) TS.

B. Boil 0.2 g with 4 ml of sodium hydroxide ($\sim$80 g/l) TS for about 3 minutes, cool, and add 5 ml of sulfuric acid ($\sim$100 g/l) TS; a white, crystalline precipitate is formed. Filter (keep the filtrate for test C), wash the precipitate with water and dry at 105 °C. Melting temperature, about 159 °C (salicylic acid).

C.   Heat the filtrate from test B with 2 ml of ethanol (~750 g/l) TS and 2 ml of sulfuric acid (~1760 g/l) TS; ethyl acetate, perceptible by its odour (proceed with caution), is produced.

Heavy metals.   Use 1.0 g and 25 ml of acetone R for the preparation of the test solution as described under "Limit test for heavy metals", procedure 2 (vol. 1, p. 118); determine the heavy metal content according to Method A (vol. 1, p. 119); not more than 20 μg/g.

Solution in ethanol.   A solution of 1.0 g in 10 ml of ethanol (~750 g/l) TS is clear and colourless.

Solution in alkali.   A solution of 0.5 g in 10 ml of warm sodium carbonate (50 g/l) TS is clear.

Sulfated ash.   Not more than 1.0 mg/g.

Loss on drying.   Dry to constant weight at ambient temperature under reduced pressure (not exceeding 0.6 kPa or about 5 mm of mercury) over silica gel, desiccant, R; it loses not more than 5.0 mg/g.

Salicylic acid.   Dissolve 0.50 g in sufficient ethanol (~750 g/l) TS to produce 25 ml and transfer 10 ml to a comparison tube. Dissolve separately 0.040 g of salicylic acid R in sufficient water to produce 100 ml. Transfer 1 ml of this solution to a second comparison tube and add to it 10 ml of ethanol (~750 g/l) TS. Add water to both tubes to make 50 ml, followed by 1 ml of ferric ammonium sulfate TS1, mix and allow to stand for 1 minute. The violet colour of the test solution is not more intense than that of the reference solution when compared as described under "Colour of liquids" (vol. 1, p. 50); the salicylic acid content is not more than 2.0 mg/g.

Assay.   To about 0.20 g, accurately weighed, add 50 ml of carbonate-free sodium hydroxide (0.1 mol/l) VS, and boil under reflux for 10 minutes. Titrate the excess of alkali with sulfuric acid (0.05 mol/l) TS, using phenolphthalein/ethanol TS as indicator. Repeat the operation without the substance being examined and make any necessary corrections. Each ml of carbonate-free sodium hydroxide (0.1 mol/l) VS is equivalent to 9.008 mg of $C_9H_8O_4$.

ACIDUM ASCORBICUM

Ascorbic acid

Molecular formula. $C_6H_8O_6$

Relative molecular mass. 176.1

Graphic formula.

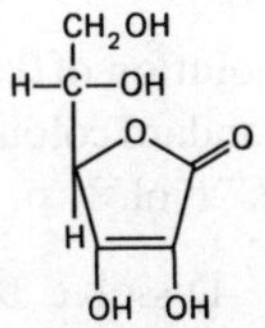

```
        CH₂OH
         |
   H—C—OH
       O.      O
   H
    OH  OH
```

Chemical name. L-Ascorbic acid; CAS Reg. No. 50-81-7.

Description. Colourless crystals or a white or almost white, crystalline powder; odourless or almost odourless.

Solubility. Freely soluble in water; soluble in ethanol (~750 g/l) TS; practically insoluble in ether R and chloroform R.

Category. Antiscorbutic.

Storage. Ascorbic acid should be kept in a tightly closed, non-metallic container, protected from light.

Additional information. Ascorbic acid in solution deteriorates rapidly in contact with air; it has an acid taste. Even in the absence of light, Ascorbic acid is gradually degraded on exposure to a humid atmosphere, the decomposition being faster at higher temperatures.

REQUIREMENTS

General requirement. Ascorbic acid contains not less than 99.0% and not more than 100.5% of $C_6H_8O_6$.

Identity tests

A.   Dissolve 0.1 g in 2 ml of water, add a few drops of nitric acid (~130 g/l) TS and a few drops of silver nitrate (40 g/l) TS; a dark grey precipitate is produced.

B.   Dissolve 0.04 g in 4 ml of water, add 0.1 g of sodium hydrogen carbonate R and about 20 mg of ferrous sulfate R, shake and allow to stand; a deep violet colour is produced, which disappears on the addition of 5 ml of sulfuric acid (~100 g/l) TS.

C.   Melting temperature, about 190 °C with decomposition.

Specific optical rotation.   Use a 50 mg/ml solution; $[\alpha]_D^{20\,°C} = +20.5$ to $+21.5°$.

Heavy metals.   Use 1.0 g for the preparation of the test solution as described under "Limit test for heavy metals", Procedure 3 (vol. 1, p. 118); determine the heavy metals content according to Method A (vol. 1, p. 119); not more than 20 μg/g.

Clarity and colour of solution.   A solution of 0.50 g in 10 ml of water is clear and not more intensely coloured than standard colour solution Rd1 when compared as described under "Colour of liquids" (vol. 1, p. 50).

Readily carbonizable substances.   Dissolve 0.10 g in 10 ml of sulfuric acid (~1760 g/l) TS.   After 15 minutes the solution is not more intensely coloured than standard colour solutions Yw1 or Gn1 when compared as described under "Colour of liquids" (vol. 1, p. 50).

Sulfated ash.   Not more than 1.0 mg/g.

Assay.   Dissolve about 0.20 g, accurately weighed, in a mixture of 25 ml of carbon-dioxide-free water R and 25 ml of sulfuric acid (~100 g/l) TS. Titrate the solution at once with iodine (0.1 mol/l) VS using starch TS as indicator, added towards the end of the titration, until a persistent blue colour is obtained. Each ml of iodine (0.1 mol/l) VS is equivalent to 8.806 mg of $C_6H_8O_6$.

ACIDUM BENZOICUM

Benzoic acid

Molecular formula. $C_7H_6O_2$

Relative molecular mass.   122.1

Graphic formula.

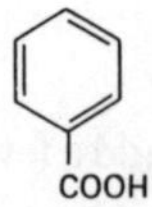

Chemical name.   Benzenecarboxylic acid; CAS Reg. No. 65-85-0.

Description.   Colourless, light, feathery crystals or a white, microcrystalline powder; odour, characteristic, faint.

Solubility. Slightly soluble in water; freely soluble in ethanol (~750 g/l) TS, ether R, and chloroform R.

Category. Dermatological agent.

Storage. Benzoic acid should be kept in a well-closed container.

REQUIREMENTS

General requirement. Benzoic acid contains not less than 99.0% and not more than 100.5% of $C_7H_6O_2$, calculated with reference to the anhydrous substance.

Identity test

Boil 0.1 g with 0.1 g of calcium carbonate R1 and 5 ml of water, and filter; add a few drops of ferric chloride (25 g/l) TS to the filtrate; a beige coloured precipitate is produced.

Melting range. 121–124°C.

Heavy metals. For the preparation of the test solution use 1.0 g dissolved in 25 ml of acetone R, add 2 ml of water and dilute to 40 ml with acetone R and mix; determine the heavy metal content as described under "Limit test for heavy metals", according to Method A (vol. 1, p. 119); not more than 20 μg/g.

Chlorinated compounds and chlorides. Dissolve 0.35 g in 5 ml of sodium carbonate (50 g/l) TS, evaporate to dryness, and heat the residue until completely charred, keeping the temperature below 400 °C. Extract the residue with a mixture of 10 ml of water and 12 ml of nitric acid (~130 g/l) TS, and filter. Proceed with the filtrate as described under "Limit test for chlorides" (vol. 1, p. 116); the chloride content is not more than 0.7 mg/g.

Sulfated ash. Not more than 1.0 mg/g.

Water. Determine as described under "Determination of water by the Karl Fischer method", Method A (vol. 1, p. 135), using about 1 g of the substance and 25 ml of a solution composed of 1 volume of methanol R and 2 volumes of pyridine R as the solvent; the water content is not more than 7.0 mg/g.

Readily oxidizable substances. Add 1.5 ml of sulfuric acid (~1760 g/l) TS to 100 ml of water, heat to boiling, and add, drop by drop, potassium permanganate (0.02 mol/l) VS until the pink colour persists for 30 seconds. Dissolve 1.0 g of the substance being examined in the hot solution and titrate with potassium permanganate (0.02 mol/l) VS to a pink colour that persists for 15 seconds; not more than 0.5 ml of potassium permanganate (0.02 mol/l) VS is required.

Assay. Dissolve about 0.25 g, accurately weighed, in 15 ml of ethanol (~750 g/l) TS, previously neutralized to phenol red/ethanol TS, add 20 ml of water and titrate with sodium hydroxide (0.1 mol/l) VS, using phenol red/ethanol TS as indicator. Repeat the operation without the substance being examined and make any necessary corrections. Each ml of sodium hydroxide (0.1 mol/l) VS is equivalent to 12.21 mg of $C_7H_6O_2$.

ACIDUM FOLICUM

Folic acid

Molecular formula. $C_{19}H_{19}N_7O_6$

Relative molecular mass. 441.4

Graphic formula.

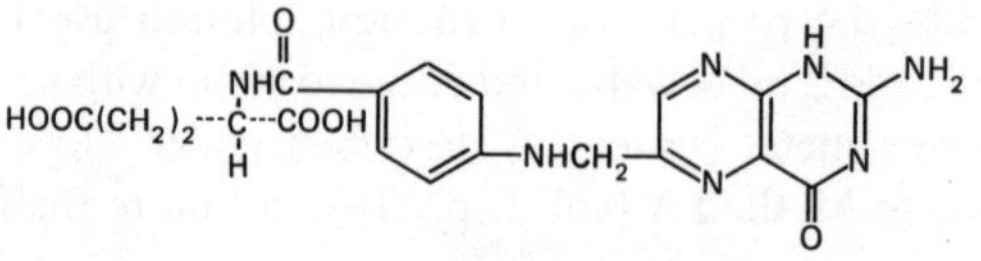

Chemical name. N-[p-[[(2-Amino-4-hydroxy-6-pteridinyl)methyl]amino]-benzoyl]-L-glutamic acid; N-[4-[[(2-amino-1,4-dihydro-4-oxo-6-pteridinyl)-methyl]amino]benzoyl]-L-glutamic acid; CAS Reg. No. 59-30-3.

Description. A yellow or yellowish orange, crystalline powder; odourless or almost odourless.

Solubility. Very slightly soluble in water; practically insoluble in ethanol (~750 g/l) TS, acetone R, chloroform R, and ether R.

Category. Haemopoietic.

Storage. Folic acid should be kept in a well-closed container, protected from light.

REQUIREMENTS

General requirement. Folic acid contains not less than 96.0% and not more than 102.0% of $C_{19}H_{19}N_7O_6$, calculated with reference to the anhydrous substance.

Identity tests

A. The absorption spectrum of a 15 μg/ml solution in sodium hydroxide (0.1 mol/l) VS, when observed between 230 nm and 380 nm, exhibits 3 maxima at about 256 nm, 283 nm, and 365 nm. The absorbances at these wavelengths are about 0.82, 0.80 and 0.28, respectively (preferably use 2-cm cells for the measurements and calculate the absorbances of 1-cm layers). The ratio of the absorbance of a 1-cm layer at 256 nm to that at 365 nm is between 2.80 and 3.00.

B. Carry out the test as described under "Thin-layer chromatography" (vol. 1, p. 83), using silica gel R1 as the coating substance and a mixture of 2 volumes of 1-propanol R, 1 volume of ethanol (~750 g/l) TS, and 2 volumes of ammonia (~260 g/l) TS as the mobile phase. Apply separately to the plate 2 μl of each of 2 solutions in a mixture of 9 volumes of methanol R and 1 volume of ammonia (~260 g/l) TS containing (A) 0.50 mg of the test substance per ml and (B) 0.50 mg of folic acid RS per ml. After removing the plate from the chromatographic chamber, allow it to dry in air, and examine the chromatogram in ultraviolet light (365 nm). The principal spot obtained with solution A corresponds in position, appearance, and intensity with that obtained with solution B.

Sulfated ash. Not more than 2.0 mg/g.

Water. Determine as described under "Determination of water by the Karl Fischer method", Method A (vol. 1, p. 135), using about 0.15 g of the substance; the water content is not less than 70 mg/g and not more than 90 mg/g.

Free amines. The ratio of the absorbance A_T of the test solution T_2 to the absorbance A_B of the blank solution B_1, as measured in the assay, should be larger than 6.

Assay. Prepare the test solution T by dissolving about 0.050 g, accurately weighed, in 50 ml of sodium hydroxide (~80 g/l) TS, mixing and diluting with sodium hydroxide (~80 g/l) TS to 100 ml.

Transfer 30.0 ml of the test solution to a 100-ml volumetric flask (test solution T_1), and a second aliquot of 30.0 ml of the test solution to a second 100-ml volumetric flask (blank B_1). To both solutions, T_1 and blank B_1, add 20 ml of hydrochloric acid (~70 g/l) TS and dilute them both with water to volume. Retain blank solution B_1. To 60 ml of the test solution T_1 add 0.5 g of zinc R powder, and allow to stand, shaking frequently, for 20 minutes. Filter the mixture through a dry filter paper, discard the first 10 ml of the filtrate, and dilute 10 ml of the subsequent filtrate with water to 100 ml (test solution T_2).

Into three separate 25-ml volumetric flasks place 5.0 ml each of test solution T_2, of blank solution B_1, and of water (solution B_2), add to each of them 1 ml of water, 1 ml of hydrochloric acid (~70 g/l) TS, and 1 ml of sodium nitrite (1 g/l) TS, mix well and allow to stand for 2 minutes. Then add to each of them 1 ml of ammonium sulfamate (5 g/l) TS, mix thoroughly, allow to stand for 2 minutes, add

1 ml of N-(1-naphthyl)ethylenediamine hydrochloride (1 g/l) TS, shake, allow to stand for 10 minutes, and dilute with water to volume.

Measure the absorbance of the test solution T_2 and of the blank solution B_1 against a solvent cell containing solution B_2 at the maximum of about 550 nm; designate these as A_T and A_B, respectively.

Carry out a similar procedure using folic acid RS and designate the respective absorbances as A_S and A_{BS}.

Calculate the content of $C_{19}H_{19}N_7O_6$ in terms of the percentage of anhydrous substance in the test substance, using the formula: $100 (10 A_T - A_B)/(10A_S - A_{BS})$, if necessary multiplying the result by the declared content (%) of $C_{19}H_{19}N_7O_6$ in the chemical reference substance.

ACIDUM NICOTINICUM

Nicotinic acid

Molecular formula. $C_6H_5NO_2$

Relative molecular mass.   123.1

Graphic formula.

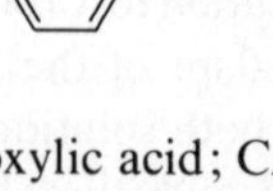

Chemical name.   3-Pyridinecarboxylic acid; CAS Reg. No. 59-67-6.

Description.   Colourless crystals or a white, crystalline powder; odourless or almost odourless.

Solubility.   Sparingly soluble in water; freely soluble in boiling water; soluble in 100 parts of ethanol (~750 g/l) TS; practically insoluble in ether R.

Category.   Component of vitamin B complex; vasodilator.

Storage.   Nicotinic acid should be kept in a well-closed container, protected from light.

REQUIREMENTS

General requirement. Nicotinic acid contains not less than 99.0% and not more than 101.0% of $C_6H_5NO_2$, calculated with reference to the dried substance.

Identity tests

• Either test A alone or all 3 tests B, C and D may be applied.

A. Carry out the examination as described under "Spectrophotometry in the infrared region" (vol. 1, p. 40). The infrared absorption spectrum is concordant with the spectrum obtained from nicotinic acid RS or with the *reference spectrum* of nicotinic acid.

B. Heat 0.1 g with 0.4 g of anhydrous sodium carbonate R; pyridine, perceptible by its odour, is produced.

C. Dissolve 10 mg in 10 ml of water. To 2 ml add 2 ml of thiocyanate reagent, obtained by adding, drop by drop, ammonium thiocyanate (0.1 mol/l) VS to bromine TS1 until the yellow coloration disappears. Then add 3 ml of aniline (25 g/l) TS and shake; a yellow colour is produced.

D. Melting temperature, about 235 °C.

Heavy metals. Use 1.0 g for the preparation of the test solution as described under "Limit test for heavy metals", Procedure 3 (vol. 1, p. 118); determine the heavy metals content according to Method A (vol. 1, p. 119); not more than 20 μg/g.

Chlorides. Dissolve 1.25 g in a mixture of 2 ml of nitric acid ($\sim$130 g/l) TS and 20 ml of water, filter if necessary, and proceed as described under "Limit test for chlorides" (vol. 1, p. 116); the chloride content is not more than 0.2 mg/g.

Sulfated ash. Not more than 1.0 mg/g.

Loss on drying. Dry to constant weight at 105 °C; it loses not more than 10 mg/g.

pH value. pH of a 13 mg/ml solution, 3.0–3.5.

Related substances. Carry out the test as described under "Thin-layer chromatography" (vol. 1, p. 83), using silica gel R2 as the coating substance and a mixture of 85 volumes of 1-propanol R, 10 volumes of anhydrous formic acid R, and 5 volumes of water as the mobile phase. For the test solution, dissolve 75 mg in 5.0 ml of water with gentle heating; this constitutes solution A. Prepare a reference solution containing 0.12 mg/ml of nicotinic acid RS; this constitutes solution B. Apply to the plate 10 μl of solution A using two 5-μl aliquots, allowing the plate to dry in a current of cold air after the first application; then apply separately 5 μl of solution B. After removing the plate from the chromatographic chamber, allow it to dry in a current of warm air, and examine the chromatogram in ultraviolet light (254 nm). Beside the principal spot, not more than 3 spots are obtained with solution A, and they are not more intense than the spot obtained with solution B.

Assay. Dissolve about 0.25 g, accurately weighed, in 50 ml of carbon-dioxide-free water R, and titrate with carbonate-free sodium hydroxide (0.1 mol/l) VS, using phenolphthalein/ethanol TS as indicator. Each ml of carbonate-free sodium hydroxide (0.1 mol/l) VS is equivalent to 12.31 mg of $C_6H_5NO_2$.

ACIDUM SALICYLICUM

Salicylic acid

Molecular formula. $C_7H_6O_3$

Relative molecular mass. 138.1

Graphic formula.

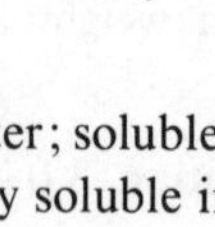

Chemical name. 2-Hydroxybenzoic acid; CAS Reg. No. 69-72-7.

Description. Colourless crystals, usually needle-like, or a white, crystalline powder; odourless.

Solubility. Slightly soluble in water; soluble in 4 parts of ethanol (~750 g/l) TS and in 3 parts of ether R; sparingly soluble in chloroform R.

Category. Keratolytic.

Storage. Salicylic acid should be kept in a well-closed container.

REQUIREMENTS

General requirement. Salicylic acid contains not less than 99.0% and not more than 101.0% of $C_7H_6O_3$, calculated with reference to the dried substance.

Identity test

Dissolve 0.14 g in 1 ml of sodium hydroxide (1 mol/l) VS and add 5 ml of water; this solution yields the reaction described under "General identification tests" as characteristic of salicylates (vol. 1, p. 114).

Melting range. 158–161 °C.

Heavy metals. Use 2.0 g and 15 ml of ethanol (~750 g/l) TS for the preparation of the test solution as described under "Limit test for heavy metals", Procedure 2 (vol. 1, p. 118); determine the heavy metals content according to Method A (vol. 1, p. 119); not more than 20 μg/g.

Chlorides. Dissolve 1.7 g in 40 ml of boiling water, cool and filter. Add 2 ml of nitric acid (~130 g/l) TS to the filtrate and proceed as described under "Limit test for chlorides" (vol. 1, p. 112); the chloride content is not more than 0.15 mg/g.

Sulfates. Dissolve 2.5 g in 40 ml of boiling water, cool, filter, and proceed with the filtrate as described under "Limit test for sulfates" (vol. 1, p. 116); the sulfate content is not more than 0.2 mg/g.

Solution in ethanol. A solution of 1.0 g in 10 ml of ethanol (~750 g/l) TS is clear and colourless.

Sulfated ash. Not more than 1.0 mg/g.

Loss on drying. Dry to constant weight over silica gel, desiccant, R at ambient temperature; it loses not more than 5.0 mg/g.

Assay. Dissolve about 0.3 g, accurately weighed, in 15 ml of neutralized ethanol TS and add 20 ml of water. Titrate with carbonate-free sodium hydroxide (0.1 mol/l) VS, using phenolphthalein/ethanol TS as indicator. Repeat the operation without the substance being examined and make any necessary corrections. Each ml of carbonate-free sodium hydroxide (0.1 mol/l) VS is equivalent to 13.81 mg of $C_7H_6O_3$.

ALLOPURINOLUM
Allopurinol

Molecular formula. $C_5H_4N_4O$

Relative molecular mass. 136.1

Graphic formula.

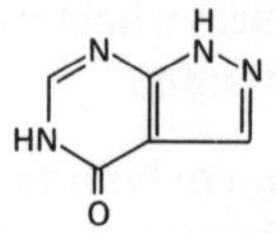

Chemical name. 1,5-Dihydro-4*H*-pyrazolo[3,4-*d*]pyrimidin-4-one; 1-*H*-pyra-zolo[3,4-*d*]pyrimidin-4-ol; CAS Reg. No. 315-30-0.

Description. A white or almost white, microcrystalline powder; odourless or almost odourless.

Solubility. Very slightly soluble in water and in ethanol (~750 g/l) TS; practically insoluble in chloroform R and ether R.

Category. Xanthine oxidase inhibitor.

Storage. Allopurinol should be kept in a well-closed container.

REQUIREMENTS

General requirement. Allopurinol contains not less than 98.0% and not more than 101.0% of $C_5H_4N_4O$, calculated with reference to the dried substance.

Identity tests

A. Carry out the examination as described under "Spectrophotometry in the infrared region" (vol. 1, p. 40). The infrared absorption spectrum is concordant with the spectrum obtained from allopurinol RS or with the *reference spectrum* of allopurinol.

B. Dissolve 0.1 g in 10 ml of sodium hydroxide (0.1 mol/l) VS and add sufficient hydrochloric acid (0.1 mol/l) VS to produce 100 ml; dilute 10 ml to 100 ml with hydrochloric acid (0.1 mol/l) VS and dilute 10 ml of this solution again to 100 ml with hydrochloric acid (0.1 mol/l) VS. The absorption spectrum of the resulting solution, when observed between 230 nm and 350 nm, exhibits a maximum at about 250 nm and a minimum at about 231 nm. The absorbance at the maximum wavelength is about 0.55. The ratio of the absorbance of a 1-cm layer at 231 nm to that at 250 nm is between 0.52 and 0.62.

C. Dissolve 0.05 g in 5 ml of sodium hydroxide (~80 g/l) TS, add 1 ml of alkaline potassio-mercuric iodide TS, heat to boiling, and allow to stand; a yellow, flocculent precipitate is produced.

Heavy metals. Use 1.0 g for the preparation of the test solution as described under "Limit test for heavy metals", Procedure 3 (vol. 1, p. 118); determine the heavy metals content according to Method A (vol. 1, p. 119); not more than 20 μg/g.

Sulfated ash. Not more than 1.0 mg/g.

Loss on drying. Dry to constant weight at 105 °C; it loses not more than 5.0 mg/g.

Related substances. Carry out the test as described under "Thin-layer chromatography" (vol. 1, p. 83), using cellulose R3 as the coating substance. Prepare the mobile phase by shaking 200 ml of 1-butanol R with 200 ml of ammonia (~100 g/l) TS. Apply separately to the plate 10 μl of each of 2 freshly prepared solutions in diethylamine R containing (A) 25 mg of the test substance per ml and (B) 0.050 mg of 3-aminopyrazole-4-carboxamide hemisulfate RS per ml. After removing the plate from the chromatographic chamber, allow it to dry in air, and examine the chromatogram in ultraviolet light (254 nm). Any spot obtained with solution A, other than the principal spot, is not more intense than that obtained with solution B.

Assay. Dissolve about 0.25 g, accurately weighed, in 50 ml of dimethylformamide R, add 2 drops of thymol blue/dimethylformamide TS and titrate with sodium methoxide (0.1 mol/l) VS to a blue endpoint, as described under "Non-aqueous titration", Method B (vol. 1, p. 132). Each ml of sodium methoxide (0.1 mol/l) VS is equivalent to 13.61 mg of $C_5H_4N_4O$.

AMINOPHYLLINUM

Aminophylline

Molecular formula. $(C_7H_8N_4O_2)_2,C_2H_8N_2$ (anhydrous) or $C_{16}H_{24}N_{10}O_4$

Relative molecular mass. 420.4 (anhydrous)

Graphic formula.

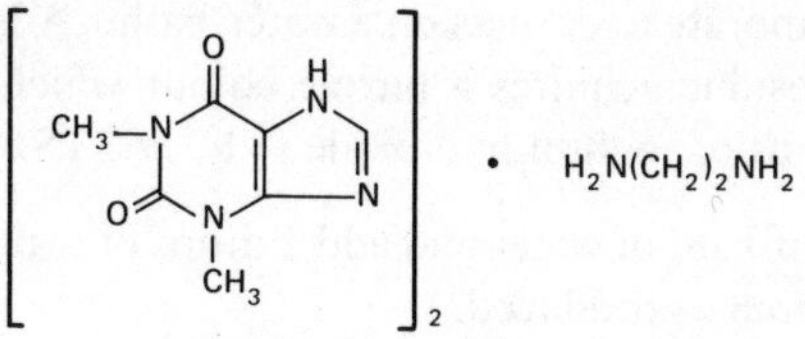

Chemical name. Theophylline compound with ethylenediamine (2:1); 3,7-dihydro-1,3-dimethyl-1H-purine-2,6-dione compound with 1,2-ethanediamine (2:1); CAS Reg. No. 317-34-0 (anhydrous).

Description. White or slightly yellowish granules or powder; odour, slightly ammoniacal.

Solubility. Freely soluble in water (the solution may become cloudy in the presence of carbon dioxide); slightly soluble in ethanol (~750 g/l) TS; practically insoluble in ether R.

Category. Antispasmodic; diuretic; coronary vasodilator.

Storage. Aminophylline should be kept in a tightly closed container, protected from light.

Additional information. Aminophylline contains a variable quantity of water of hydration. Upon exposure to air Aminophylline gradually loses ethylenediamine and absorbs carbon dioxide with the liberation of free theophylline. Even in the absence of light, Aminophylline is gradually degraded on exposure to a humid atmosphere, the decomposition being faster at higher temperatures.

REQUIREMENTS

General requirement. Aminophylline contains not less than 78.0% and not more than 86.0% of theophylline ($C_7H_8N_4O_2$), and not less than 12.8% and not more than 15.0% of ethylenediamine ($C_2H_8N_2$), both calculated with reference to the anhydrous substance.

Identity tests

A.   Dissolve 1 g in 10 ml of water and add, drop by drop, while shaking 2 ml of hydrochloric acid (~70 g/l) TS. Collect the precipitate on a filter, wash it with water and dry at 105 °C; melting temperature, about 272 °C (theophylline). Keep the precipitate for test B.

B.   To 10 mg of the precipitate obtained from test A, contained in a porcelain dish, add 1 ml of hydrochloric acid (~250 g/l) TS and 0.5 ml of hydrogen peroxide (~60 g/l) TS, and evaporate to dryness on a water-bath. Add 1 drop of ammonia (~100 g/l) TS; the residue acquires a purple colour which is destroyed by the addition of a few drops of sodium hydroxide (~80 g/l) TS.

C.   Dissolve 0.05 g in 1 ml of water and add 2 drops of copper(II) sulfate (80 g/l) TS; a deep violet colour is produced.

D. Warm 0.05 g with 2 ml of sodium hydroxide (~80 g/l) TS and 2 drops of chloroform R; an isocyanide, perceptible by its characteristic odour (proceed with caution), is produced.

Clarity of solution. A solution of 1.0 g in 10 ml of boiling water is clear or is not more than slightly opalescent.

Sulfated ash. Not more than 1.5 mg/g.

Water. Determine as described under "Determination of water by the Karl Fischer method", Method A (vol. 1, p. 135), using about 0.15 g of the substance and 25 ml of pyridine R as the solvent; the water content is not more than 80 mg/g.

Alkalinity. Add 1 drop of thymol blue/ethanol TS to a 10 mg/ml solution prepared in carbon-dioxide-free water R; a green or blue colour is produced.

Assay.

For theophylline. Place about 0.25 g, accurately weighed, in a 250-ml conical flask, add 50 ml of water and 8 ml of ammonia (~100 g/l) TS and gently warm the mixture on a water-bath until complete solution is effected. Add 20.0 ml of silver nitrate (0.1 mol/l) VS, mix, heat to boiling and boil for 15 minutes. Cool to between 5°C and 10°C for 20 minutes, then filter through a filtering crucible under reduced pressure and wash the precipitate 3 times with 10-ml portions of water. Acidify the combined filtrate and washings with nitric acid (~1000 g/l) TS, and add an excess of 3 ml of the acid. Cool, add 2 ml of ferric ammonium sulfate (45 g/l) TS, and titrate the excess of silver nitrate with ammonium thiocyanate (0.1 mol/l) VS. Each ml of silver nitrate (0.1 mol/l) VS is equivalent to 18.02 mg of $C_7H_8N_4O_2$.

For ethylenediamine. Dissolve about 0.5 g, accurately weighed, in 30 ml of water and titrate with hydrochloric acid (0.1 mol/l) VS, using bromocresol green/ethanol TS as indicator. Repeat the operation without the substance being examined and make any necessary corrections. Each ml of hydrochloric acid (0.1 mol/l) VS is equivalent to 3.005 mg of $C_2H_8N_2$.

AMITRIPTYLINI HYDROCHLORIDUM

Amitriptyline hydrochloride

Molecular formula. $C_{20}H_{23}N$, HCl

Relative molecular mass. 313.9

Graphic formula.

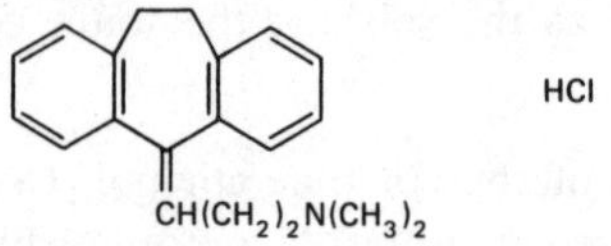

HCl

CH(CH₂)₂N(CH₃)₂

Chemical name. 10,11-Dihydro-N,N-dimethyl-5H-dibenzo[a,d]cycloheptene-$\Delta^{5,\gamma}$-propylamine hydrochloride; 3-(10,11-dihydro-5H-dibenzo[a,d]cyclohepten-5-ylidene)-N,N-dimethyl-1-propanamine hydrochloride; CAS Reg. No. 549-18-8.

Description. Colourless crystals or a white or almost white powder; odourless or almost odourless.

Solubility. Soluble in 1 part of water and in 1.5 parts of ethanol ($\sim$750 g/l) TS; freely soluble in chloroform R; practically insoluble in ether R.

Category. Antidepressant.

Storage. Amitriptyline hydrochloride should be kept in a tightly closed container, protected from light.

Additional information. Amitriptyline hydrochloride has a bitter and burning taste that is followed by a sensation of numbness. Even in the absence of light, Amitriptyline hydrochloride is gradually degraded on exposure to a humid atmosphere, the decomposition being faster at higher temperatures.

REQUIREMENTS

General requirement. Amitriptyline hydrochloride contains not less than 99.0% and not more than 101.5% of $C_{20}H_{23}N$,HCl, calculated with reference to the dried substance.

Identity tests

A. Carry out the examination as described under "Spectrophotometry in the infrared region" (vol. 1, p. 40). The infrared absorption spectrum is concordant

with the spectrum obtained from amitriptyline hydrochloride RS or with the *reference spectrum* of amitriptyline hydrochloride.

B.   A 20 mg/ml solution yields reaction B described under "General identification tests" as characteristic of chlorides (vol. 1, p. 113).

C.   Melting temperature, about 197 °C.

Sulfated ash.   Not more than 1.0 mg/g.

Loss on drying.   Dry to constant weight at 60 °C under reduced pressure (not exceeding 0.6 kPa or about 5 mm of mercury); it loses not more than 5.0 mg/g.

pH value.   pH of a 10 mg/ml solution, 4.5–6.0.

Related substances.   Carry out the test as described under "Thin-layer chromatography" (vol. 1, p. 83), using silica gel R2 as the coating substance and a mixture of 85 volumes of cyclohexane R, 15 volumes of ethyl acetate R and 3 volumes of diethylamine R as the mobile phase.   Apply separately to the plate 10 μl of each of 2 solutions in chloroform R containing (A) 20 mg of the test substance per ml and (B) 0.20 mg of the test substance per ml.   After removing the plate from the chromatographic chamber, allow it to dry in air, and examine the chromatogram in ultraviolet light (254 nm).   Any spot obtained with solution A, other than the principal spot, is not more intense than that obtained with solution B.

Assay.   Dissolve about 0.3 g, accurately weighed, in 30 ml of glacial acetic acid R1, add 10 ml of dioxan R and 10 ml of mercuric acetate/acetic acid TS, and titrate with perchloric acid (0.1 mol/l) VS as described under "Non-aqueous titration", Method A (vol. 1, p. 131).   Each ml of perchloric acid (0.1 mol/l) VS is equivalent to 31.39 mg of $C_{20}H_{23}N,HCl$.

AMODIAQUINI HYDROCHLORIDUM

Amodiaquine hydrochloride

Molecular formula. $C_{20}H_{22}ClN_3O,2HCl,2H_2O$

Relative molecular mass.   464.8

Graphic formula.

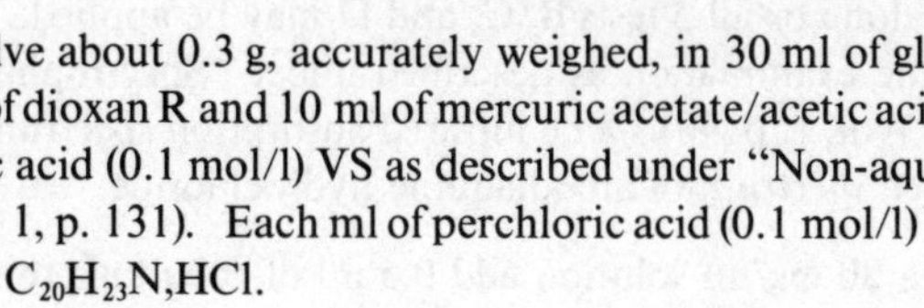

Chemical name. 4-[(7-Chloro-4-quinolyl)amino]-α-(diethylamino)-o-cresol di-hydrochloride dihydrate; 4-[(7-chloro-4-quinolinyl)amino]-2-[(diethylamino)-methyl]phenol dihydrochloride dihydrate; CAS Reg. No. 6398-98-7.

Description. A yellow, crystalline powder; odourless.

Solubility. Soluble in about 22 parts of water; sparingly soluble in ethanol (~750 g/l) TS; practically insoluble in chloroform R and ether R.

Category. Antimalarial.

Storage. Amodiaquine hydrochloride should be kept in a tightly closed container.

REQUIREMENTS

General requirement. Amodiaquine hydrochloride contains not less than 98.0% and not more than 101.5% of $C_{20}H_{22}ClN_3O,2HCl$, calculated with reference to the anhydrous substance.

Identity tests

• Either test A alone or all 3 tests B, C, and D may be applied.

A. Carry out the examination as described under "Spectrophotometry in the infrared region" (vol. 1, p. 40). The infrared absorption spectrum is concordant with the *reference spectrum* of amodiaquine hydrochloride.

B. To 1 ml of a 20 mg/ml solution add 0.5 ml of cobaltous thiocyanate TS; a green precipitate is produced.

C. A 20 mg/ml solution yields reaction B described under "General identification tests" as characteristic of chlorides (vol. 1, p. 113).

D. Melting temperature, determined without previous drying, about 158 °C with decomposition.

Sulfated ash. Not more than 2.0 mg/g.

Water. Determine as described under "Determination of water by the Karl Fischer method", Method A (vol. 1, p. 135), using about 0.15 g of the substance; the water content is not less than 70 mg/g and not more than 90 mg/g.

pH value. pH of a 20 mg/ml solution, 4.0–4.8.

Related substances. Carry out the test as described under "Thin-layer chromatography" (vol. 1, p. 83). Prepare a solution of chloroform saturated with ammonia by shaking chloroform R with ammonia (~260 g/l) TS and separate the chloroform-layer. Use silica gel R2 as the coating substance and a mixture of

9 volumes of chloroform saturated with ammonia, and 1 volume of dehydrated ethanol R as the mobile phase. For the preparation of the test solutions transfer 0.20 g of the substance being examined to a glass-stoppered test-tube, add 10 ml of chloroform saturated with ammonia, shake vigorously for 2 minutes, allow the solids to settle, and decant the solution to a second tube; this constitutes solution A. Dilute 1.0 ml of solution A with sufficient chloroform saturated with ammonia to 200 ml; this constitutes solution B. Apply separately to the plate 10 μl of each of solutions A and B. After removing the plate from the chromatographic chamber, allow it to dry in air, and examine the chromatogram in ultraviolet light (254 nm). Any spot obtained with solution A, other than the principal spot, is not more intense than that obtained with solution B.

Assay. Dissolve about 0.3 g, accurately weighed, in 50 ml of water, make the solution alkaline with ammonia (~100 g/l) TS, and allow to stand for 30 minutes. Filter, wash the residue with water until the washings are free from chlorides, and dry to constant weight at 105 °C. Each g of residue is equivalent to 1.205 g of $C_{20}H_{22}ClN_3O,2HCl$.

AMPICILLINUM

Ampicillin

Ampicillin anhydrous
Ampicillin trihydrate

Molecular formula. $C_{16}H_{19}N_3O_4S$ (anhydrous); $C_{16}H_{19}N_3O_4S,3H_2O$ (trihydrate).

Relative molecular mass. 349.4 (anhydrous); 403.5 (trihydrate).

Graphic formula.

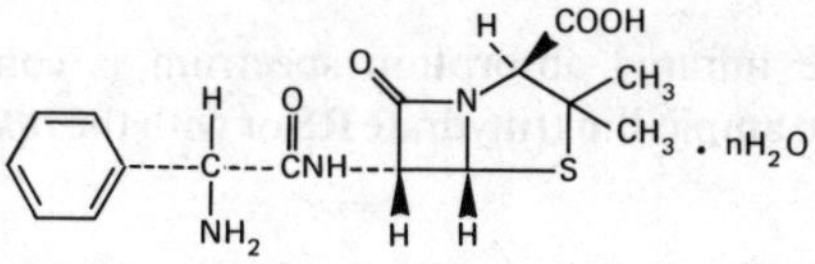

$n = 0$ (anhydrous)
$n = 3$ (trihydrate)

Chemical name. (2S,5R,6R)-6-[(R)-2-Amino-2-phenylacetamido]-3,3-dimethyl-7-oxo-4-thia-1-azabicyclo[3.2.0]heptane-2-carboxylic acid; [2S-[2α,5α,6β(S*)]]-6-[(aminophenylacetyl)amino]-3,3-dimethyl-7-oxo-4-thia-1-azabicyclo [3.2.0]-heptane-2-carboxylic acid; CAS Reg. No. 69-53-4 (anhydrous).
(2S,5R,6R)-6-[(R)-2-Amino-2-phenylacetamido]-3,3-dimethyl-7-oxo-4-thia-1-azabicyclo[3.2.0]heptane-2-carboxylic acid trihydrate; [2S-[2α,5α,6β(S*)]]-6-[(aminophenylacetyl)amino]-3,3-dimethyl-7-oxo-4-thia-1-azabicyclo[3.2.0]hep-tane-2-carboxylic acid trihydrate; CAS Reg. No. 7177-48-2 (trihydrate).

Description. A white or almost white, crystalline powder; odourless or almost odourless.

Solubility. Slightly soluble in water; practically insoluble in ethanol (~750 g/l) TS, chloroform R, and ether R.

Category. Antibiotic.

Storage. Ampicillin should be kept in a tightly closed container, protected from light and stored at a temperature not exceeding 25 °C.

Labelling. The designation on the container of Ampicillin should state whether the substance is in the anhydrous form or is the trihydrate.

Additional information. Even in the absence of light, Ampicillin is gradually degraded on exposure to a humid atmosphere, the decomposition being faster at higher temperatures.

REQUIREMENTS

General requirement. Ampicillin contains not less than 95.0% and not more than 102.0% of $C_{16}H_{19}N_3O_4S$, calculated with reference to the anhydrous substance.

Identity tests

• Either test A or test B may be applied.
A. Carry out the examination as described under "Spectrophotometry in the infrared region" (vol. 1, p. 40). For the anhydrous form the infrared absorption spectrum is concordant with the spectrum obtained from ampicillin RS or with the *reference spectrum* of ampicillin.

For the trihydrate the infrared absorption spectrum is concordant with the spectrum obtained from ampicillin trihydrate RS or with the *reference spectrum* of ampicillin trihydrate.

B. To 2 mg in a test-tube add 1 drop of water followed by 2 ml of sulfuric acid (~1760 g/l) TS and mix; the solution is colourless. Immerse the test-tube for

1 minute in a water-bath; the solution remains colourless. Place 2 mg in a second test-tube, add 1 drop of water and 2 ml of formaldehyde/sulfuric acid TS and mix; the solution is colourless to slightly pink. Immerse the test-tube for 1 minute in a water-bath; an orange-yellow colour is produced.

Specific optical rotation. Use a 2.5 mg/ml solution and calculate with reference to the anhydrous substance: $[\alpha]_D^{20\,°C} = +280$ to $+305°$.

Water. Determine as described under "Determination of water by the Karl Fischer method", Method A (vol. 1, p. 135).

For the anhydrous form use about 0.8 g of the substance; the water content is not more than 15 mg/g.

For the trihydrate use about 0.1 g of the substance; the water content is not less than 120 mg/g and not more than 150 mg/g.

pH value. pH of a 2.5 mg/ml solution, 3.5–6.0.

Assay. Dissolve about 0.12 g, accurately weighed, in sufficient water to produce 500 ml. Transfer 10.0 ml of this solution to a 100-ml volumetric flask, add 10 ml of buffer borate, pH 9.0, TS, 1 ml of acetic anhydride/dioxan TS, allow to stand for 5 minutes at room temperature and dilute to volume with water.

Transfer two 2.0-ml aliquots of this solution into separate stoppered tubes. To one tube add 10.0 ml of imidazole/mercuric chloride TS, mix, stopper the tube, and place in a water-bath at 60 °C for exactly 25 minutes. Cool the tube rapidly to 20 °C (solution A).

To the second tube add 10.0 ml of water and mix (solution B).

Without delay, measure the absorbance of a 1-cm layer at the maximum at about 325 nm, against a solvent cell containing a mixture of 2.0 ml of water and 10.0 ml of imidazole/mercuric chloride TS for solution A and water for solution B.

From the difference between the absorbance of solution A and that of solution B, calculate the amount of $C_{16}H_{19}N_3O_4S$ in the substance being tested by comparison with ampicillin RS similarly and concurrently examined. In an adequate calibrated spectrophotometer the absorbance of the reference solution should be 0.29 ± 0.02.

———————————

AMPICILLINUM NATRICUM

Ampicillin sodium

Ampicillin sodium (non-injectable)
Ampicillin sodium, sterile

Molecular formula. $C_{16}H_{18}N_3NaO_4S$

Relative molecular mass.   371.4

Graphic formula.

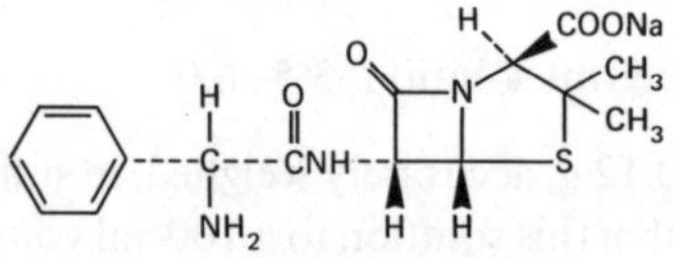

Chemical name.   Sodium $(2S,5R,6R)$-6-[(R)-2-amino-2-phenylacetamido]-3,3-dimethyl-7-oxo-4-thia-1-azabicyclo[3.2.0]heptane-2-carboxylate; sodium [$2S$-[$2\alpha,5\alpha,6\beta(S^*)$]]-6-[(aminophenylacetyl)amino]-3,3-dimethyl-7-oxo-4-thia-1-aza-bicyclo[3.2.0]heptane-2-carboxylate; CAS Reg. No. 69-52-3.

Description.   A white or almost white powder; odourless.

Solubility.   Soluble in about 2 parts of water; slightly soluble in chloroform R; practically insoluble in ether R.

Category.   Antibiotic.

Storage.   Ampicillin sodium should be kept in a tightly closed container, protected from light, and stored at a temperature not exceeding 25 °C.

Labelling.   The designation sterile Ampicillin sodium indicates that the substance complies with the requirements for sterile Ampicillin sodium and may be used for parenteral administration or for other sterile applications.

Additional information.   Ampicillin sodium is a crystalline or amorphous powder; it is very hygroscopic and is deliquescent in air with a relative humidity of 60% or more.   Even in the absence of light, Ampicillin sodium is gradually degraded on exposure to a humid atmosphere, the decomposition being faster at higher temperatures.

REQUIREMENTS

General requirement.   Ampicillin sodium contains not less than 85.0% and not more than 96.0% of $C_{16}H_{19}N_3O_4S$, calculated with reference to the anhydrous substance. Furthermore, the sum of the percentage of $C_{16}H_{19}N_3O_4S$ determined in the assay and the percentage of iodine-absorbing compounds, both calculated with reference to the anhydrous substance, is not less than 90.0%.

Identity tests

• Either tests A and C or tests B and C may be applied.

A. Carry out the examination as described under "Spectrophotometry in the infrared region" (vol. 1, p. 40). The infrared absorption spectrum is concordant with the spectrum obtained from ampicillin sodium RS or with the *reference spectrum* of ampicillin sodium.

B. To 2 mg in a test-tube add 1 drop of water followed by 2 ml of sulfuric acid (~1760 g/l) TS and mix; the solution is colourless. Immerse the test-tube for 1 minute in a water-bath; the solution remains colourless. Place 2 mg in a second test-tube, add 1 drop of water and 2 ml of formaldehyde/sulfuric acid TS and mix; the solution is colourless. Immerse the test-tube for 1 minute in a water-bath; a dark yellow colour is produced.

C. When tested for sodium as described under "General identification tests" (vol. 1, p. 115) yields the characteristic reactions. If reaction B is to be used, ignite a small quantity and dissolve the residue in acetic acid (~60 g/l) TS.

Specific optical rotation. Use a 5.0 mg/ml solution in acetate standard buffer TS and calculate with reference to the anhydrous substance; $[\alpha]_D^{20\,°C} = +260$ to $+290°$.

Clarity of solution. A freshly prepared solution of 1.0 g in 10 ml of water is clear. A solution of 1.0 g in 10 ml of hydrochloric acid (1 mol/l) VS is also clear.

Water. Determine as described under "Determination of water by the Karl Fischer method", Method A (vol. 1, p. 135), using about 0.5 g of the substance; the water content is not more than 20 mg/g.

pH value. pH of a 0.10 g/ml solution in carbon-dioxide-free water R, 8.0–10.0.

Iodine-absorbing compounds. Dissolve 0.25 g in sufficient water to produce 100 ml. To 10 ml of this solution add 0.5 ml of hydrochloric acid (1 mol/l) VS and 10 ml of iodine (0.02 mol/l) VS and titrate with sodium thiosulfate (0.02 mol/l) VS, using starch TS as indicator, added towards the end of the titration. Repeat the operation without the substance being examined; the difference between the titrations represents the amount of iodine-absorbing compounds. Calculate as a percentage the amount of these compounds in the examined substance, taking into account that each ml of sodium thiosulfate (0.02 mol/l) VS is equivalent to 0.7368 mg of iodine-absorbing compounds expressed as $C_{16}H_{19}N_3O_4S$.

Assay. Dissolve about 0.12 g, accurately weighed, in sufficient water to produce 500 ml. Transfer 10.0 ml of this solution to a 100-ml volumetric flask, add 10 ml of buffer borate, pH 9.0, TS, 1 ml of acetic anhydride/dioxan TS, allow to stand for 5 minutes at room temperature and dilute to volume with water.

Transfer two 2.0-ml aliquots of this solution into separate stoppered tubes. To one tube add 10.0 ml of imidazole/mercuric chloride TS, mix, stopper the tube and place in a water-bath at 60 °C for exactly 25 minutes. Cool the tube rapidly to 20 °C (solution A).

To the second tube add 10.0 ml of water and mix (solution B).

Without delay measure the absorbance of a 1-cm layer at the maximum at about 325 nm against a solvent cell containing a mixture of 2.0 ml of water and 10.0 ml of imidazole/mercuric chloride TS for solution A and water for solution B.

From the difference between the absorbance of solution A and that of solution B, calculate as a percentage the amount of $C_{16}H_{19}N_3O_4S$ in the substance being tested by comparison with ampicillin RS similarly and concurrently examined. In an adequately calibrated spectrophotometer the absorbance of the reference solution should be 0.29 ± 0.02.

Additional Requirements for Sterile Ampicillin Sodium

Pyrogens. Carry out the test as described under "Test for pyrogens" (vol. 1, p. 155) injecting, per kg of the rabbit's weight, a solution containing 10 mg of the substance to be examined in 5 ml of sterile water R.

Sterility. Complies with the "Sterility testing of antibiotics" (vol. 1, p. 152), applying either the membrane filtration test procedure with added penicillinase TS or the direct test procedure.

———————

ATROPINI SULFAS

Atropine sulfate

Molecular formula. $(C_{17}H_{23}NO_3)_2,H_2SO_4,H_2O$

Relative molecular mass. 694.8

Graphic formula.

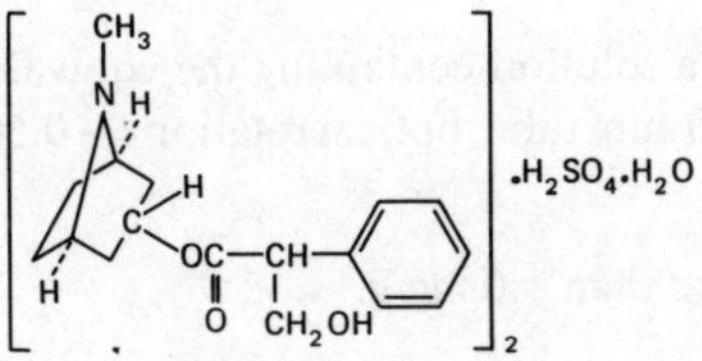

Chemical name. $1\alpha H,5\alpha H$-Tropan-3α-ol ($\pm$)-tropate (ester) sulfate (2:1) (salt) monohydrate; ($\pm$)-endo-8-methyl-8-azabicyclo[3.2.1]oct-3-yl α-(hydroxymethyl)benzeneacetate sulfate (2:1) (salt) monohydrate; CAS Reg. No. 5908-99-6.

Description. Colourless crystal or a white, crystalline powder; odourless.

Solubility. Soluble in less than 1 part of water; freely soluble in ethanol (~750 g/l) TS; practically insoluble in ether R and benzene R.

Category. Cholinergic blocking agent (parasympatholytic).

Storage. Atropine sulfate should be kept in a tightly closed container, protected from light.

Additional information. Atropine sulfate is very poisonous; it effloresces in dry air; it is slowly affected by light.

REQUIREMENTS

General requirement. Atropine sulfate contains not less than 98.5% and not more than 101.0% of $(C_{17}H_{23}NO_3)_2,H_2SO_4$, calculated with reference to the dried substance.

Identity tests

• Either test A alone or all 3 tests B, C, and D may be applied.

A. Carry out the examination as described under "Spectrophotometry in the infrared region" (vol. 1, p. 40). The infrared absorption spectrum is concordant with the spectrum obtained from atropine sulfate RS or with the *reference spectrum* of atropine sulfate.

B. Mix 1 mg with 5 drops of fuming nitric acid R and evaporate to dryness on a water-bath. To the cooled residue add 2 ml of acetone R and 3–4 drops of potassium hydroxide/methanol TS; a deep violet colour is produced.

C. A 20 mg/ml solution yields reaction A described under "General identification tests" as characteristic of sulfates (vol. 1, p. 115).

D. Dissolve 0.6 g in 30 ml of carbon-dioxide-free water R and add 2 ml of sodium hydroxide (~80 g/l) TS. Filter, wash the precipitate with water and dry at 100 °C. Melting temperature, about 116 °C (atropine base).

Optical rotation. Use a solution containing the equivalent of 0.10 g/ml of the dried substance, in a 200-mm tube; optical rotation = − 0.50 to + 0.10° (distinction from hyoscyamine).

Sulfated ash. Not more than 1.0 mg/g.

Loss on drying. Dry to constant weight at 120 °C; it loses not less than 25 mg/g and not more than 40 mg/g.

Acidity. Dissolve 1.0 g in 20 ml of carbon-dioxide-free water R and titrate with sodium hydroxide (0.02 mol/l) VS, using methyl red/ethanol TS as indicator; not more than 0.3 ml is required to obtain the midpoint of the indicator (orange).

Readily oxidizable substances. To 10 ml of a 10 mg/ml solution add 0.1 ml of potassium permanganate (0.02 mol/l) VS; the colour is not completely discharged at the end of 3 minutes.

Related substances. Carry out the test as described under "Thin-layer chromatography" (vol. 1, p. 83), using silica gel R1 as the coating substance and a mixture of 6 volumes of ethylmethylketone R, 3 volumes of methanol R and 1 volume of ammonia (~100 g/l) TS as the mobile phase. Apply to the plate 10 μl of a solution in methanol R containing 12.5 mg/ml of the test substance. After removing the plate from the chromatographic chamber, allow it to dry in air, spray with potassium iodobismuthate TS2 and examine the chromatogram in daylight. No spot is obtained, other than the principal spot.

Assay. Dissolve about 0.6 g, accurately weighed, in 30 ml of glacial acetic acid R1, and titrate with perchloric acid (0.1 mol/l) VS as described under "Non-aqueous titration", Method A (vol. 1, p. 131). Each ml of perchloric acid (0.1 mol/l) VS is equivalent to 67.68 mg of $(C_{17}H_{23}NO_3)_2,H_2SO_4$.

BENZOCAINUM

Benzocaine

Molecular formula. $C_9H_{11}NO_2$

Relative molecular mass. 165.2

Graphic formula.

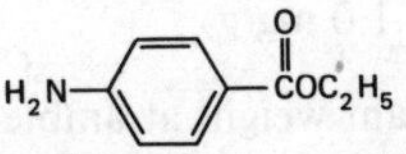

Chemical name. Ethyl p-aminobenzoate; ethyl 4-aminobenzoate; CAS Reg. No. 94-09.7.

Other name. Ethyl aminobenzoate.

Description. Colourless crystals or a white, crystalline powder; odourless.

Solubility. Very slightly soluble in water; soluble in 6 parts of ethanol ($\sim$750 g/l) TS, 3 parts of chloroform R, and 5.5 parts of ether R.

Category. Local anaesthetic.

Storage. Benzocaine should be kept in a well-closed container, protected from light.

Additional information. Benzocaine causes local numbness after being placed on the tongue.

REQUIREMENTS

General requirement. Benzocaine contains not less than 98.0% and not more than 101.0% of $C_9H_{11}NO_2$, calculated with reference to the dried substance.

Identity tests

A. Dissolve 0.10 g in 5 ml of water, add 3 drops of hydrochloric acid ($\sim$70 g/l) TS and 5 drops of iodine TS; a brown precipitate is produced.

B. Heat 0.05 g with 2 drops of acetic acid ($\sim$300 g/l) TS and 4 drops of sulfuric acid ($\sim$1760 g/l) TS; ethyl acetate, perceptible by its odour (proceed with caution), is produced.

C. About 0.05 g yields the reaction described for the identification of primary aromatic amines under "General identification tests" (vol. 1, p. 111), producing an orange-red precipitate.

Melting range. 88–92 °C.

Heavy metals. Use 1.0 g and ethanol (~750 g/l) TS for the preparation of the test solution as described under "Limit test for heavy metals", Procedure 2 (vol. 1, p. 118); determine the heavy metals content according to Method A (vol. 1, p. 119); not more than 10 μg/g.

Solution in ethanol. A solution of 1.0 g in 10 ml of ethanol (~750 g/l) TS is clear and colourless.

Sulfated ash. Not more than 1.0 mg/g.

Loss on drying. Dry to constant weight at ambient temperature under reduced pressure (not exceeding 0.6 kPa or about 5 mm of mercury) over silica gel, desiccant, R or phosphorus pentoxide R; it loses not more than 10 mg/g.

Acidity or alkalinity. To a solution of 0.5 g in 10 ml of neutralized ethanol TS add 10 ml of carbon-dioxide-free water R and 2 drops of phenolphthalein/ethanol TS; no pink colour is produced. Add 0.5 ml of carbonate-free sodium hydroxide (0.01 mol/l) VS; a pink colour is produced.

Assay. Carry out the assay as described under "Nitrite titration" (vol. 1, p. 133), using about 0.3 g, accurately weighed, dissolved in 50 ml of hydrochloric acid (~70 g/l) TS and titrate with sodium nitrite (0.1 mol/l) VS. Each ml of sodium nitrite (0.1 mol/l) VS is equivalent to 16.52 mg of $C_9H_{11}NO_2$.

BENZYLIS BENZOAS

Benzyl benzoate

Molecular formula. $C_{14}H_{12}O_2$

Relative molecular mass. 212.3

Graphic formula.

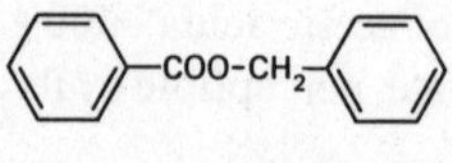

Chemical name. Phenylmethyl benzoate; CAS Reg. No. 120-51-4.

Description. A clear, colourless, oily liquid; odour, faintly aromatic.

Miscibility. Practically immiscible with water and glycerol R; miscible with ethanol (~750 g/l) TS, chloroform R, and ether R.

Category. Scabicide (topical use).

Storage. Benzyl benzoate should be kept in a tightly closed and well-filled container, protected from light.

Additional information. Benzyl benzoate may slowly decompose on contact with air.

REQUIREMENTS

General requirement. Benzyl benzoate contains not less than 98.0% and not more than 100.5% of $C_{14}H_{12}O_2$.

Identity tests

Boil 2 g with 25 ml of potassium hydroxide/ethanol TS2 for 10 minutes, evaporate the ethanol on a water-bath, cool, extract with 2 successive quantities, each of 15 ml of ether R, and proceed as follows:

A. Evaporate the ethereal layer on a water-bath; heat 1 drop of the oily liquid with 5 ml of sodium carbonate (50 g/l) TS and 1 ml of potassium permanganate (0.02 mol/l) VS; an odour of benzaldehyde is discernible.

B. To the aqueous layer add 10 ml of sulfuric acid (~100 g/l) TS; a white, crystalline precipitate is produced. Wash and dry the precipitate; melting temperature, about 123 °C (benzoic acid).

Congealing temperature. Not below 17.0 °C.

Refractive index. n_D^{20} = 1.568–1.570.

Mass density. ρ_{20} = 1.116–1.120 g/ml.

Chlorinated compounds. For the preparation of the test solution dissolve 0.30 g in 15 ml of ethanol (~750 g/l) TS and add 6 ml of sodium hydroxide (~80 g/l) TS. Warm the solution for 5 minutes on a water-bath. Cool, transfer to a comparison tube, and add 3 ml of nitric acid (~130 g/l) TS. For the reference solution transfer separately 2.0 ml of hydrochloric acid ClTS and 4 ml of nitric acid (~130 g/l) TS to a comparison tube, and dilute to 25 ml with water. To both tubes add 0.5 ml of silver nitrate (40 g/l) TS. Stir immediately with a glass rod and set aside for 5 minutes, protected from direct sunlight. The opalescence produced from the test liquid is not stronger than that produced from the reference solution; not more than 0.33 mg/g of chlorine.

Acidity. Add 5 ml of the test liquid to 5 ml of neutralized ethanol TS, and titrate with carbonate-free sodium hydroxide (0.1 mol/l) VS, phenolphthalein/ethanol TS being used as indicator; not more than 0.3 ml is required to obtain the midpoint of the indicator (pink).

Assay. Add about 2.0 g, accurately weighed, to 40 ml of potassium hydroxide/ethanol (0.5 mol/l) VS and boil under reflux for 1 hour. Cool, and titrate with hydrochloric acid (0.5 mol/l) VS, using phenolphthalein/ethanol TS as indicator. Repeat the operation without the test liquid being examined and make any necessary corrections. Each ml of potassium hydroxide/ethanol (0.5 mol/l) VS is equivalent to 106.1 mg of $C_{14}H_{12}O_2$.

BENZYLPENICILLINUM KALICUM

Benzylpenicillin potassium

Benzylpenicillin potassium (non-injectable)
Benzylpenicillin potassium, sterile

Molecular formula. $C_{16}H_{17}KN_2O_4S$

Relative molecular mass. 372.5

Graphic formula.

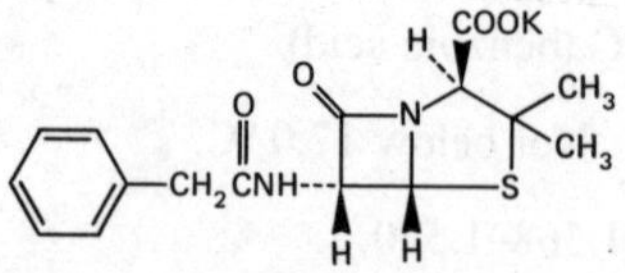

Chemical name. Potassium $(2S,5R,6R)$-3,3-dimethyl-7-oxo-6-(2-phenylacet-amido)-4-thia-1-azabicyclo[3.2.0]heptane-2-carboxylate; potassium [2S-$(2\alpha,5\alpha,6\beta)$]-3,3-dimethyl-7-oxo-6-[(phenylacetyl)amino]-4-thia-1-azabicyclo-[3.2.0]heptane-2-carboxylate; CAS Reg. No. 113-98-4.

Description. A white or almost white, crystalline powder; odourless or with a faint characteristic odour.

Solubility. Very soluble in water; practically insoluble in chloroform R and ether R.

Category. Antibiotic.

Storage. Benzylpenicillin potassium should be kept in a tightly closed container, protected from light, and stored at a temperature not exceeding 25 °C.

Labelling. The designation sterile Benzylpenicillin potassium indicates that the substance complies with the additional requirements for sterile Benzylpenicillin potassium and may be used for parenteral administration or for other sterile applications.

Additional information. Benzylpenicillin potassium is moderately hygroscopic; it is readily decomposed by acids, alkalis and oxidizing agents. Even in the absence of light, Benzylpenicillin potassium is gradually degraded on exposure to a humid atmosphere, the decomposition being faster at higher temperatures.

REQUIREMENTS

General requirement. Benzylpenicillin potassium contains not less than 96.0% and not more than 102.0% of $C_{16}H_{17}KN_2O_4S$, calculated with reference to the dried substance.

Identity tests

• Either tests A and C or tests B and C may be applied.

A. Carry out the examination as described under "Spectrophotometry in the infrared region" (vol. 1, p. 40). The infrared absorption spectrum is concordant with the spectrum obtained from benzylpenicillin potassium RS or with the *reference spectrum* of benzylpenicillin potassium.

B. To 2 mg in a test-tube add 1 drop of water followed by 2 ml of sulfuric acid (~1760 g/l) TS and mix; the solution is colourless. Immerse the test-tube for 1 minute in a water-bath; the solution remains colourless. Place 2 mg in a second test-tube, add 1 drop of water and 2 ml of formaldehyde/sulfuric acid TS and mix; the solution is brownish yellow. Immerse the test-tube for 1 minute in a water-bath; a reddish brown colour is produced.

C. Ignite a small quantity, dissolve the residue in water and filter; on addition of 2 ml of sodium hydroxide (~80 g/l) TS to the filtrate it yields the reaction described under "General identification tests", as characteristic of potassium (vol. 1, p. 114).

Specific optical rotation. Use a 20 mg/ml solution; $[\alpha]_D^{20\,°C}$ = +270 to +300 °.

Clarity and colour of solution. A solution of 0.20 g in 10 ml of water is clear and colourless.

Loss on drying. Dry to constant weight at 105 °C; it loses not more than 10 mg/g.

pH value. pH of a 20 mg/ml solution in carbon-dioxide-free water R, 5.0–7.5.

Light-absorbing impurities. Using a freshly prepared 1.9 mg/ml solution in water, measure the absorbances at 280 nm and at 325 nm; the absorbance at each of these wavelengths does not exceed 0.10.

Assay. Dissolve about 50 mg, accurately weighed, in sufficient water to produce 1000 ml. Transfer two 2.0-ml aliquots of this solution into separate stoppered tubes. To one tube add 10.0 ml of imidazole/mercuric chloride TS, mix, stopper the tube and place in a water-bath at 60 °C for exactly 25 minutes. Cool the tube rapidly to 20 °C (solution A).

To the second tube add 10.0 ml of water and mix (solution B).

Without delay measure the absorbance of a 1-cm layer at the maximum at about 325 nm against a solvent cell containing a mixture of 2.0 ml of water and 10.0 ml of imidazole/mercuric chloride TS for solution A and water for solution B.

From the difference between the absorbance of solution A and that of solution B, calculate the amount of $C_{16}H_{17}KN_2O_4S$ in the substance being tested by comparison with benzylpenicillin sodium RS similarly and concurrently examined, taking into account that each mg of benzylpenicillin sodium RS ($C_{16}H_{17}N_2NaO_4S$) is equivalent to 1.045 mg of benzylpenicillin potassium ($C_{16}H_{17}KN_2O_4S$). In an adequately calibrated spectrophotometer the absorbance of the reference solution should be 0.62 ± 0.03.

Additional Requirements for Sterile Benzylpenicillin Potassium

Pyrogens. Carry out the test as described under "Test for pyrogens" (vol. 1, p. 155) injecting, per kg of the rabbit's weight, a solution containing 1.5 mg of the substance to be examined in 5 ml of sterile water R.

Sterility. Complies with the "Sterility testing of antibiotics" (vol. 1, p. 152), applying either the membrane filtration test procedure with added penicillinase TS or the direct test procedure.

BENZYLPENICILLINUM NATRICUM

Benzylpenicillin sodium

Benzylpenicillin sodium (non-injectable)

Benzylpenicillin sodium, sterile

Molecular formula. $C_{16}H_{17}N_2NaO_4S$

Relative molecular mass. 356.4

Graphic formula.

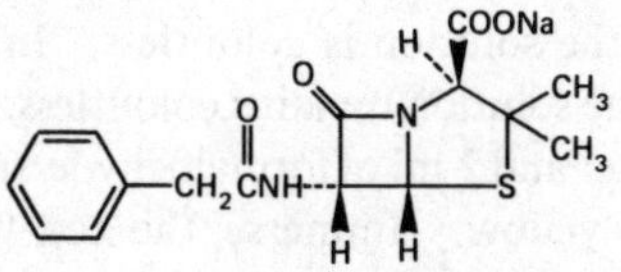

Chemical name. Sodium (2S,5R,6R)-3,3-dimethyl-7-oxo-6-(2-phenylacet-amido)-4-thia-1-azabicyclo[3.2.0]heptane-2-carboxylate; sodium [2S-(2α,5α, 6β)]-3,3-dimethyl-7-oxo-6-[(phenylacetyl)amino]-4-thia-1-azabicyclo[3.2.0]-heptane-2-carboxylate; CAS Reg. No. 69-57-8.

Description. A white or almost white, crystalline powder; odourless or with a faint characteristic odour.

Solubility. Soluble in about 0.5 part of water; practically insoluble in chloroform R and ether R.

Category. Antibiotic.

Storage. Benzylpenicillin sodium should be kept in a tightly closed container, protected from light, and stored at a temperature not exceeding 25 °C.

Labelling. The designation sterile Benzylpenicillin sodium indicates that the substance complies with the additional requirements for sterile Benzylpenicillin sodium and may be used for parenteral administration or for other sterile applications.

Additional information. Benzylpenicillin sodium is hygroscopic; it is readily decomposed by acid, alkalis and oxidizing agents. Even in the absence of light, Benzylpenicillin sodium is gradually degraded on exposure to a humid atmos-phere, the decomposition being faster at higher temperatures.

REQUIREMENTS

General requirement. Benzylpenicillin sodium contains not less than 96.0% and not more than 102.0% of $C_{16}H_{17}N_2NaO_4S$, calculated with reference to the dried substance.

Identity tests

• Either tests A and C or tests B and C may be applied.

A.   Carry out the examination as described under "Spectrophotometry in the infrared region" (vol. 1, p. 40).   The infrared absorption spectrum is concordant with the spectrum obtained from benzylpenicillin sodium RS or with the *reference spectrum* of benzylpenicillin sodium.

B.   To 2 mg in a test-tube add 1 drop of water followed by 2 ml of sulfuric acid (~ 1760 g/l) TS and mix; the solution is colourless.   Immerse the test-tube for 1 minute in a water-bath; the solution remains colourless.   Place 2 mg in a second test-tube, add 1 drop of water and 2 ml of formaldehyde/sulfuric acid TS and mix; the solution is brownish yellow.   Immerse the test-tube for 1 minute in a water-bath; a reddish brown colour is produced.

C.   When tested for sodium as described under "General identification tests" (vol. 1, p. 115) yields the characteristic reaction.   If reaction B is to be used, ignite a small quantity and dissolve the residue in acetic acid (~ 60 g/l) TS.

Specific optical rotation.   Use a 20 mg/ml solution; $[\alpha]_D^{20\,°C} = +280$ to $+310°$.

Clarity and colour of solution.   A solution of 0.20 g in 10 ml of water is clear and colourless.

Loss on drying.   Dry to constant weight at 105 °C; it loses not more than 10 mg/g.

pH value.   pH of a 20 mg/ml solution in carbon-dioxide-free water R, 5.0–7.5.

Light-absorbing impurities.   Using a freshly prepared 1.8 mg/ml solution in water, measure the absorbances at 280 nm and at 325 nm; the absorbance at each of these wavelengths does not exceed 0.10.

Assay.   Dissolve about 50 mg, accurately weighed, in sufficient water to produce 1000 ml.   Transfer two 2.0-ml aliquots of this solution into separate stoppered tubes.   To one tube add 10.0 ml of imidazole/mercuric chloride TS, mix, stopper the tube and place in a water-bath at 60 °C for exactly 25 minutes.   Cool the tube rapidly to 20 °C (solution A).

To the second tube add 10.0 ml of water and mix (solution B).

Without delay measure the absorbance of a 1-cm layer at the maximum at about 325 nm against a solvent cell containing a mixture of 2.0 ml of water and

10.0 ml of imidazole/mercuric chloride TS for solution A and water for solution B.

From the difference between the absorbance of solution A and that of solution B, calculate the amount of $C_{16}H_{17}N_2NaO_4S$ in the substance being tested by comparison with benzylpenicillin sodium RS similarly and concurrently examined. In an adequately calibrated spectrophotometer the absorbance of the reference solution should be 0.62 ± 0.03.

Additional Requirements for Sterile Benzylpenicillin Sodium

Pyrogens. Carry out the test as described under "Test for pyrogens" (vol. 1, p. 155) injecting, per kg of the rabbit's weight, a solution containing 1.5 mg of the substance to be examined in 5 ml of sterile water R.

Sterility. Complies with the "Sterility testing of antibiotics", (vol. 1, p. 152) applying either the membrane filtration test procedure with added penicillinase TS or the direct test procedure.

BEPHENII HYDROXYNAPHTHOAS
Bephenium hydroxynaphthoate

Molecular formula. $C_{28}H_{29}NO_4$

Relative molecular mass. 443.5

Graphic formula.

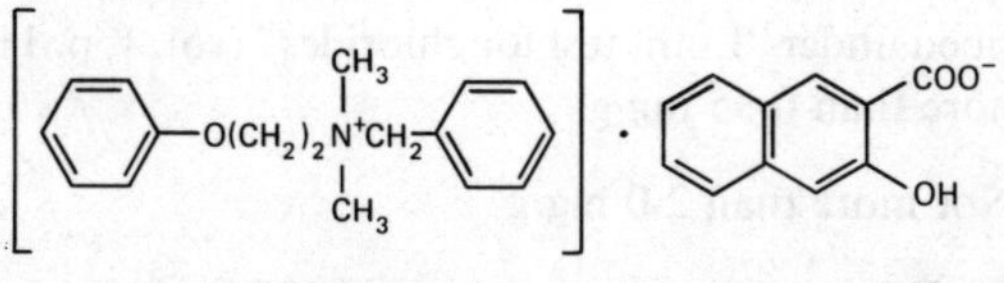

Chemical name. Benzyldimethyl(2-phenoxyethyl)ammonium 3-hydroxy-2-naphthoate (1:1); N,N-dimethyl-N-(2-phenoxyethyl)benzenemethanaminium salt with 3-hydroxy-2-naphthalenecarboxylic acid (1:1); CAS Reg. No. 3818-50-6.

Description. A yellow to greenish yellow, crystalline powder; odourless or almost odourless.

Solubility. Practically insoluble in water, ether R, benzene R, and chloroform R; soluble in 50 parts of ethanol (~750 g/l) TS.

Category. Anthelmintic.

Storage. Bephenium hydroxynaphthoate should be kept in a tightly closed container.

Additional information. Even in the absence of light. Bephenium hydroxynaphthoate is gradually degraded on exposure to a humid atmosphere, the decomposition being faster at higher temperatures.

REQUIREMENTS

General requirement. Bephenium hydroxynaphthoate contains not less than 99.0% and not more than 101.0%, of $C_{28}H_{29}NO_4$, calculated with reference to the dried substance.

Identity tests

• Either test A alone or tests B and C may be applied.

A. Carry out the examination as described under "Spectrophotometry in the infrared region" (vol. 1, p. 40). The infrared absorption spectrum is concordant with the spectrum obtained from bephenium hydroxynaphthoate RS or with the *reference spectrum* of bephenium hydroxynaphthoate.

B. See the test described below under "Related substances". The principal spots obtained with solution B at 254 nm correspond in position, appearance, and intensity with those obtained with solution C.

C. Melting temperature, about 170 °C with decomposition.

Chlorides. For the preparation of the test solution, boil 0.7 g with 30 ml of water, cool in ice and filter. Add 10 ml of nitric acid (~130 g/l) TS to the filtrate, and proceed as described under "Limit test for chlorides" (vol. 1, p. 116); the chloride content is not more than 0.35 mg/g.

Sulfated ash. Not more than 2.0 mg/g.

Loss on drying. Dry to constant weight at 105 °C; it loses not more than 10 mg/g.

Related substances. Carry out the test described under "Thin-layer chromatography" (vol. 1, p. 83), using silica gel R4 as the coating substance and a mixture of 5 volumes of 1-butanol R, 4 volumes of water and 1 volume of acetic acid (~300 g/l) TS as the mobile phase. Apply separately to the plate 5 µl of each of 3 solutions in methanol R containing (A) 40 mg of the test substance per ml, (B) 0.40 mg of the test substance per ml, and (C) 0.40 mg of bephenium hydroxy-naphthoate RS per ml. After removing the plate from the chromatographic chamber, allow it to dry in air, and examine the chromatogram in ultraviolet light (254 nm and 365 nm). At 254 nm two principal spots are visible with each of the solutions A, B, and C, whereas at 365 nm only the spots closer to the solvent front fluoresce. Any additional spot visible with solution A other than the two principal spots, is not more intense in appearance in both lights than the spot obtained closer to the starting line of solution B.

Afterwards, spray the plate first with sodium molybdotungstophosphate TS, then with sodium carbonate (200 g/l) TS, and examine the chromatogram in daylight. Two principal spots are obtained with each of the solutions A, B, and C. Any additional spot obtained with solution A, disregarding those that may have been visible in ultraviolet light, is not more intense than the principal spot closer to the solvent front obtained with solution B.

Assay. Dissolve about 0.4 g, accurately weighed, in 30 ml of glacial acetic acid R1, and titrate with perchloric acid (0.1 mol/l) VS as described under "Non-aqueous titration", Method A (vol. 1, p. 131). Each ml of perchloric acid (0.1 mol/l) VS is equivalent to 44.35 mg of $C_{28}H_{29}NO_4$.

BETAMETHASONUM

Betamethasone

Molecular formula. $C_{22}H_{29}FO_5$

Relative molecular mass. 392.5

Graphic formula.

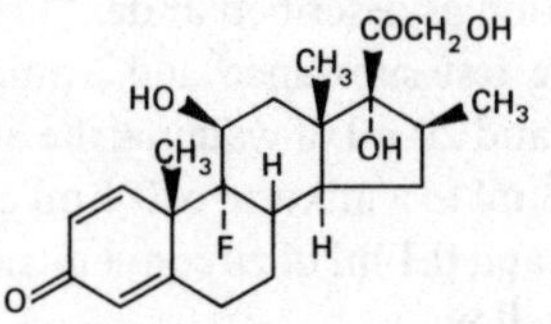

Chemical name. 9-Fluoro-11β,17,21-trihydroxy-16β-methylpregna-1,4-diene-3,20-dione; CAS Reg. No. 378-44-9.

Description. A white or creamy white powder; odourless.

Solubility. Practically insoluble in water; sparingly soluble in ethanol (~750 g/l) TS; very slightly soluble in chloroform R.

Category. Adrenoglucocorticoid.

Storage. Betamethasone should be kept in a tightly closed container, protected from light.

REQUIREMENTS

General requirement. Betamethasone contains not less than 96.0% and not more than 104.0% of $C_{22}H_{29}FO_5$, calculated with reference to the dried substance.

Identity tests

• Either tests A, B and C, or tests B, C and D may be applied.

A.   Carry out the examination as described under "Spectrophotometry in the infrared region" (vol. 1, p. 40). The infrared absorption spectrum is concordant with the spectrum obtained from betamethasone RS or with the *reference spectrum* of betamethasone (recrystallization from chloroform R of the test substance and the reference substance might be necessary to obtain the same crystalline form).

B.   Dissolve 20 mg in 20 ml of ethanol (~750 g/l) TS and dilute 2 ml to 20 ml with the same solvent. To 2 ml of this solution placed in a stoppered test-tube add 10 ml of phenylhydrazine/sulfuric acid TS, mix, heat in a water-bath at 60 °C for 20 minutes, and cool immediately. The absorbance of a 1-cm layer at the maximum at about 450 nm is not more than 0.30 (preferably use 2-cm cells for the measurement and calculate the absorbance of a 1-cm layer).

C.   See the test described below under "Related steroids". The principal spots obtained with solutions A and C correspond in position with that obtained with solution B. In addition the appearance and intensity of the principal spot obtained with solution A corresponds with that obtained with solution B.

D.   Carry out the combustion as described under "Oxygen flask method" (vol. 1, p. 125), using 7 mg of the test substance and a mixture of 0.5 ml of sodium hydroxide (0.01 mol/l) VS and 20 ml of water as the absorbing liquid. When the process is complete, add 0.1 ml to a mixture of 0.1 ml of a freshly prepared sodium alizarinsulfonate (1 g/l) TS and 0.1 ml of zirconyl nitrate TS; the red colour of the solution changes to clear yellow.

Specific optical rotation. Use a 5.0 mg/ml solution in dioxan R; $[\alpha]_D^{20\,°C} = +114$ to $+122°$.

Sulfated ash. Weigh 0.1 g and use a platinum dish; not more than 5.0 mg/g.

Loss on drying. Dry to constant weight at 100 °C under reduced pressure (not exceeding 0.6 kPa or about 5 mm of mercury); it loses not more than 5.0 mg/g.

Related steroids. Carry out the test as described under "Thin-layer chromatography" (vol. 1, p. 83), using silica gel R1 as the coating substance and a mixture of 77 volumes of dichloromethane R, 15 volumes of ether R, 8 volumes of methanol R, and 1.2 volumes of water as the mobile phase. Apply separately to the plate 1 µl of each of 2 solutions in a mixture of 9 volumes of chloroform R and 1 volume of methanol R containing (A) 15 mg of the test substance per ml and (B) 15 mg of betamethasone RS per ml; also apply to the plate 2 µl of a third solution (C) composed of a mixture of equal volumes of solutions A and B and 1 µl of a fourth solution (D) containing 0.15 mg of the test substance per ml in the same solvent mixture used for solutions A and B. After removing the plate from the chromatographic chamber, allow it to dry in air until the solvents have evaporated and heat at 105 °C for 10 minutes, allow to cool, spray with blue tetrazolium/sodium hydroxide TS, and examine the chromatogram in daylight. Any spot obtained with solution A, other than the principal spot, is not more intense than that obtained with solution D.

Assay.

• The solutions must be protected from light throughout the assay.

Dissolve about 20 mg, accurately weighed, in sufficient aldehyde-free ethanol (~750 g/l) TS to produce 100 ml. Dilute 20 ml of this solution with sufficient aldehyde-free ethanol (~750 g/l) TS to produce 100 ml. Transfer 10.0 ml of the diluted solution to a 25-ml volumetric flask, add 2.0 ml of blue tetrazolium/ethanol TS, and displace the air in the flask with oxygen-free nitrogen R. Immediately add 2.0 ml of tetramethylammonium hydroxide/ethanol TS and again displace the air with oxygen-free nitrogen R. Stopper the flask, mix the contents by gentle swirling and allow to stand for 1 hour in a water-bath at 30 °C. Cool rapidly, add sufficient aldehyde-free ethanol (~750 g/l) TS to produce 25 ml and mix. Measure the absorbance of a 1-cm layer at the maximum at about 525 nm against a solvent cell containing a solution prepared by treating 10 ml of aldehyde-free ethanol (~750 g/l) in a similar manner. Calculate the amount of $C_{22}H_{29}FO_5$ in the substance being tested by comparison with betamethasone RS, similarly and concurrently examined.

BUPIVACAINI HYDROCHLORIDUM
Bupivacaine hydrochloride

Molecular formula. $C_{18}H_{28}N_2O,HCl,H_2O$

Relative molecular mass. 342.9

Graphic formula.

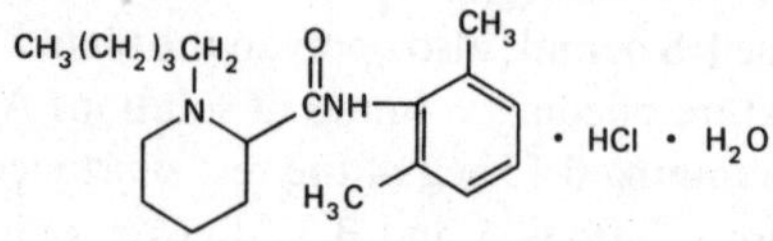

Chemical name. 1-Butyl-2′,6′-pipecoloxylidide monohydrochloride monohydrate; 1-butyl-N-(2,6-dimethylphenyl)-2-piperidinecarboxamide monohydrochloride monohydrate; CAS Reg. No. 73360-54-0.

Description. A white, crystalline powder; odourless.

Solubility. Soluble in 25 parts of water and in 8 parts of ethanol (~750 g/l) TS; slightly soluble in ether R and chloroform R.

Category. Local anaesthetic.

Storage. Bupivacaine hydrochloride should be kept in a well-closed container.

REQUIREMENTS

General requirement. Bupivacaine hydrochloride contains not less than 98.5% and not more than 101.0% of $C_{18}H_{28}N_2O,HCl$, calculated with reference to the dried substance.

Identity tests

A. Carry out the examination as described under "Spectrophotometry in the infrared region" (vol. 1, p. 40). The infrared absorption spectrum is concordant with the spectrum obtained from bupivacaine hydrochloride RS or with the *reference spectrum* of bupivacaine hydrochloride.

B. Dissolve 0.15 g in 10 ml of water and add 20 ml of trinitrophenol (7 g/l) TS. Heat the mixture to boiling, allow to cool and, if necessary, scrape the inner surface of the beaker to induce crystallization; wash the precipitate rapidly with a small quantity of water, followed by successive quantities of methanol R and ether R, using 2 ml each time; melting temperature about 194 °C (bupivacaine picrate).

C.   A 2 mg/ml solution yields reaction B, described under "General identification tests" as characteristic of chlorides (vol. 1, p. 113).

Copper.   To 0.25 g in 10 ml of water, add 0.25 ml of disodium edetate (0.05 mol/l) VS, and allow to stand for 2 minutes; add 0.2 g of copper-free citric acid R, 1 ml of ammonia (~100 g/l) TS and 1 ml of sodium diethyldithiocarbamate (0.8 g/l) TS and extract with 10 ml of carbon tetrachloride R for 2 minutes.   The colour of the extract is not deeper than that of the extract obtained when 10 ml of a mixture of 3 volumes of copper(II) sulfate (80 g/l) TS and 397 volumes of water are similarly treated.

Iron.   Ignite 1.0 g with 1 g of anhydrous sodium carbonate FeR; cool and dissolve the residue in 5 ml of hydrochloric acid (~250 g/l) FeTS and 30 ml of water.   Treat the solution as described under "Limit test for iron" (vol. 1, p. 121), using 0.5 ml of iron standard FeTS; the iron content is not more than 10 μg/g.

Sulfated ash.   Not more than 1.0 mg/g.

Loss on drying.   Dry to constant weight at 105 °C; it loses not less than 45 mg/g and not more than 60 mg/g.

pH value.   pH of a 10 mg/ml solution, 4.5–6.0.

Absorption in the ultraviolet region.   The absorption spectrum of a 0.4 mg/ml solution in hydrochloric acid (0.01 mol/l) VS, when observed between 230 nm and 350 nm, exhibits 2 maxima at about 263 nm and 271 nm.   The absorbance of a 1-cm layer at the maximum wavelength of 263 nm is not less than 0.53 and not more than 0.58, and at the maximum wavelength of 271 nm is not less than 0.43 and not more than 0.48 (preferably use 2-cm cells for the measurements and calculate the absorbances of 1-cm layers).

Related substances.   Carry out the test as described under "Thin-layer chromatography" (vol. 1, p. 83), using silica gel R1 as the coating substance and ethanol (~750 g/l) TS as the mobile phase.   Apply separately to the plate 2 μl of each of 2 solutions in methanol R containing (A) 50 mg of the test substance per ml and (B) 0.50 mg of the test substance per ml.   After removing the plate from the chromatographic chamber, allow it to dry in air, spray with potassium iodobismuthate TS2, and examine the chromatogram in daylight.   Any spot obtained with solution A, other than the principal spot, is not more intense than that obtained with solution B.

Assay.   Dissolve about 0.65 g, accurately weighed, in 30 ml of glacial acetic acid R1, add 10 ml of mercuric/acetic acid TS, and titrate with perchloric acid (0.1 mol/l) VS as described under "Non-aqueous titration", Method A (vol. 1, p. 131).   Each ml of perchloric acid (0.1 mol/l) VS is equivalent to 32.49 mg of $C_{18}H_{28}N_2O,HCl$.

CALCII GLUCONAS
Calcium gluconate

Molecular formula. $(C_6H_{11}O_7)_2Ca,H_2O$

Relative molecular mass. 448.4

Graphic formula.

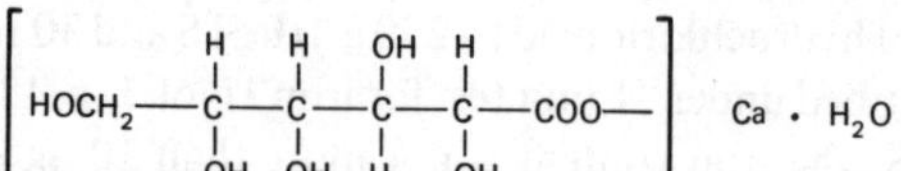

$$\left[HOCH_2 - \overset{\overset{\displaystyle H}{|}}{\underset{\underset{\displaystyle OH}{|}}{C}} - \overset{\overset{\displaystyle H}{|}}{\underset{\underset{\displaystyle OH}{|}}{C}} - \overset{\overset{\displaystyle OH}{|}}{\underset{\underset{\displaystyle H}{|}}{C}} - \overset{\overset{\displaystyle H}{|}}{\underset{\underset{\displaystyle OH}{|}}{C}} - COO - \right]_2 \quad Ca \cdot H_2O$$

Chemical name. Calcium D-gluconate (1:2) monohydrate; CAS Reg. No. 299-28-5.

Description. White, crystalline granules or a white, crystalline powder; odourless.

Solubility. Slowly soluble in water; freely soluble in boiling water; practically insoluble in dehydrated ethanol R, ether R, and chloroform R.

Category. Calcium source.

Storage. Calcium gluconate should be kept in a tightly closed container, protected from light.

Additional information. Even in the absence of light, Calcium gluconate is gradually degraded on exposure to a humid atmosphere, the decomposition being faster at higher temperatures.

REQUIREMENTS

General requirement. Calcium gluconate contains not less than 98.0% and not more than 102.0% of $(C_6H_{11}O_7)_2Ca,H_2O$, calculated as the monohydrate.

Identity tests

A.   A 20 mg/ml solution yields the reactions described under "General identification tests" as characteristic of calcium (vol. 1, p. 112).

B.   To 1 ml of a 30 mg/ml solution add 1 drop of ferric chloride (25 g/l) TS; a yellow colour is produced.

C. To 5 ml of a warm 0.1 g/ml solution add 0.7 ml of glacial acetic acid R and 1 ml of freshly distilled phenylhydrazine R, heat on a water-bath for 30 minutes, allow to cool, and scrape the inner surface of the tube to induce crystallization. Collect the crystals, dissolve in 10 ml of hot water, add a small amount of charcoal R, and filter. Allow the filtrate to cool, and scrape the inner surface of the tube; a white, crystalline precipitate is produced; melting temperature, about 200 °C with decomposition (phenylhydrazide of gluconic acid).

Heavy metals. Use 1.0 g for the preparation of the test solution as described under "Limit test for heavy metals", Procedure 3 (vol. 1, p. 118); determine the heavy metals content according to Method A (vol. 1, p. 119); not more than 20 μg/g.

Chlorides and other halides. Dissolve 0.50 g in a mixture of 2 ml of nitric acid ($\sim$130 g/l) TS and 20 ml of water, and proceed as described under "Limit test for chlorides" (vol. 1, p. 116); the chloride content is not more than 0.5 mg/g.

Magnesium and alkaline metals. Dissolve 1.0 g in 100 ml of boiling water, add 10 ml of ammonium chloride (100 g/l) TS, 1 ml of ammonia ($\sim$260 g/l) TS and, drop by drop, 50 ml of hot ammonium oxalate (25 g/l) TS. Allow to stand for 4 hours, dilute to 200 ml with water and filter. Evaporate 100 ml of the filtrate to dryness and ignite; the residue weighs not more than 2.0 mg.

Sulfates. Dissolve 5.0 g in 40 ml of boiling water, cool and filter. Proceed with the filtrate as described under "Limit test for sulfates" (vol. 1, p. 116); the sulfate content is not more than 0.1 mg/g.

Glucose and sucrose. Dissolve 0.5 g in 10 ml of hot water, add 2 ml of hydrochloric acid ($\sim$70 g/l) TS, and boil for about 2 minutes. Cool, add 15 ml of sodium carbonate (50 g/l) TS, allow to stand for 5 minutes, and filter. Add 5 ml of the clear filtrate to about 2 ml of potassio-cupric tartrate TS, and boil for 1 minute; neither a red turbidity nor any precipitate is produced.

Clarity and colour of solution. A solution of 0.50 g in 10 ml of water is clear and not more intensely coloured than standard colour solution Ywl when compared as described under "Colour of liquids" (vol. 1, p. 50).

Assay. Dissolve about 0.5 g, accurately weighed, in 20 ml of hot water containing 2 ml of hydrochloric acid ($\sim$70 g/l) TS, allow to cool and dilute to 100 ml with water. Proceed with the titration as described under "Complexometric titrations" (vol. 1, p. 128). Each ml of disodium edetate (0.05 mol/l) VS is equivalent to 22.42 mg of $(C_6H_{11}O_7)_2Ca,H_2O$.

CARBO ACTIVATUS

Charcoal, activated

Description.   Fine, black powder, free from grittiness; odourless.

Solubility.   Practically insoluble in water and in all usual solvents.

Category.   General-purpose antidote; pharmaceutic aid.

Storage.   Activated Charcoal should be kept in a well-closed container.

Additional information.   Activated Charcoal is a tasteless powder.

REQUIREMENTS

Identity test.   Heat a small quantity of the test substance to redness; it burns slowly without a flame.

Heavy metals.   Boil 1 g with a mixture of 20 ml of hydrochloric acid ($\sim$70 g/l) TS and 5 ml of bromine TS1 for 5 minutes, filter, and wash with 50 ml of boiling water. Evaporate the combined filtrates to dryness on a water-bath and add to the residue 1 ml of hydrochloric acid (1 mol/1) VS, 20 ml of water, and 5 ml of sulfurous acid TS.   Boil the solution until all the sulfur dioxide has been expelled, filter if necessary, and dilute with water to 50 ml.   Use 10 ml as the test solution and determine the content of heavy metals as described under "Limit test for heavy metals", according to Method A (vol. 1, p. 119); not more than 100 μg/g.

Cyanides.   In a distillation apparatus, heat 5 g carefully with 50 ml of water and 2 g of tartaric acid R.   Collect about 25 ml of distillate in a mixture of 10 ml of water and 2 ml of sodium hydroxide (1 mol/l) VS and dilute to 50 ml with water. To 25 ml add 0.05 g of ferrous sulfate R and heat until boiling starts. Cool in a water-bath at 70 °C and acidify with 10 ml of hydrochloric acid ($\sim$250 g/l) TS; no green or blue colour develops.

Sulfides.   To 1 g in a small conical flask, add 20 ml of water and 5 ml of hydrochloric acid ($\sim$250 g/l) TS; the escaping vapours do not darken a strip of filter paper moistened with lead acetate (80 g/l) TS.

Zinc.   To 1 g add 25 ml of nitric acid ($\sim$130 g/l) TS and heat to boiling for 5 minutes; filter through sintered glass and wash with 10 ml of hot water. Determine the content of zinc either by a dithizone method (A) or by atomic absorption spectrophotometry (B):

A.   To 10 ml of the clear solution obtained as described above add successively 3.0 ml of water, 3.0 ml of sodium acetate (60 g/l) TS, 5.0 ml of cyanide/

oxalate/thiosulfate TS, and 5.0 ml of a freshly prepared 30 mg/ml solution of dithizone R in carbon tetrachloride R. Mix thoroughly for 2–3 minutes. Separate the dithizone-layer and place in a suitable comparison tube. To 0.5 ml of zinc standard (20 μg/ml Zn) TS add 9.5 ml of water and treat it in the same manner as above. The solution of the test substance shows by reflection a more intense violet colour and, by transmitted light, a not more intense violet colour than the reference solution.

B. Dilute appropriately the solution obtained as described above and proceed as described under "Atomic absorption spectrophotometry" (vol. 1, p. 45).

Fluorescent substances. In an apparatus for intermittent extraction, treat 10 g with 100 ml of cyclohexane R1 for 2 hours. Collect the cyclohexane extract, adjust the volume to 100 ml, and examine in ultraviolet light (365 nm). The fluorescence of the solution is not more intense than that of a solution containing 0.083 mg of quinine R in 1000 ml of sulfuric acid (0.005 mol/l) VS.

Ethanol-soluble substances. In a flask fitted with a reflux condenser, heat 2 g with 50 ml of ethanol (~750 g/l) TS. Boil for 10 minutes, filter immediately, cool, and readjust the volume to 50 ml with ethanol (~750 g/l) TS; the filtrate is not more intensely coloured than reference solution Yw1. Evaporate 40 ml of the filtrate, dry the residue at 105 °C, and weigh; not more than 8 mg (5 mg/g).

Acid-soluble substances. Boil 1 g with a mixture of 20 ml of water and 5 ml of hydrochloric acid (~420 g/l) TS for 5 minutes, filter into a tared porcelain crucible, and wash the residue with 10 ml of hot water, adding the washings to the filtrate. To the combined filtrate and washings add 1 ml of sulfuric acid (~1760 g/l) TS, evaporate to dryness, and ignite to constant weight; not more than 35 mg/g.

Alkali-soluble coloured matter. Heat 0.25 g with 10 ml of sodium hydroxide (~80 g/l) TS for 1 minute, cool and filter. Dilute the filtrate to 10 ml with water; the colour is not more intense than reference solution Gn2.

Sulfated ash. Not more than 50 mg/g.

Loss on drying. Dry for 4 hours at 120 °C; it loses not more than 150 mg/g.

Acidity or alkalinity. To 2 g add 40 ml of water and heat to boiling for 5 minutes. Cool, restore to the original volume with freshly boiled and cooled water and filter. Reject the first 20 ml of filtrate. The filtrate does not induce any colour change in red or blue litmus paper R. To 10 ml of the filtrate add 0.25 ml of bromothymol blue/ethanol TS and 0.25 ml of sodium hydroxide (0.02 mol/l) VS; the solution is blue. Add 0.75 ml of hydrochloric acid (0.02 mol/l) VS; the solution turns yellow.

Adsorbing power

A.   Place 1 g, previously dried at 120 °C for 4 hours, in a solution of 100 mg of strychnine sulfate R in 50 ml of water and shake for 5 minutes; filter, rejecting the first 10 ml of filtrate.   To a 10-ml portion of the filtrate add 1 drop of hydrochloric acid (~ 420 g/l) TS and 5 drops of potassio-mercuric iodide TS; no turbidity is produced.

B.   To each of two glass-stoppered 100-ml flasks transfer 50 ml of methylthioninium chloride (1 g/l) TS.   To one of the flasks add 0.250 g, accurately weighed, of the test substance, insert the stopper in the flask, and shake for 5 minutes.   Filter the contents of each flask, rejecting the first 20 ml of each filtrate.   Transfer 25-ml portions of the filtrates to two 250-ml volumetric flasks.   Add to each flask 50 ml of sodium acetate (60 g/l) TS, mix, and add from a burette 35.0 ml of iodine (0.1 mol/l) VS, swirling the mixture during the addition. Stopper the flasks, and allow them to stand for 50 minutes, shaking them vigorously at 10-minute intervals. Dilute each mixture with water to volume, mix, allow to stand for 10 minutes, and filter, rejecting the first 30 ml of each filtrate.   Titrate the excess iodine in a 100-ml aliquot of each filtrate with sodium thiosulfate (0.1 mol/l) VS, adding 3 ml of starch TS towards the end of the titration.   Calculate the number of ml of iodine (0.1 mol/l) VS consumed in each titration; the difference between the two volumes is not less than 0.7 ml.

––––––––––––

CHLORAMPHENICOLUM

Chloramphenicol

Molecular formula. $C_{11}H_{12}Cl_2N_2O_5$

Relative molecular mass.   323.1

Graphic formula.

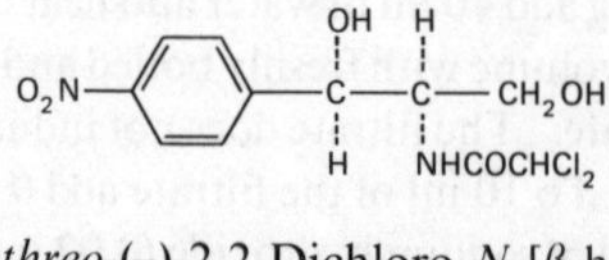

$$O_2N-\text{(benzene ring)}-\overset{\overset{OH}{|}}{\underset{\underset{H}{|}}{C}}-\overset{\overset{H}{|}}{\underset{\underset{NHCOCHCl_2}{|}}{C}}-CH_2OH$$

Chemical   name.   D-*threo*-(–)-2,2-Dichloro-*N*-[β-hydroxy-α-(hydroxymethyl)-*p*-nitrophenethyl]acetamide;   [*R*-(*R**,*R**)]-2,2-dichloro-*N*-[2-hydroxy-1-(hydroxymethyl)-2-(4-nitrophenyl)ethyl]acetamide; CAS Reg. No. 56–75–7.

Description. Colourless to greyish white or yellowish white, needle-like crystals or elongated plates or a crystalline powder; odourless.

Solubility. Slightly soluble in water; freely soluble in ethanol (~750 g/l) TS and propylene glycol R; slightly soluble in chloroform R and ether R.

Category. Antibiotic.

Storage. Chloramphenicol should be kept in a well-closed container, protected from light.

Additional information. Chloramphenicol has a bitter taste. A solution in dehydrated ethanol R is dextrorotatory and a solution in ethyl acetate R is levorotatory.

REQUIREMENTS

General requirement. Chloramphenicol contains not less than 97.0% and not more than 102.0% of $C_{11}H_{12}Cl_2N_2O_5$, calculated with reference to the dried substance.

Identity tests

● Either test A alone or tests B and C may be applied.
A. Carry out the examination as described under "Spectrophotometry in the infrared region" (vol. 1, p. 40). The infrared absorption spectrum is concordant with the spectrum obtained from chloramphenicol RS or with the *reference spectrum* of chloramphenicol.

B. See the test described below under "Related substances". The principal spot obtained with solution B corresponds in position, appearance, and intensity with that obtained with solution C.

C. Melting temperature, about 151 °C.

Specific optical rotation. Use a 50 mg/ml solution in dehydrated ethanol R; $[\alpha]_D^{20\,°C} = +18.5$ to $+21.5°$.

Free chlorides. For the preparation of the test solution shake 0.50 g with 20 ml of water and 10 ml of nitric acid (~130 g/l) TS for 1 minute, filter, and wash the filter with 5 ml of water. Proceed with the filtrate as described under "Limit test for chlorides" (vol. 1, p. 116); the chloride content is not more than 0.5 mg/g.

Solution in ethanol. A solution of 0.50 g in 10 ml of ethanol (~750 g/l) TS is clear.

Sulfated ash. Not more than 1.0 mg/g.

Loss on drying. Dry to constant weight at 105°C; it loses not more than 10 mg/g.

pH value. Shake 0.05 g with 10 ml of carbon-dioxide-free water R; pH of the suspension, 5.0–7.5.

Related substances. Carry out the test as described under "Thin-layer chromatography" (vol. 1, p. 83), using silica gel R2 as the coating substance and a mixture of 9 volumes of chloroform R and 1 volume of methanol R as the mobile phase. Apply separately to the plate 5 μl of each of 3 freshly prepared solutions in ethanol (~750 g/l) TS containing (A) 20 mg of the test substance per ml, (B) 0.20 mg of the test substance per ml, and (C) 0.20 mg of chloramphenicol RS per ml. After removing the plate from the chromatographic chamber, allow it to dry in air until the solvents have evaporated, heat at 105 °C for 5 minutes, and examine the chromatogram in ultraviolet light (254 nm). Any spot obtained with solution A, other than the principal spot, is not more intense than that obtained with solution B.

Assay. Dissolve about 20 mg, accurately weighed, in sufficient water to produce 100 ml; dilute 10.0 ml of this solution to 100 ml with the same solvent. Measure the absorbance of a 1-cm layer of the diluted solution at the maximum at about 278 nm. Calculate the amount of $C_{11}H_{12}Cl_2N_2O_5$ in the substance being tested by comparison with chloramphenicol RS, similarly and concurrently examined. In an adequately calibrated spectrophotometer, the absorbance of the reference solution should be 0.60 ± 0.03.

———————

CHLORMETHINI HYDROCHLORIDUM
Chlormethine hydrochloride

Molecular formula. $C_5H_{11}Cl_2N,HCl$

Relative molecular mass. 192.5

Graphic formula.

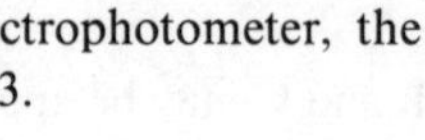

$$Cl(CH_2)_2N(CH_2)_2Cl \cdot HCl$$
$$\overset{|}{CH_3}$$

Chemical name. 2,2'-Dichloro-N-methyldiethylamine hydrochloride; 2-chloro-N-(2-chloroethyl)-N-methylethanamine hydrochloride; CAS Reg. No. 55-86-7.

Description.   A white or almost white, crystalline powder.

Solubility.   Very soluble in water; soluble in ethanol (~750 g/l) TS.

Category.   Antineoplastic.

Storage.   Chlormethine hydrochloride should be kept in a tightly closed container and stored at a cool temperature.

Additional information.   CAUTION: Chlormethine hydrochloride is vesicant, it must be handled with care avoiding contact with the skin and inhaling airborne particles.   It is hygroscopic.

REQUIREMENTS

General requirement.   Chlormethine hydrochloride contains not less than 98.0% and not more than 101.0% of $C_5H_{11}Cl_2N, HCl$, calculated with reference to the anhydrous substance.

Identity tests

A.   Dissolve 0.05 g in 5 ml of water and add 0.02 ml of potassio-mercuric iodide TS; a cream-coloured precipitate is produced.

B.   Add 0.1 g to 1 ml of sodium thiosulfate (0.1 mol/1) VS contained in a test-tube. Shake, allow to stand for 2 hours, and add 1 drop of iodine TS; the colour of free iodine remains.

C.   Melting temperature, about 110 °C with decomposition.

Clarity of solution.   A solution of 0.10 g in 10 ml of carbon-dioxide-free water R is clear.

Sulfated ash.   Not more than 1.0 mg/g.

Water.   Determine as described under "Determination of water by the Karl Fischer method", Method A (vol. 1, p. 135), using about 1 g of the substance; the water content is not more than 5.0 mg/g.

pH value.   pH of a 2.0 mg/ml solution, 3.0–5.0.

Assay.   To about 0.20 g, accurately weighed, add 15 ml of potassium hydroxide/ ethanol (1 mol/1) VS and 15 ml of water. Boil under a reflux condenser for 2 hours, and evaporate the solution to half its volume on a water-bath. Dilute to 150 ml with water, add 3 ml of nitric acid (~1000 g/l) TS and 50 ml of silver nitrate (0.1 mol/1) VS. Shake vigorously and filter. Wash the precipitate with water and titrate the excess of silver nitrate in the combined filtrate and washings with ammonium thiocyanate (0.1 mol/1) VS, using 2.5 ml of ferric ammonium sulfate (45 g/l) TS as indicator. Each ml of silver nitrate (0.1 mol/1) VS is equivalent to 6.417 mg of $C_5H_{11}Cl_2N, HCl$.

CHLOROQUINI PHOSPHAS

Chloroquine phosphate

Molecular formula. $C_{18}H_{26}ClN_3, 2H_3PO_4$

Relative molecular mass. 515.9

Graphic formula.

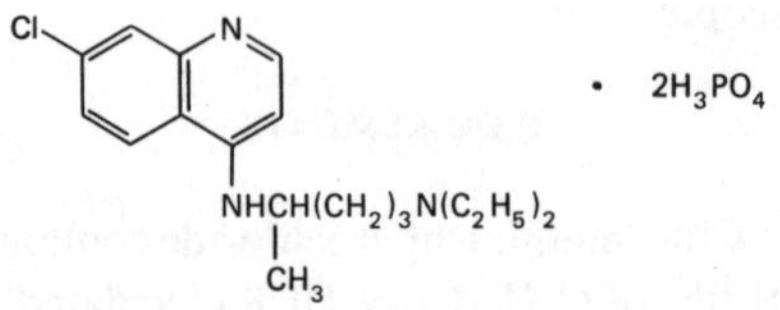

$\cdot$ $2H_3PO_4$

NHCH(CH$_2$)$_3$N(C$_2$H$_5$)$_2$

CH$_3$

Chemical name. 7-Chloro-4-[[4-(diethylamino)-1-methylbutyl]amino]quino-line phosphate (1:2); N^4-(7-chloro-4-quinolinyl)-N^1,N^1-diethyl-1,4-pentanedi-amine phosphate (1:2); CAS Reg. No. 50-63-5.

Description. A white or almost white, crystalline powder; odourless or almost odourless.

Solubility. Soluble in 4 parts of water; very slightly soluble in ethanol (~750 g/l) TS, chloroform R, and ether R.

Category. Antimalarial; antiamoebic.

Storage. Chloroquine phosphate should be kept in a well-closed container, protected from light.

Additional information. Chloroquine phosphate has a bitter taste; it is slowly discoloured by light. Chloroquine phosphate may exist in 2 polymorphic forms differing in melting temperature, one of which melts at about 194°C, the other at about 215°C; mixtures of the 2 forms melt between 194°C and 215°C.

REQUIREMENTS

General requirement. Chloroquine phosphate contains not less than 98.0% and not more than 101.0% of $C_{18}H_{26}ClN_3, 2H_3PO_4$, calculated with reference to the dried substance.

Identity tests

A. The absorption spectrum of a 10 μg/ml solution in hydrochloric acid (0.01 mol/l) VS, when observed between 240 nm and 360 nm, exhibits 3 maxima at about 257 nm, 329 nm, and 343 nm. The absorbances at those wavelengths are about 0.29, 0.32, and 0.37, respectively (preferably use 2-cm cells for the measurements and calculate the absorbances of 1-cm layers). The ratio of the absorbance of a 1-cm layer at 257 nm to that at 343 nm is between 0.77 and 0.85, and the ratio of the absorbance at 329 nm to that at 343 nm is between 0.86 and 0.95.

B. To 1 ml of a 20 mg/ml solution add 3 ml of nitric acid (~130 g/l) TS; yields reaction A described under "General identification tests" as characteristic of orthophosphates (vol. 1, p. 114).

C. To a solution of 0.05 g in 20 ml of water add 5 ml of trinitrophenol (7 g/l) TS. Filter, wash the precipitate with water until the filtrate is colourless, and dry the precipitate over silica gel, desiccant, R. Melting temperature, about 207 °C (picrate).

Loss on drying. Dry to constant weight at 105 °C; it loses not more than 20 mg/g.

pH value. pH of a 0.10 g/ml solution, 3.5–4.5.

Related substances. Carry out the test as described under "Thin-layer chromatography" (vol. 1, p. 83), using silica gel R2 as the coating substance and a mixture of 5 volumes of chloroform R, 4 volumes of cyclohexane R, and 1 volume of diethylamine R as the mobile phase. Apply separately to the plate 5 μl of each of 2 solutions containing (A) 40 mg of the test substance per ml and (B) 0.80 mg of the test substance per ml. After removing the plate from the chromatographic chamber, allow it to dry in air, and examine the chromatogram in ultraviolet light (254 nm). Any spot obtained with solution A, other than the principal spot, is not more intense than that obtained with solution B.

Assay. Dissolve about 0.23 g, accurately weighed, in 20 ml of glacial acetic acid R1 with the aid of heat (preferably heat under reflux condenser), cool and add 20 ml of dioxan R. Titrate with perchloric acid (0.1 mol/l) VS as described under "Non-aqueous titration", Method A (vol. 1, p. 131). Each ml of perchloric acid (0.1 mol/l) VS is equivalent to 25.79 mg of $C_{18}H_{26}ClN_3, 2H_3PO_4$.

CHLOROQUINI SULFAS

Chloroquine sulfate

Molecular formula. $C_{18}H_{26}ClN_3, H_2SO_4, H_2O$

Relative molecular mass. 436.0

Graphic formula.

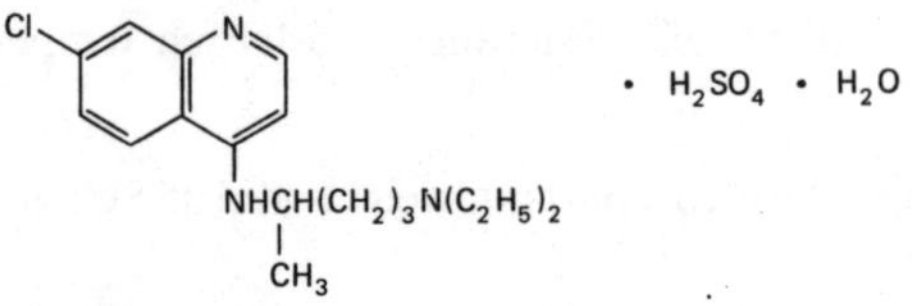

$\cdot\ H_2SO_4\ \cdot\ H_2O$

Chemical name. 7-Chloro-4-[[4-(diethylamino)-1-methylbutyl]amino]quinoline sulfate (1:1) monohydrate; N^4-(7-chloro-4-quinolinyl)-N^1,N^1-diethyl-1,4-pentanediamine sulfate (1:1) monohydrate; CAS Reg. No. 6823-83-2.

Description. A white or almost white, crystalline powder; odourless.

Solubility. Soluble in 3 parts of water; practically insoluble in ethanol (~750 g/l) TS; sparingly soluble in chloroform R and ether R.

Category. Antimalarial.

Storage. Chloroquine sulfate should be kept in a well-closed container protected from light.

Additional information. Chloroquine sulfate has a bitter taste.

REQUIREMENTS

General requirement. Chloroquine sulfate contains not less than 98.0% and not more than 101.0% of $C_{18}H_{26}ClN_3, H_2SO_4$, calculated with reference to the dried substance.

Identity tests

A. The absorption spectrum of a 10 μg/ml solution in hydrochloric acid (0.01 mol/l) VS, when observed between 240 nm and 360 nm, exhibits 3 maxima at about 257 nm, 329 nm, and 343 nm. The absorbances at those wavelengths are about 0.39, 0.44, and 0.46, respectively (preferably use 2-cm cells for the measurements and calculate the absorbances of 1-cm layers). The ratio of the absorbance of a 1-cm layer at 257 nm to that at 343 nm is between 0.83 and 0.98 and the ratio of the absorbance at 329 nm to that at 343 nm is between 0.94 and 1.03.

B.   A 0.05 g/ml solution yields reaction A described under "General identification tests" as characteristic of sulfates (vol. 1, p. 115).

C.   To a solution of 0.05 g in 20 ml of water add 5 ml of trinitrophenol (7 g/l) TS. Filter, wash the precipitate with water until the filtrate is colourless and dry the precipitate over silica gel, desiccant, R. Melting temperature, about 207 °C (picrate).

Sulfated ash.   Not more than 1.0 mg/g.

Loss on drying.   Dry to constant weight at 105 °C under reduced pressure (not exceeding 0.6 kPa or about 5 mm of mercury); it loses not less than 30 mg/g and not more than 50 mg/g.

pH value.   pH of a 0.10 g/ml solution, 4.0–5.0.

Related substances.   Carry out the test as described under "Thin-layer chromatography" (vol. 1, p. 83), using silica gel R2 as the coating substance and a mixture of 5 volumes of chloroform R, 4 volumes of cyclohexane R, and 1 volume of diethylamine R as the mobile phase. Apply separately to the plate 5 μl of each of 2 solutions containing (A) 40 mg of the test substance per ml and (B) 0.80 mg of the test substance per ml. After removing the plate from the chromatographic chamber, allow it to dry in air, and examine the chromatogram in ultraviolet light (254 nm). Any spot obtained with solution A, other than the principal spot, is not more intense than that obtained with solution B.

Assay.   Dissolve about 0.4 g, accurately weighed, in 20 ml of glacial acetic acid R1 with the aid of heat (preferably heat under a reflux condenser), cool and add 20 ml of dioxan R. Titrate with perchloric acid (0.1 mol/l) VS as described under "Non-aqueous titration", Method A (vol. 1, p. 131). Each ml of perchloric acid (0.1 mol/l) VS is equivalent to 20.90 mg of $C_{18}H_{26}ClN_3, H_2SO_4$.

CHLORPHENAMINI HYDROGENOMALEAS

Chlorphenamine hydrogen maleate

Molecular formula. $C_{16}H_{19}ClN_2, C_4H_4O_4$ or $C_{20}H_{23}ClN_2O_4$

Relative molecular mass. 390.9

Graphic formula.

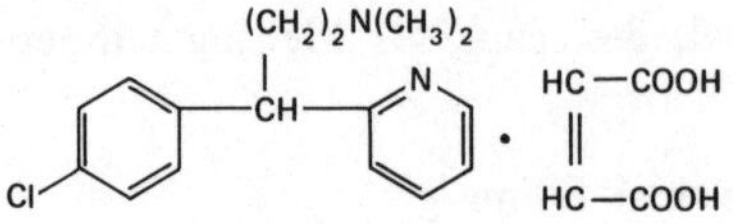

Chemical name. 2-[p-Chloro-α-[2-(dimethylamino)ethyl]benzyl]pyridine maleate (1:1); γ-(4-chlorophenyl)-N,N-dimethyl-2-pyridinepropanamine (Z)-2-butenedioate (1:1); CAS Reg. No. 113-92-8.

Other name. Chlorpheniramine hydrogen maleate.

Description. A white, crystalline powder; odourless.

Solubility. Soluble in 4 parts of water; soluble in ethanol ($\sim$750 g/l) TS and chloroform R; slightly soluble in ether R.

Category. Antihistaminic.

Storage. Chlorphenamine hydrogen maleate should be kept in a tightly closed container, protected from light.

Additional information. Even in the absence of light, Chlorphenamine hydrogen maleate is gradually degraded on exposure to a humid atmosphere, the decomposition being faster at higher temperatures.

REQUIREMENTS

General requirement. Chlorphenamine hydrogen maleate contains not less than 98.0% and not more than 101.0% of $C_{16}H_{19}ClN_2, C_4H_4O_4$, calculated with reference to the dried substance.

Identity tests

• Either tests A and C or tests B and C may be applied.
A. Carry out the examination as described under "Spectrophotometry in the infrared region" (vol. 1, p. 40). The infrared absorption spectrum is concordant

with the spectrum obtained from chlorphenamine hydrogen maleate RS or with the *reference spectrum* of chlorphenamine hydrogen maleate.

B.   Dissolve 1 mg in 5 ml of water.   To 1 ml of this solution add 1 ml of buffer phthalate, pH 3.5, TS and 1 ml of cyanogen bromide TS.   Allow to stand for 10 minutes with intermittent, gentle shaking.   Add 2 ml of a solution composed of 1 ml of aniline R diluted to 25 ml with dichloroethane R, and shake; an orange-yellow colour is produced in the lower layer.

C.   Dissolve 0.5 g in 5 ml of water, add 0.2 ml of sulfuric acid (~100 g/l) TS and extract 4 times with ether R, using 25 ml each time.   Combine the ethereal extracts, dry them over anhydrous sodium sulfate R, filter, and evaporate the filtrate in a current of warm air; melting temperature of the residue, about 132°C (maleic acid).

Sulfated ash.   Not more than 1.5 mg/g.

Loss on drying.   Dry to constant weight at 105 °C; it loses not more than 5.0 mg/g.

pH value.   pH of a 20 mg/ml solution, 4.0–5.2.

Related substances.   Carry out the test as described under "Thin-layer chromatography" (vol. 1, p. 83), using silica gel R2 as the coating substance and a mixture of 5 volumes of ethyl acetate R, 3 volumes of methanol R, and 2 volumes of acetic acid (~60 g/l) TS as the mobile phase.   Apply separately to the plate 2 μl of each of 2 solutions in chloroform R containing (A) 50 mg of the test substance per ml and (B) 0.10 mg of the test substance per ml.   After removing the plate from the chromatographic chamber, allow it to dry in air, and examine the chromatogram in ultraviolet light (254 nm).   Any spot obtained with solution A, other than the two principal spots due to chlorphenamine and maleic acid, is not more intense than that obtained with solution B.

Assay.   Dissolve about 0,4 g, accurately weighed, in 30 ml of glacial acetic acid R1, and titrate with perchloric acid (0.1 mol/l) VS as described under "Non-aqueous titration", Method A (vol. 1, p. 131).   Each ml of perchloric acid (0.1 mol/l) VS is equivalent to 19.54 mg of $C_{16}H_{19}ClN_2,C_4H_4O_4$.

CHLORPROMAZINI HYDROCHLORIDUM

Chlorpromazine hydrochloride

Molecular formula. $C_{17}H_{19}ClN_2S, HCl$

Relative molecular mass.   355.3

Graphic formula.

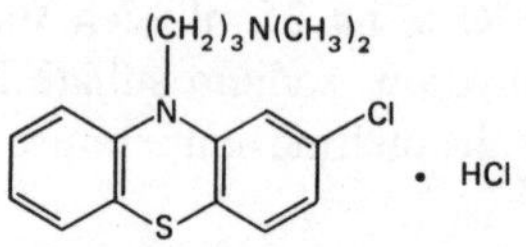

Chemical name.   2-Chloro-10-[3-(dimethylamino)propyl]phenothiazine mono-hydrochloride;   2-chloro-N,N-dimethyl-10H-phenothiazine-10-propanamine monohydrochloride; CAS Reg. No. 69-09-0.

Description.   A white or slightly creamy white, crystalline powder; odour, slight.

Solubility.   Soluble in 0.4 part of water; freely soluble in ethanol (~750 g/l) TS and chloroform R; practically insoluble in ether R.

Category.   Neuroleptic.

Storage.   Chlorpromazine hydrochloride should be kept in a tightly closed container, protected from light.

Additional information.   Chlorpromazine hydrochloride has a very bitter taste. It darkens on prolonged exposure to light.   Even in the absence of light, Chlorpromazine hydrochloride is gradually degraded on exposure to a humid atmosphere, the decomposition being faster at higher temperature.

REQUIREMENTS

General requirement.   Chlorpromazine hydrochloride contains not less than 98.0% and not more than 101.0% of $C_{17}H_{19}ClN_2S, HCl$, calculated with reference to the dried substance.

Identity tests

● Either test A alone or all 3 tests B, C, and D may be applied.

A.   Carry out the examination as described under "Spectrophotometry in the infrared region" (vol. 1, p. 40).   The infrared absorption spectrum is concordant

with the spectrum obtained from chlorpromazine hydrochloride RS or with the *reference spectrum* of chlorpromazine hydrochloride.

B.   Carry out the test as described under "Thin-layer chromatography" (vol. 1, p. 83), using kieselguhr R1 as the coating substance and a mixture of 10 volumes of 2-phenoxyethanol R, 5 volumes of macrogol 400R, and 85 volumes of acetone R to impregnate the plate. After the solvent has reached the top of the plate, remove the plate from the chromatographic chamber, and use it immediately. As the mobile phase use a mixture of 2 volumes of diethylamine R and 100 volumes of light petroleum R1 saturated with 2-phenoxyethanol R. Apply separately to the plate 2 μl of each of 2 solutions in chloroform R containing (A) 2.0 mg of the test substance per ml and (B) 2.0 mg of chlorpromazine hydrochloride RS per ml. After removing the plate from the chromatographic chamber, allow it to dry in air, and examine the chromatogram in ultraviolet light (365 nm), observing the fluorescence produced after about 2 minutes. Spray the plate with sulfuric acid/ethanol TS and examine the chromatogram in daylight. The principal spot obtained with solution A corresponds in position, appearance, and intensity with that obtained with solution B.

C.   A 0.1 g/ml solution yields reaction B described under "General identification tests" as characteristic of chlorides (vol. 1, p. 113).

D.   Melting temperature, about 196 °C.

Sulfated ash.   Not more than 1.0 mg/g.

Loss on drying.   Dry to constant weight at 105 °C; it loses not more than 5.0 mg/g.

pH value.   pH of a freshly prepared 0.10 g/ml solution, 4.0–5.0.

Related substances.   Carry out the test as described under "Thin-layer chromatography" (vol. 1, p. 83), using silica gel R2 as the coating substance and a mixture of 80 volumes of cyclohexane R, 10 volumes of acetone R, and 10 volumes of diethylamine R as the mobile phase. Apply separately to the plate 10 μl of each of 2 freshly prepared solutions in a mixture of 95 volumes of methanol R and 5 volumes of diethylamine R containing (A) 20 mg of the test substance per ml and (B) 0.50 mg of the test substance per ml. After removing the plate from the chromatographic chamber allow it to dry in air, and examine the chromatogram in ultraviolet light (254 nm). Ignore any spot on the base line. Any spot obtained with solution A, other than the principal spot, is not more intense than that obtained with solution B.

Assay.   Dissolve about 0.7 g, accurately weighed, in 200 ml of acetone R, add 10 ml of mercuric acetate/acetic acid TS and 3 ml of methyl orange/acetone TS, and titrate with perchloric acid (0.1 mol/l) VS as described under "Non-aqueous titration", Method A (vol. 1, p. 131). Each ml of perchloric acid (0.1 mol/l) VS is equivalent to 35.53 mg of $C_{17}H_{19}ClN_2S,HCl$.

CHLORTALIDONUM

Chlortalidone

Molecular formula. $C_{14}H_{11}ClN_2O_4S$

Relative molecular mass. 338.8

Graphic formula.

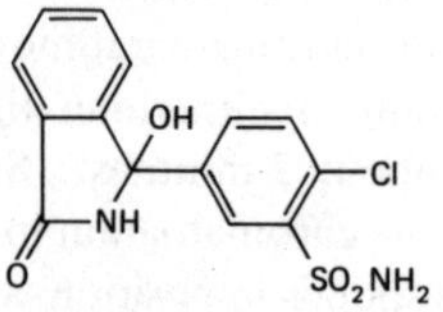

Chemical name. 2-Chloro-5-(l-hydroxy-3-oxo-1-isoindolinyl)benzenesulfon-amide; 2-chloro-5-(2,3-dihydro-1-hydroxy-3-oxo-1H-isoindol-1-yl)benzenesul-fonamide; CAS Reg. No. 77-36-1.

Description. A white to yellowish white, crystalline powder; odourless or almost odourless.

Solubility. Practically insoluble in water, ether R, and chloroform R; soluble in methanol R; slightly soluble in ethanol (~750 g/l) TS.

Category. Diuretic.

Storage. Chlortalidone should be kept in a well-closed container.

REQUIREMENTS

General requirement. Chlortalidone contains not less than 98.0% and not more than 102.0% of $C_{14}H_{11}ClN_2O_4S$, calculated with reference to the dried substance.

Identity tests

● Either tests A and B or tests B and C may be applied.

A. Carry out the examination as described under "Spectrophotometry in the infrared region" (vol. 1, p. 40). The infrared absorption spectrum is concordant

with the spectrum obtained from chlortalidone RS or with the *reference spectrum* of chlortalidone.

B. See the test described below under "Related substances". The principal spot obtained with solution A corresponds in position, appearance, and intensity with that obtained with solution B.

C. Dissolve 20 mg in 1 ml of sulfuric acid (~1760 g/l) TS; an intense yellow colour is produced. Warm the mixture in a water-bath and add 10 mg of 1-naphthol R; a red-violet colour is produced.

Solution in alkali. A solution of 1.0 g in 10 ml of sodium hydroxide (~200 g/l) TS is clear and not more intensely coloured than standard colour solution Yw2 when compared as described under "Colour of liquids" (vol. 1, p. 50).

Sulfated ash. Not more than 1.0 mg/g.

Loss on drying. Dry to constant weight at 105 °C; it loses not more than 5.0 mg/g.

Related substances. Carry out the test as described under "Thin-layer chromatography" (vol. 1, p. 83), using silica gel R2 as the coating substance and a mixture of 15 volumes of 1-butanol R and 3 volumes of ammonia (~17 g/l) TS as the mobile phase. Apply separately to the plate 10 μl of each of 3 solutions in methanol R containing (A) 10 mg of the test substance per ml, (B) 10 mg of chlortalidone RS per ml, and (C) 0.10 mg of 2-(4-chloro-3-sulfamoylbenzoyl)benzoic acid RS per ml. After removing the plate from the chromatographic chamber, allow it to dry in air, and examine the chromatogram in ultraviolet light (254 nm). Any spot obtained with solution A, other than the principal spot, is not more intense than that obtained with solution C.

Assay. Dissolve about 0.3 g, accurately weighed, in 50 ml of pyridine R and titrate with tetrabutylammonium hydroxide (0.1 mol/l) VS, determining the endpoint potentiometrically as described under "Non-aqueous titration", Method B (vol. 1, p. 132). Each ml of tetrabutylammonium hydroxide (0.1 mol/l) VS is equivalent to 33.88 mg of $C_{14}H_{11}ClN_2O_4S$.

CLOXACILLINUM NATRICUM

Cloxacillin sodium

Cloxacillin sodium (non-injectable)
Cloxacillin sodium, sterile

Molecular formula. $C_{19}H_{17}ClN_3NaO_5S, H_2O$

Relative molecular mass. 475.9

Graphic formula.

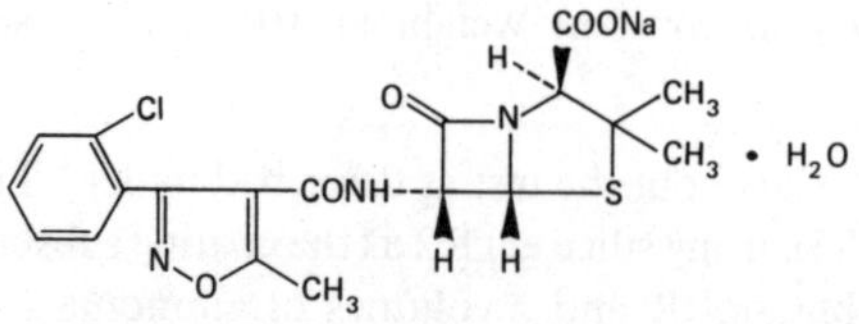

Chemical name. Sodium (2S,5R,6R)-6-[3-(o-chlorophenyl)-5-methyl-4-isoxazolecarboxamido]-3,3-dimethyl-7-oxo-4-thia-1-azabicyclo[3.2.0]heptane-2-carboxylate monohydrate;   sodium [2S-(2α,5α,6β)]-6-[[[3-(2-chlorophenyl)-5 methyl-4-isoxazolyl]carbonyl]amino]-3,3-dimethyl-7-oxo-4-thia-1-azabicyclo-[3.2.0]heptane-2-carboxylate monohydrate; monosodium [3-(o-chlorophenyl)-5-methyl-4-isoxazolyl]penicillin monohydrate; CAS Reg. No. 7081-44-9.

Description. A white, crystalline powder; odourless.

Solubility. Soluble in 2.5 parts of water, in 30 parts of ethanol (~750 g/l) TS and in 500 parts of chloroform R.

Category. Antibiotic.

Storage. Cloxacillin sodium should be kept in a tightly closed container, protected from light, and stored at a temperature not exceeding 25 °C.

Labelling. The designation sterile Cloxacillin sodium indicates that the substance complies with the additional requirements for sterile Cloxacillin sodium and may be used for parenteral administration or for other sterile applications.

Additional information. Cloxacillin sodium is hygroscopic. Even in the absence of light, Cloxacillin sodium is gradually degraded on exposure to a humid atmosphere, the decomposition being faster at higher temperatures.

REQUIREMENTS

General requirement. Cloxacillin sodium contains not less than 90.0% of total penicillins calculated as $C_{19}H_{18}ClN_3O_5S$, and with reference to the anhydrous substance.

Identity tests

• Either tests A and C or tests B and C may be applied.

A. Carry out the examination as described under "Spectrophotometry in the infrared region" (vol. 1, p. 40). The infrared absorption spectrum is concordant with the spectrum obtained from cloxacillin sodium RS or with the *reference spectrum* of cloxacillin sodium.

B. Place 2 mg into a test-tube, add 2 mg of disodium chromotropate R and 2 ml of sulfuric acid (~1760 g/l) TS. Immerse the tube in a suitable bath at 150 °C for 3–4 minutes; a purple colour is produced.

C. Ignite 20 mg and dissolve the residue in acetic acid (~60 g/l) TS. The solution yields reaction B described under "General identification tests" as characteristic of sodium (vol. 1, p. 115).

Specific optical rotation. Use a 10 mg/ml solution, and calculate with reference to the anhydrous substance; $[\alpha]_D^{20\,°C} = +163$ to $+172°$.

Water. Determine as described under "Determination of water by the Karl Fischer method", Method A (vol. 1, p. 135), using about 0.25 g of the substance; the water content is not less than 35 mg/g and not more than 45 mg/g.

pH value. pH of a 0.10 g/ml solution in carbon-dioxide-free water R, 5.0–7.0.

Chlorine. Carry out the combustion as described under the "Oxygen flask method" (vol. 1, p. 124), but using 0.040 g of the test substance and 20 ml of sodium hydroxide (1 mol/l) VS as the absorbing liquid. When the process is complete, add 2.5 ml of nitric acid (~130 g/l) TS, 2.5 ml of water, and 20 ml of silver nitrate (0.01 mol/l) VS and titrate with ammonium thiocyanate (0.01 mol/l) VS, using ferric ammonium sulfate (45 g/l) TS as indicator. Repeat the operation without the substance being tested. Each ml of silver nitrate (0.01 ml/l) VS is equivalent to 0.3546 mg of Cl; the chlorine content is 70–75 mg/g.

Assay. Dissolve about 50 mg, accurately weighed, in sufficient water to produce 1000 ml. Transfer two 2.0-ml aliquots of this solution into separate stoppered tubes. To one tube add 10 ml of imidazole/mercuric chloride TS, mix, stopper the tube and place in a water-bath at 60 °C for exactly 25 minutes. Cool the tube rapidly to 20 °C (solution A).

To the second tube add 10.0 ml of water and mix (solution B).

Without delay measure the absorbance of a 1-cm layer at the maximum at about 343 nm against a solvent cell containing a mixture of 2.0 ml of water and

10.0 ml of imidazole/mercuric chloride TS for solution A and water for solution B.

From the difference between the absorbance of solution A and that of solution B, calculate the amount of $C_{19}H_{17}ClN_3NaO_5S$ in the substance being tested by comparison with cloxacillin sodium RS, similarly and concurrently examined. In an adequately calibrated spectrophotometer the absorbance of the reference solution should be 0.40 ± 0.02.

Additional Requirements for Sterile Cloxacillin Sodium

Undue toxicity.   Carry out the test as described under "Test for undue toxicity" (vol. 1, p. 154) using 0.5 ml of a solution in saline TS containing a quantity equivalent to 20 mg/ml.

Pyrogens.   Carry out the test as described under "Test for pyrogens" (vol. 1, p. 155) injecting, per kg of the rabbit's weight, a solution containing 6 mg of the substance to be examined in 5 ml of sterile water R.

Sterility.   Complies with the "Sterility testing of antibiotics" (vol. 1, p. 152), applying either the membrane filtration test procedure with added penicillinase TS or the direct test procedure.

CODEINUM MONOHYDRICUM

Codeine monohydrate

Molecular formula. $C_{18}H_{21}NO_3, H_2O$

Relative molecular mass.   317.4

Graphic formula.

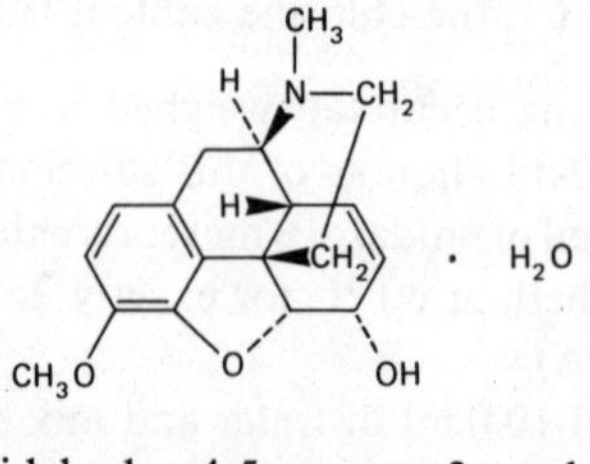

Chemical name.   7,8-Didehydro-4,5α-epoxy-3-methoxy-17-methylmorphinan-6α-ol monohydrate; CAS Reg. No. 6059-47-8.

Description. Colourless crystals or a white, crystalline powder; odourless.

Solubility. Slightly soluble in water; freely soluble in ethanol (~750 g/l) TS and ether R.

Category. Antitussive; analgesic.

Storage. Codeine monohydrate should be kept in a tightly closed container, protected from light.

Additional information. Codeine monohydrate effloresces slowly in dry air.

REQUIREMENTS

General requirement. Codeine monohydrate contains not less than 99.0% and not more than 101.0% of $C_{18}H_{21}NO_3$, calculated with reference to the dried substance.

Identity tests

A. Dissolve 5 mg in 1 ml of sulfuric acid (~1760 g/l) TS, add 1 drop of ferric chloride (25 g/l) TS, and warm on a water-bath; a blue colour is produced, which changes to red on the addition of 1 drop of nitric acid (~130 g/l) TS.

B. Dissolve 1 mg in 0.5 ml of selenious acid/sulfuric acid TS; a green colour is produced, which rapidly changes to blue, then slowly to dark yellow-green.

C. Melting temperature, about 156°C.

Specific optical rotation. Use a 20 mg/ml solution in ethanol (~750 g/l) TS and calculate with reference to the dried substance; $[\alpha]_D^{20\,°C} = -142$ to $-146°$.

Clarity and colour of solution. A solution of 0.050 g in 10 ml of water is clear and colourless.

Sulfated ash. Not more than 1.0 mg/g.

Loss on drying. Dry to constant weight at 105°C; it loses not less than 50 mg/g and not more than 60 mg/g.

pH value. pH of a 5.0 mg/ml solution in carbon-dioxide-free water R, not less than 9.0.

Related alkaloids. Carry out the test as described under "Thin-layer chromatography" (vol. 1, p. 83), using silica gel R1 as the coating substance and a mixture of 72 volumes of ethanol (~750 g/l) TS, 30 volumes of cyclohexane R, and 6 volumes of ammonia (~260 g/l) TS as the mobile phase. Apply separately to the plate 10 μl of each of 2 solutions in a mixture of 4 volumes of hydrochloric acid (0.01 mol/l) VS and 1 volume of ethanol (~750 g/l) TS containing (A) 50 mg of the test substance per ml and (B) 0.66 mg of the test substance per ml. After removing the plate from the chromatographic chamber, allow it to dry in air, spray with potassium iodobismuthate TS2, and examine the chromatogram in daylight. Any spot obtained with solution A, other than the principal spot, is not more intense than that obtained with solution B.

Assay. Dissolve about 0.25 g, accurately weighed, in 30 ml of glacial acetic acid R1, add 10 ml of acetic anhydride R, and titrate with perchloric acid (0.1 mol/l) VS as described under "Non-aqueous titration", Method A (vol. 1, p. 131). Each ml of perchloric acid (0.1 mol/l) VS is equivalent to 29.94 mg of $C_{18}H_{21}NO_3$.

CODEINI PHOSPHAS

Codeine phosphate

Codeine phosphate hemihydrate
Codeine phosphate sesquihydrate

Molecular formula. $C_{18}H_{21}NO_3,H_3PO_4,\frac{1}{2}H_2O$ (hemihydrate);
$C_{18}H_{21}NO_3,H_3PO_4,1\frac{1}{2}H_2O$ (sesquihydrate).

Relative molecular mass. 406.4 (hemihydrate); 424.4 (sesquihydrate).

Graphic formula.

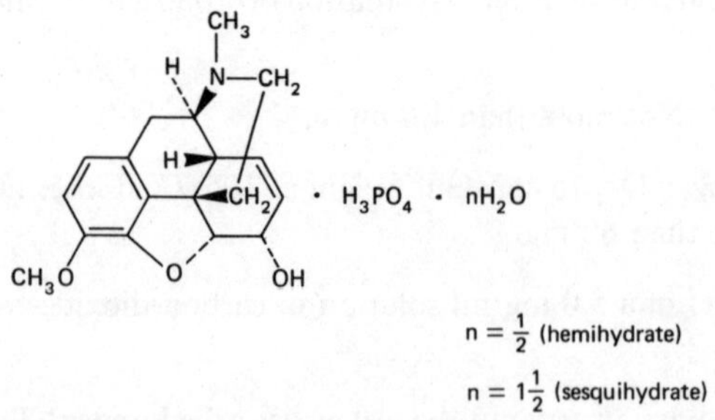

$\cdot\ H_3PO_4\ \cdot\ nH_2O$

$n = \frac{1}{2}$ (hemihydrate)

$n = 1\frac{1}{2}$ (sesquihydrate)

Chemical name. 7,8-Didehydro-4,5α-epoxy-3-methoxy-17-methylmorphinan-6α-ol phosphate (1:1) (salt) hemihydrate; CAS Reg. No. 41444-62-6 (hemihydrate).   7,8-Didehydro-4,5α-epoxy-3-methoxy-17-methylmorphinan-6α-ol phosphate (1:1) (salt) sesquihydrate; CAS Reg. No.5913-76-8 (sesquihydrate).

Description. Small, colourless crystals or a white, crystalline powder; odourless.

Solubility. Soluble in 4 parts of water; slightly soluble in ethanol (~750 g/l) TS; practically insoluble in chloroform R and ether R.

Category. Antitussive; analgesic.

Storage. Codeine phosphate should be kept in a tightly closed container, protected from light.

Labelling. The designation on the container should state if the Codeine phosphate is the hemihydrate or the sesquihydrate.

Additional information. Codeine phosphate effloresces in dry air.

REQUIREMENTS

General requirement. Codeine phosphate contains not less than 98.0% and not more than 101.0% of $C_{18}H_{21}NO_3, H_3PO_4$, calculated with reference to the dried substance.

Identity tests

A. Dissolve 5 mg in 1 ml of sulfuric acid (~1760 g/l) TS, add 1 drop of ferric chloride (25 g/l) TS, and warm on a water-bath; a blue colour is produced, which changes to red on the addition of 1 drop of nitric acid (~130 g/l) TS.

B. Dissolve 1 mg in 0.5 ml of selenious acid/sulfuric acid TS; a green colour is produced, which rapidly changes to blue, then slowly to dark yellow-green.

C. Neutralize a 20 mg/ml solution with ammonia (~100 g/l) TS; it yields reaction B described under "General identification tests" as characteristic of orthophosphates (vol. 1, p. 114).

D. To 5 ml of a 0.2 g/ml solution add 1 ml of ammonia (~100 g/l) TS, cool and scratch the inside of the test-tube to induce crystallization. Wash the precipitate with ethanol (~750 g/l) TS and dry at 105°C. Melting temperature, about 156°C (codeine base).

Specific optical rotation.   Use a 20 mg/ml solution and calculate with reference to the dried substance; $[\alpha]_D^{20\,°C} = -98$ to $-102\,°$.

Chlorides.   Dissolve 0.70 g in a mixture of 2 ml of nitric acid ($\sim$130 g/l) TS and 20 ml of water, and proceed as described under "Limit test for chlorides" (vol. 1, p. 116); the chloride content is not more than 0.35 mg/g.

Sulfates.   Dissolve 0.50 g in 20 ml of water and proceed as described under "Limit test for sulfates" (vol. 1, p. 116); the sulfate content is not more than 1 mg/g.

Clarity and colour of solution.   A solution of 0.40 g in 10 ml of water is clear and not more intensely coloured than standard colour solution Yw2 when compared as described under "Colour of liquids" (vol. 1, p. 50).

Loss on drying.   Dry to constant weight at 105 °C: Codeine phosphate (hemihydrate) loses not more than 30 mg/g.   Codeine phosphate sesquihydrate loses not less than 50 mg/g and not more than 70 mg/g.

pH value.   pH of a 0.04 g/ml solution, 4.2–5.0.

Related alkaloids.   Carry out the test as described under "Thin-layer chromatography" (vol. 1, p. 83), using silica gel R1 as the coating substance and a mixture of 72 volumes of ethanol ($\sim$750 g/l) TS, 30 volumes of cyclohexane R and 6 volumes of ammonia ($\sim$260 g/l) TS as the mobile phase.   Apply separately to the plate 10 μl of each of 2 solutions in a mixture of 4 volumes of hydrochloric acid (0.01 mol/l) VS and 1 volume of ethanol ($\sim$750 g/l) TS containing (A) 50 mg of the test substance per ml and (B) 0.66 mg of the test substance per ml.   After removing the plate from the chromatographic chamber, allow it to dry in air, spray with potassium iodobismuthate TS2, and examine the chromatogram in daylight.   Any spot obtained with solution A, other than the principal spot, is not more intense than that obtained with solution B.

Assay.   Dissolve about 0.35 g, accurately weighed, in 30 ml of glacial acetic acid R1, and titrate with perchloric acid (0.1 mol/l) VS as described under "Non-aqueous titration", Method A (vol. 1, p. 131).   Each ml of perchloric acid (0.1 mol/l) VS is equivalent to 39.74 mg of $C_{18}H_{21}NO_3,H_3PO_4$.

COFFEINUM

Caffeine

Caffeine anhydrous
Caffeine monohydrate

Molecular formula. $C_8H_{10}N_4O_2$ (anhydrous); $C_8H_{10}N_4O_2,H_2O$ (monohydrate).

Relative molecular mass. 194.2 (anhydrous); 212.2 (monohydrate).

Graphic formula.

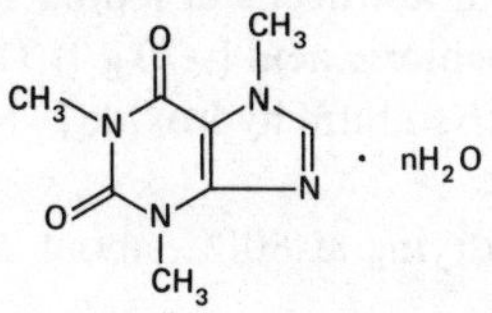

$\cdot \; nH_2O$

n = 0 (anhydrous)
n = 1 (monohydrate)

Chemical name. 3,7-Dihydro-1,3,7-trimethyl-1H-purine-2,6-dione; CAS Reg. No. 58-08-2 (anhydrous). 3,7-Dihydro-1,3,7-trimethyl-1H-purine-2,6-dione monohydrate; CAS Reg. No. 5743-12-4 (monohydrate).

Description. Silky, colourless crystals or a white, crystalline powder; odourless.

Solubility. Soluble in 60 parts of water and in 100 parts of ethanol (~750 g/l) TS; freely soluble in chloroform R; slightly soluble in ether R.

Category. Central nervous stimulant.

Storage. Caffeine should be kept in a well-closed container.

Labelling. The designation on the container of Caffeine should state whether the substance is the monohydrate or is in the anhydrous form .

Additional information. Caffeine monohydrate is efflorescent in air.

REQUIREMENTS

General requirement. Caffeine contains not less than 98.5% and not more than 101.0% of $C_8H_{10}N_4O_2$, calculated with reference to the dried substance.

Identity tests

• Either test A alone or all 3 tests B, C, and D may be applied.

A. Carry out the examination as described under "Spectrophotometry in the infrared region" (vol. 1, p. 40). For Caffeine monohydrate, the substance must be previously dried to constant weight at 80 °C. The infrared absorption spectrum is concordant with the spectrum obtained from caffeine RS or with the *reference spectrum* of caffeine.

B. To 10 mg, contained in a porcelain dish, add 1 ml of hydrochloric acid (~250 g/l) TS and 0.5 ml of hydrogen peroxide (~60 g/l) TS, and evaporate to dryness on a water-bath. Add 1 drop of ammonia (~100 g/l) TS; the residue acquires a purple colour, which disappears upon the addition of 2–3 drops of sodium hydroxide (~80 g/l) TS.

C. To a saturated solution add a few drops of iodine TS; the solution remains clear. Add a few drops of hydrochloric acid (~70 g/l) TS; a brown precipitate is produced. On neutralization with sodium hydroxide (~80 g/l) TS, the precipitate dissolves.

D. Melting temperature, after drying at 80 °C, about 236 °C.

Clarity and colour of solution. A solution of 5.0 g in 10 ml of boiling water is clear and colourless.

Sulfated ash. Not more than 1.0 mg/g.

Loss on drying. Dry to constant weight at 80 °C: Caffeine (anhydrous) loses not more than 5.0 mg/g. Caffeine monohydrate loses not less than 50 mg/g and not more than 90 mg/g.

pH value. pH of a 10 mg/ml solution in carbon-dioxide-free water R, 4.8–6.6.

Related substances. Carry out the test as described under "Thin-layer chromatography" (vol. 1, p. 83), using silica gel R2 as the coating substance and a mixture of 4 volumes of 1-butanol R, 3 volumes of chloroform R, and 1 volume of ammonia (~260 g/l) TS as the mobile phase. Prepare 2 solutions in a mixture of 6 volumes of chloroform R and 4 volumes of methanol R containing (A) 20 mg of the test substance per ml and (B) 0.20 mg of the test substance per ml. Apply separately to the plate 10 µl of solution A and 5 µl of solution B. After removing the plate from the chromatographic chamber, allow it to dry in air, and examine the chromatogram in ultraviolet light (254 nm). Any spot obtained with solution A, other than the principal spot, is not more intense than that obtained with solution B.

Assay. Dissolve about 0.18 g, accurately weighed, in 10 ml of acetic anhydride R and 20 ml of toluene R, and titrate with perchloric acid (0.1 mol/l) VS as described under "Non-aqueous titration", Method A (vol. 1, p. 131). Each ml of perchloric acid (0.1 mol/l) VS is equivalent to 19.42 mg of $C_8H_{10}N_4O_2$.

COLECALCIFEROLUM

Colecalciferol

Molecular formula. $C_{27}H_{44}O$

Relative molecular mass. 384.7

Graphic formula.

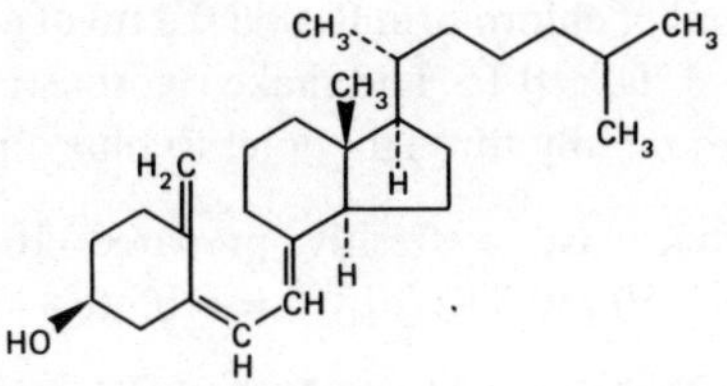

Chemical name. (5Z,7E)-9,10-Secocholesta-5,7,10(19)-trien-3β-ol; CAS Reg. No. 67-97-0.

Other name. Cholecalciferol.

Description. Colourless crystals or a white, crystalline powder; odourless.

Solubility. Practically insoluble in water; soluble in ethanol (~750 g/l) TS, ether R, and chloroform R.

Category. Vitamin, antirachitic.

Storage. Colecalciferol should be kept in a hermetically closed container, in an inert atmosphere, protected from light and stored in a cool place.

Additional information. Even in the absence of light, Colecalciferol is gradually degraded on exposure to a humid atmosphere, the decomposition being faster at higher temperatures.

REQUIREMENTS

General requirement. Colecalciferol contains not less than 95.0% and not more than 105.0% of $C_{27}H_{44}O$.

Identity tests

• Either test A alone or tests B and C may be applied.

A.   Carry out the examination as described under "Spectrophotometry in the infrared region" (vol. 1, p. 40). The infrared absorption spectrum is concordant with the spectrum obtained from colecalciferol RS or with the *reference spectrum* of colecalciferol.

B.   Dissolve 1 mg in 1 ml of dichloroethane R and add 4 ml of antimony trichloride TS; a yellowish orange colour is produced.

C.   Dissolve 5 mg in 5 ml of chloroform R, add 0.3 ml of acetic anhydride R and 0.1 ml of sulfuric acid (~1760 g/l) TS, and shake vigorously; a bright red colour is produced which changes rapidly through violet to blue and finally to green.

Specific optical rotation. Use a freshly prepared 10 mg/ml solution in aldehyde-free ethanol (~750 g/l) TS; $[\alpha]_D^{20\,°C} = +105$ to $+112°$.

7-Dehydrocholesterol.   Dissolve 0.04 g in 2 ml of ethanol (~750 g/l) TS, using a glass-stoppered test-tube, and add 1 ml of digitonin TS; the solution produced remains clear for 12 hours.

Assay. With the aid of heat, dissolve about 20 mg, accurately weighed, in sufficient aldehyde-free ethanol (~750 g/l) TS to produce 100 ml; dilute 5.0 ml of this solution to 100 ml with the same solvent. Measure without delay the absorbance of a 1-cm layer of the diluted solution at the maximum at about 265 nm. Calculate the amount of $C_{27}H_{44}O$ in the substance being tested by comparison with colecalciferol RS, similarly and concurrently examined. In an adequately calibrated spectrophotometer the absorbance of the reference solution should be 0.54 ± 0.03.

CYANOCOBALAMINUM

Cyanocobalamin

Molecular formula. $C_{63}H_{88}CoN_{14}O_{14}P$

Relative molecular mass. 1355

Graphic formula.

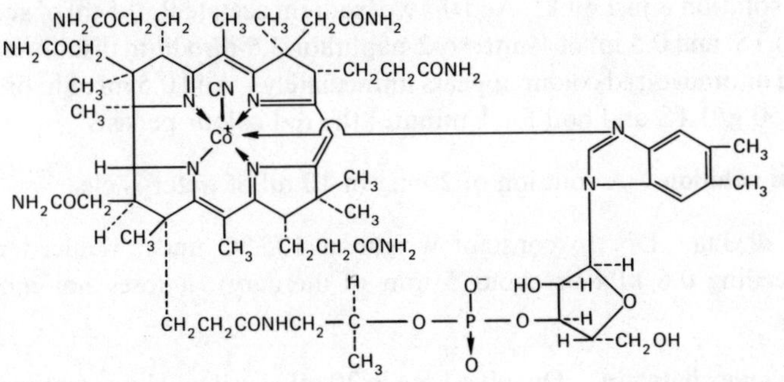

Chemical name. α-(5,6-Dimethylbenzimidazol-2-yl)cobamide cyanide; CAS Reg. No. 68-19-9.

Other name. Vitamin B_{12}.

Description. Dark red crystals or a red, crystalline powder; odourless.

Solubility. Soluble in 80 parts of water; soluble in ethanol (~750 g/l) TS; practically insoluble in acetone R, chloroform R, and ether R.

Category. Haemopoietic.

Storage. Cyanocobalamin should be kept in a tightly closed container, protected from light.

Additional information. The anhydrous form of Cyanocobalamin is highly hygroscopic.

REQUIREMENTS

General requirement. Cyanocobalamin contains not less than 96.0% and not more than 102.0% of $C_{63}H_{88}CoN_{14}O_{14}P$, calculated with reference to the dried substance.

Identity tests

A.   The absorption spectrum of a 20 $\mu g/ml$ solution, when observed between 230 nm and 600 nm, exhibits 3 maxima at about 278 nm, 361 nm and 550 nm; the ratio of the absorbance of a 1-cm layer at 361 nm to that at 278 nm is between 1.70 and 1.90, and the ratio of the absorbance at 361 nm to that at 550 nm is between 3.15 and 3.45.

B.   Mix 1 mg with about 10 mg of potassium sulfate R and 2 drops of sulfuric acid ($\sim$100 g/l) TS, heat the mixture carefully to redness until fused. Cool, break up the mass with a glass rod, and dissolve in 3 ml of water by boiling. Add 1 drop of phenolphthalein/ethanol TS and, drop by drop, sodium hydroxide ($\sim$80 g/l) TS until the solution is just pink. Add 0.5 g of sodium acetate R, 0.5 ml of acetic acid ($\sim$ 60 g/l) TS, and 0.5 ml of 1-nitroso-2-naphthol-3,6-disodium disulfonate (2 g/l) TS; a red or orange-red colour appears immediately. Add 0.5 ml of hydrochloric acid ($\sim$250 g/l) TS and boil for 1 minute; the red colour persists.

Clarity of solution.   A solution of 20 mg in 10 ml of water is clear.

Loss on drying.   Dry to constant weight at 105 $^{\circ}$C under reduced pressure (not exceeding 0.6 kPa or about 5 mm of mercury); it loses not more than 120 mg/g.

Pseudocyanocobalamin.   Dissolve 1 mg in 20 ml of water. Transfer the solution to a small separator, add 5 ml of a mixture of equal volumes of carbon tetrachloride R and freshly distilled o-cresol R, and shake well for about 1 minute. Allow to separate, draw off the lower layer into a second small separator, add a mixture of 2.5 ml of sulfuric acid ($\sim$570 g/l) TS and 2.5 ml of water, shake well and allow to separate completely (the separation of the layers may be facilitated by centrifuging). Prepare a reference solution containing 1.5 ml of potassium permanganate (0.002 mol/1) VS in 250 ml of water. The separated upper layer of the test solution is colourless or not more intensely coloured than the reference solution when compared as described under "Colour of liquids" (vol. 1, p. 50).

Related substances.   Carry out the test as described under "Thin-layer chromatography" (vol. 1, p. 83), using equal parts of silica gel R1 and kieselguhr R1 as the coating substance and a mixture of 15 volumes of chloroform R, 10 volumes of methanol R, and 3 volumes of ammonia ($\sim$100 g/l) TS as the mobile phase. Carry out all operations protected from light. Apply separately to the plate 10 μl of each of 3 solutions containing (A) 5.0 mg of the test substance per ml, (B) 0.20 mg of the test substance per ml, and (C) 0.10 mg of the test substance per ml. After removing the plate from the chromatographic chamber, allow it to dry in air, and examine the chromatogram in daylight. Any spot obtained with solution A, other than the principal spot is not more intense than that obtained with solution B. Not more than one spot obtained with solution A, other than the principal spot, is more intense than that obtained with solution C.

Assay. Dissolve about 0.03 g, accurately weighed, in sufficient water to produce 1000 ml. Determine the absorbance of this solution in a 1-cm layer at the maximum at about 361 nm and calculate the content of $C_{63}H_{88}CoN_{14}O_{14}P$, using the absorptivity value of 20.7 ($E_{1\,cm}^{1\%} = 207$).

DAPSONUM

Dapsone

Molecular formula. $C_{12}H_{12}N_2O_2S$

Relative molecular mass. 248.3

Graphic formula.

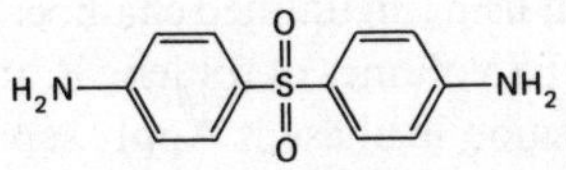

Chemical name. 4,4'-Sulfonyldianiline; 4,4'-sulfonylbis[benzenamine]; 4,4'-diaminodiphenylsulfone; CAS Reg. No. 80-08-0.

Description. A white or creamy white, crystalline powder; odourless.

Solubility. Soluble in 7000 parts of water and in 30 parts of ethanol (~750 g/l) TS; soluble in acetone R.

Category. Antileprotic.

Storage. Dapsone should be kept in a tightly closed container, protected from light.

Additional information. Even in the absence of light, Dapsone is gradually degraded on exposure to a humid atmosphere, the decomposition being faster at higher temperatures.

REQUIREMENTS

General requirement. Dapsone contains not less than 99.0% and not more than 101.0% of $C_{12}H_{12}N_2O_2S$, calculated with reference to the dried substance.

Identity tests

A. The absorption spectrum of a 5.0 μg/ml solution in methanol R, when observed between 230 nm and 350 nm, exhibits maxima at about 260 nm and 295 nm; the absorbances of a 1-cm layer at the maximum wavelength of 260 nm and 295 nm are about 0.72 and 1.20, repectively.

B. See the test described below under "Related substances". The principal spot obtained with solution A corresponds in position, appearance, and intensity with that obtained with solution B.

C. About 0.1 g yields the reaction described for the identification of primary aromatic amines under "General identification tests" (vol. 1, p. 111), producing a vivid red precipitate.

D. Melting temperature, about 178 °C.

Sulfated ash. Not more than 1.0 mg/g.

Loss on drying. Dry to constant weight at 105 °C; it loses not more than 15 mg/g.

Related substances. Carry out the test as described under "Thin-layer chromatography" (vol. 1, p. 83), but using an unlined chamber, silica gel R3 as the coating substance, and a mixture of 8 volumes of toluene R and 4 volumes of acetone R saturated with water as the mobile phase.   Apply separately to the plate 10 μl of each of 5 solutions in methanol R containing (A) 10 mg of the test substance per ml, (B) 10 mg of dapsone RS per ml, (C) 0.15 mg of the test substance per ml, (D) 20 μg of the test substance per ml and (E) 0.10 mg of 4,4'-thiodianiline RS per ml.   The solution of 4,4'-thiodianiline RS should be freshly prepared.   Pour the mobile phase into the chamber and insert the plate immediately, to avoid prior saturation of the chamber.   After removing the plate from the chromatographic chamber, spray it with 4-dimethylaminocinnamaldehyde TS2.   Heat the plate at 100 °C and examine the chromatogram in daylight.   The spot obtained with solution C is more intense than any spot obtained with solution A, other than the principal spot, and in addition, not more than 2 among those secondary spots are more intense than the spot obtained with solution D.   Moreover, there is no visible spot corresponding in position and appearance with that obtained with solution E.

Assay. Carry out the assay as described under "Nitrite titration" (vol. 1, p. 133), using about 0.25 g, accurately weighed, dissolved in a mixture of 15 ml of water and 15 ml of hydrochloric acid ($\sim$70 g/l) TS and titrate with sodium nitrite (0.1 mol/l) VS.   Each ml of sodium nitrite (0.1 mol/l) VS is equivalent to 12.42 mg of $C_{12}H_{12}N_2O_2S$.

DEXAMETHASONI ACETAS

Dexamethasone acetate

Dexamethasone acetate, anhydrous
Dexamethasone acetate monohydrate

Molecular formula. $C_{24}H_{31}FO_6$ (anhydrous); $C_{24}H_{31}FO_6,H_2O$ (monohydrate).

Relative molecular mass. 434.5

Graphic formula.

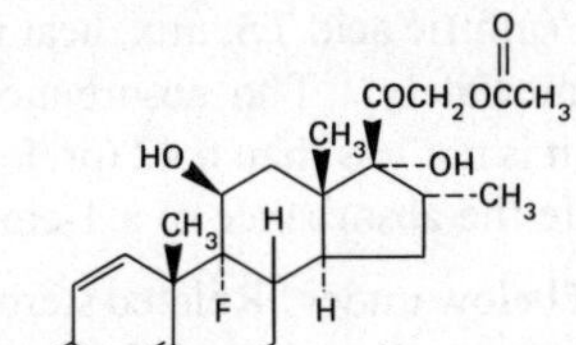

Chemical name. 9-Fluoro-11β,17,21-trihydroxy-16α-methylpregna-1,4-diene-3,20-dione 21-acetate; 21-(acetyloxy)-9-fluoro-11β,17-dihydroxy-16α-methyl-pregna-1,4-diene-3,20-dione; CAS Reg. No. 1177-87-3 (anhydrous).
9-Fluoro-11β,17,21-trihydroxy-16α-methylpregna-1,4-diene-3,20-dione 21-acetate monohydrate; 21-(acetyloxy)-9-fluoro-11β,17-dihydroxy-16α-methyl-pregna-1,4-diene-3,20-dione monohydrate; CAS Reg. No. 55812-90-3 (mono-hydrate).

Description. A white or almost white powder, odourless.

Solubility. Practically insoluble in water; soluble in 40 parts of ethanol (~750 g/l) TS; slightly soluble in ether R; sparingly soluble in chloroform R.

Category. Adrenoglucocorticoid.

Storage. Dexamethasone acetate should be kept in a tightly closed container, protected from light.

Labelling. The designation on the container of Dexamethasone acetate should state whether the substance is the monohydrate or is in the anhydrous form.

REQUIREMENTS

General requirement. Dexamethasone acetate contains not less than 96.0% and not more than 104.0% of $C_{24}H_{31}FO_6$, calculated with reference to the dried substance.

Identity tests

• Either tests A, B, C and E, or tests B, C, D and E may be applied.

A. Carry out the examination as described under "Spectrophotometry in the infrared region" (vol. 1, p. 40). For the anhydrous form the infrared absorption spectrum is concordant with the spectrum obtained from dexamethasone acetate RS or with the *reference spectrum* of dexamethasone acetate. For the monohydrate the infrared absorption spectrum is concordant with the spectrum obtained from dexamethasone acetate monohydrate RS or with the *reference spectrum* of dexamethasone acetate monohydrate.

B. Dissolve 22 mg in 20 ml of ethanol (~750 g/l) TS and dilute 2 ml to 20 ml with the same solvent. To 2 ml of this solution placed in a stoppered test-tube add 10 ml of phenylhydrazine/sulfuric acid TS, mix, heat in a water-bath at 60 °C for 20 minutes and cool immediately. The absorbance of a 1-cm layer at the maximum at about 423 nm is not less than 0.42 (preferably use 2-cm cells for the measurement and calculate the absorbance of a 1-cm layer).

C. See the test described below under "Related steroids". The principal spots obtained with solutions A and C correspond in position with that obtained with solution B. In addition the appearance and intensity of the principal spot obtained with solution A corresponds with that obtained with solution B.

D. Carry out the combustion as described under "Oxygen flask method" (vol. 1, p. 125), using 7 mg of the test substance and a mixture of 0.5 ml of sodium hydroxide (0.01 mol/l) VS and 20 ml of water as the absorbing liquid. When the process is complete, add 0.1 ml to a mixture of 0.1 ml of freshly prepared sodium alizarinsulfonate (1 g/l) TS and 0.1 ml of zirconyl nitrate TS; the red colour of the solution changes to clear yellow.

E. Heat 0.05 g with 2 ml of potassium hydroxide/ethanol (0.5 mol/l) VS in a water-bath for 5 minutes. Cool, add 2 ml of sulfuric acid (~700 g/l) TS, and boil gently for 1 minute; ethyl acetate, perceptible by its odour (proceed with caution), is produced.

Specific optical rotation. Use a 10 mg/ml solution in dioxan R; $[\alpha]_D^{20\,°C} = +82$ to $+88°$.

Sulfated ash. Weigh 0.1 g and use a platinum dish; not more than 5.0 mg/g.

Loss on drying. Dry to constant weight at 100 °C under reduced pressure (not exceeding 0.6 kPa or about 5 mm of mercury). For the anhydrous form use about 0.5 g of the substance; it loses not more than 5.0 mg/g. For the monohydrate use about 0.15 g of the substance; it loses not less than 35 mg/g and not more than 45 mg/g.

Related steroids. Carry out the test as described under "Thin-layer chromatography" (vol. 1, p. 83), using silica gel R1 as the coating substance and a mixture of 77 volumes of dichloromethane R, 15 volumes of ether R, 8 volumes of methanol R, and 1.2 volumes of water as the mobile phase. Apply separately to the plate 1 μl of each of 2 solutions in a mixture of 9 volumes of chloroform R and

1 volume of methanol R containing (A) 15 mg of the test substance per ml and (B) 15 mg of dexamethasone acetate RS per ml; also apply to the plate 2 μl of a third solution (C) composed of a mixture of equal volumes of solutions A and B and 1 μl of a fourth solution (D) containing 0.15 mg of the test substance per ml in the same solvent mixture as used for solutions A and B. After removing the plate from the chromatographic chamber, allow it to dry in air until the solvents have evaporated and heat at 105 °C for 10 minutes; allow to cool, spray with blue tetrazolium/ sodium hydroxide TS, and examine the chromatogram in daylight. Any spot obtained with solution A, other than the principal spot, is not more intense than that obtained with solution D.

Assay

• The solutions must be protected from light throughout the assay.

Dissolve about 20 mg, accurately weighed, in sufficient aldehyde-free ethanol (~750 g/l) TS to produce 100 ml. Dilute 20 ml of this solution with sufficient aldehyde-free ethanol (~750 g/l) TS to produce 100 ml. Transfer 10.0 ml of the diluted solution to a 25-ml volumetric flask, add 2.0 ml of blue tetrazolium/ ethanol TS and displace the air with oxygen-free nitrogen R. Immediately add 2.0 ml of tetramethylammonium hydroxide/ethanol TS and again displace the air with oxygen-free nitrogen R. Stopper the flask, mix the contents by gentle swirling and allow to stand for 1 hour in a water-bath at 30 °C. Cool rapidly, add sufficient aldehyde-free ethanol (~750 g/l) TS to produce 25 ml, and mix. Measure the absorbance of a 1-cm layer at the maximum at about 525 nm against a solvent cell containing a solution prepared by treating 10 ml of aldehyde-free ethanol (~750 g/l) TS in a similar manner. Calculate the amount of $C_{24}H_{31}FO_6$ in the substance being tested by comparison with dexamethasone acetate RS, similarly and concurrently examined.

DEXAMETHASONUM

Dexamethasone

Molecular formula. $C_{22}H_{29}FO_5$

Relative molecular mass.   392.5

Graphic formula.

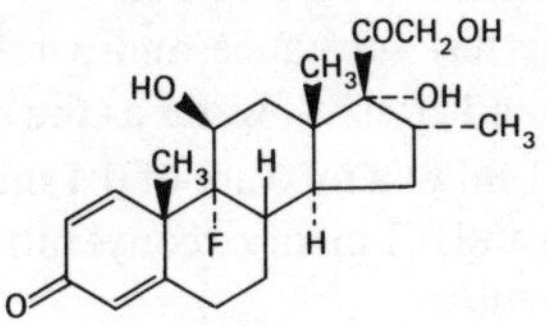

Chemical name.   9-Fluoro-11β,17,21-trihydroxy-16α-methylpregna-1,4-diene-3,20-dione; CAS Reg. No. 50-02-2.

Description.   Colourless crystals or a white or almost white, crystalline powder; odourless.

Solubility.   Practically insoluble in water; sparingly soluble in ethanol (~750 g/l) TS; slightly soluble in chloroform R.

Category.   Adrenoglucocorticoid.

Storage.   Dexamethasone should be kept in a tightly closed container, protected from light.

REQUIREMENTS

General requirement.   Dexamethasone contains not less than 96.0% and not more than 104.0% of $C_{22}H_{29}FO_5$, calculated with reference to the dried substance.

Identity tests

• Either tests A, B and C, or tests B, C and D may be applied.

A.   Carry out the examination as described under "Spectrophotometry in the infrared region" (vol. 1, p. 40).   The infrared absorption spectrum is concordant with the spectrum obtained from dexamethasone RS or with the *reference spectrum* of dexamethasone.

B.   Dissolve 20 mg in 20 ml of ethanol (~750 g/l) TS and dilute 2 ml to 20 ml with the same solvent.   To 2 ml of this solution placed in a stoppered test-tube add 10 ml of phenylhydrazine/sulfuric acid TS, mix, heat in a water-bath at 60°C for 20 minutes, and cool immediately.   The absorbance of a 1-cm layer at the maximum at about 423 nm is not less than 0.42 (preferably use 2-cm cells for the measurement and calculate the absorbance of a 1-cm layer).

C.   See the test described below under "Related steroids".   The principal spots obtained with solutions A and C correspond in position with that obtained with solution B.   In addition the appearance and intensity of the principal spot obtained with solution A corresponds with that obtained with solution B.

D.   Carry out the combustion as described under "Oxygen flask method" (vol. 1, p. 125), using 7 mg of the test substance and a mixture of 0.5 ml of sodium hydroxide (0.01 mol/l) VS and 20 ml of water as the absorbing liquid.   When the process is complete add 0.1 ml to a mixture of 0.1 ml of freshly prepared sodium alizarinsulfonate (1 g/l) TS and 0.1 ml of zirconyl nitrate TS; the red colour of the solution changes to clear yellow.

Specific optical rotation.   Use a 10 mg/ml solution in dioxan R; $[\alpha]_D^{20\ ^\circ C} = +72$ to $+80^\circ$.

Sulfated ash.   Weigh 0.1 g and use a platinum dish; not more than 5.0 mg/g.

Loss on drying.   Dry to constant weight at 100 °C under reduced pressure (not exceeding 0.6 kPa or about 5 mm of mercury); it loses not more than 5.0 mg/g.

Related steroids.   Carry out the test as described under "Thin-layer chromatography" (vol. 1, p. 83), using silica gel R1 as the coating substance and a mixture of 77 volumes of dichloromethane R, 15 volumes of ether R, 8 volumes of methanol R, and 1.2 volumes of water as the mobile phase.   Apply separately to the plate 1 μl of each of 2 solutions in a mixture of 9 volumes of chloroform R and 1 volume of methanol R containing (A) 15 mg of the test substance per ml and (B) 15 mg of dexamethasone RS per ml; also apply to the plate 2 μl of a third solution (C) composed of a mixture of equal volumes of solutions A and B and 1 μl of a fourth solution (D) containing 0.15 mg of the test substance per ml in the same solvent mixture as used for solutions A and B.   After removing the plate from the chromatographic chamber, allow it to dry in air until the solvents have evaporated and heat at 105 °C for 10 minutes; allow to cool, spray with blue tetrazolium/ sodium hydroxide TS, and examine the chromatogram in daylight.   Any spot obtained with solution A, other than the principal spot, is not more intense than that obtained with solution D.

Assay

• The solutions must be protected from light throughout the assay.

Dissolve about 20 mg, accurately weighed, in sufficient aldehyde-free ethanol (~750 g/l) TS to produce 100 ml.   Dilute 20 ml of this solution with sufficient aldehyde-free ethanol (~750 g/l) TS to produce 100 ml.   Transfer 10.0 ml of the diluted solution to a 25-ml volumetric flask, add 2.0 ml of blue tetrazolium/ ethanol TS, and displace the air in the flask with oxygen-free nitrogen R. Immediately add 2.0 ml of tetramethylammonium hydroxide/ethanol TS and again displace the air with oxygen-free nitrogen R.   Stopper the flask, mix the contents by gentle swirling, and allow to stand for 1 hour in a water-bath at 30 °C. Cool rapidly, add sufficient aldehyde-free ethanol (~750 g/l) TS to produce 25 ml, and mix.   Measure the absorbance of a 1-cm layer at the maximum at about 525 nm against a solvent cell containing a solution prepared by treating 10 ml of aldehyde-free ethanol (~750 g/l) TS in a similar manner.   Calculate the amount of $C_{22}H_{29}FO_5$ in the substance being tested by comparison with dexamethasone RS, similarly and concurrently examined.

DIAZEPAMUM

Diazepam

Molecular formula. $C_{16}H_{13}ClN_2O$

Relative molecular mass. 284.7

Graphic formula.

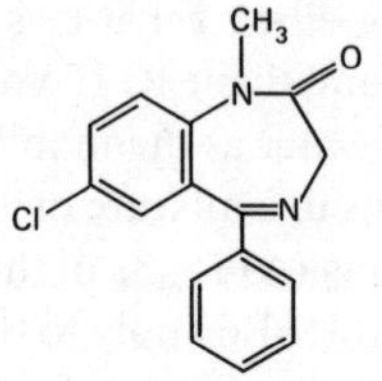

Chemical name. 7-Chloro-1,3-dihydro-1-methyl-5-phenyl-2H-1,4-benzodiaze-pin-2-one; CAS Reg. No. 439-14-5.

Description. A white or almost white, crystalline powder; odourless or almost odourless.

Solubility. Very slightly soluble in water; soluble in ethanol (~750 g/l) TS; freely soluble in chloroform R.

Category. Tranquillizer.

Storage. Diazepam should be kept in a well-closed container, protected from light.

REQUIREMENTS

General requirement. Diazepam contains not less than 99.0% and not more than 101.0% of $C_{16}H_{13}ClN_2O$, calculated with reference to the dried substance.

Identity tests

• Either tests A and D or tests B, C and D may be applied.

NOTE: For tests B and C use low-actinic glassware and measure within 30 minutes.

A.   Carry out the examination as described under "Spectrophotometry in the infrared region" (vol. 1, p. 40). The infrared absorption spectrum is concordant with the spectrum obtained from diazepam RS or with the *reference spectrum* of diazepam.

B. The absorption spectrum of an 8.0 μg/ml solution in hydrochloric acid (0.1 mol/l) VS, when observed between 230 nm and 350 nm, exhibits maxima at about 241 nm and 286 nm; the absorbances of a 1-cm layer at the maximum wavelengths of 241 nm and 286 nm are about 0.80 and 0.38, respectively (preferably use 2-cm cells for the measurements and calculate the absorbances for 1-cm layers).

C. The absorption spectrum of a 0.030 mg/ml solution in hydrochloric acid (0.1 mol/l) VS, when observed between 325 nm and 400 nm, exhibits a maximum at about 362 nm; the absorbance of a 1-cm layer at this wavelength is about 0.44 (preferably use 2-cm cells for the measurement and calculate the absorbance of a 1-cm layer).

D. Carry out the combustion as described under "Oxygen flask method" (vol. 1, p. 124), using 20 mg of the test substance and 5 ml of sodium hydroxide (~80 g/l) TS as the absorbing liquid. When the process is complete, acidify with sulfuric acid (~100 g/1) TS and boil gently for 2 minutes; the solution yields reaction A, described under "General identification tests" as characteristic of chlorides (vol. 1, p. 112).

Melting range. 131–135 °C.

Heavy metals. Use 1.0 g for the preparation of the test solution as described under "Limit test for heavy metals", Procedure 3 (vol. 1, p. 118); determine the heavy metals content according to Method A (vol. 1, p. 119); not more than 20 μg/g.

Sulfated ash. Not more than 1.0 mg/g.

Loss on drying. Dry to constant weight at 50 °C under reduced pressure (not exceeding 0.6 kPa or about 5 mm of mercury); it loses not more than 5.0 mg/g.

Related substances. Carry out the test in subdued light as described under "Thin-layer chromatography" (vol. 1, p. 83), using silical gel R2 as the coating substance and a mixture of 1 volume of dehydrated ethanol R and 24 volumes of ethyl acetate R as the mobile phase. Apply separately to the plate 10 μl of each of 2 freshly prepared solutions in chloroform R containing (A) 0.20 g of the test substance per ml and (B) 0.10 mg of 5-chloro-2-methylaminobenzophenone RS per ml. After removing the plate from the chromatographic chamber, allow it to dry in air, and examine the chromatogram in ultraviolet light (254 nm). Any spot obtained with solution A, other than the principal spot, is not more intense than that obtained with solution B.

Assay. Dissolve about 0.55 g, accurately weighed, in 30 ml of glacial acetic acid R1, and titrate with perchloric acid (0.1 mol/l) VS, determining the endpoint potentiometrically as described under "Non-aqueous titration", Method A (vol. 1, p. 131). Each ml of perchloric acid (0.1 mol/1) VS is equivalent to 28.47 mg of $C_{16}H_{13}ClN_2O$.

———————

DIAZOXIDUM

Diazoxide

Molecular formula. $C_8H_7ClN_2O_2S$

Relative molecular mass. 230.7

Graphic formula.

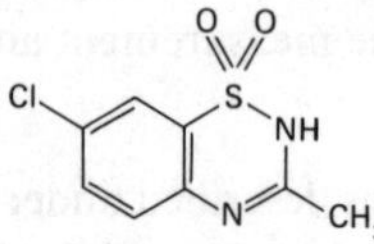

Chemical name. 7-Chloro-3-methyl-2H-1,2,4-benzothiadiazine 1,1-dioxide; CAS Reg. No. 364-98-7.

Description. A white, or almost white, crystalline powder; odourless.

Solubility. Practically insoluble in water, ether R, and chloroform R; freely soluble in dimethylformamide R; slightly soluble in ethanol (~750 g/1) TS.

Category. Antihypertensive.

Storage. Diazoxide should be kept in a well-closed container.

REQUIREMENTS

General requirement. Diazoxide contains not less than 98.0% and not more than 101.0% of $C_8H_7ClN_2O_2S$, calculated with reference to the dried substance.

Identity tests

A. Carry out the examination as described under "Spectrophotometry in the infrared region" (vol. 1, p. 40). The infrared absorption spectrum is concordant with the spectrum obtained from diazoxide RS or with the *reference spectrum* of diazoxide.

B. See the test described below under "Related substances". The principal spot obtained with solution B corresponds in position, appearance, and intensity with that obtained with solution C.

Sulfated ash. Not more than 1.0 mg/g.

Loss on drying. Dry to constant weight at 105 °C; it loses not more than 5.0 mg/g.

Related substances. Carry out the test as described under "Thin-layer chromatography" (vol. 1, p. 83), using silica gel R2 as the coating substance and a mixture of 17 volumes of ethyl acetate R, 4 volumes of methanol R, and 3 volumes of ammonia (~260 g/l) TS as the mobile phase. Apply separately to the plate 10 μl of each of 3 solutions in sodium hydroxide (0.1 mol/l) VS containing (A) 15 mg of the test substance per ml, (B) 0.15 mg of the test substance per ml and (C) 0.15 mg of diazoxide RS per ml. After removing the plate from the chromatographic chamber, allow it to dry in air until the odour of ammonia is no longer detectable, and examine the chromatogram in ultraviolet light (254 nm). Any spot obtained with solution A, other than the principal spot, is not more intense than that obtained with solution B.

Assay. Dissolve 0.45 g, accurately weighed, in 100 ml of a mixture of 2 volumes of dimethylformamide R and 1 volume of water, and titrate with sodium hydroxide (0.1 mol/l) VS, determining the endpoint potentiometrically. Each ml of sodium hydroxide (0.1 mol/l) VS is equivalent to 23.07 mg of $C_8H_7ClN_2O_2S$.

DICOUMAROLUM
Dicoumarol

Molecular formula. $C_{19}H_{12}O_6$

Relative molecular mass. 336.3

Graphic formula.

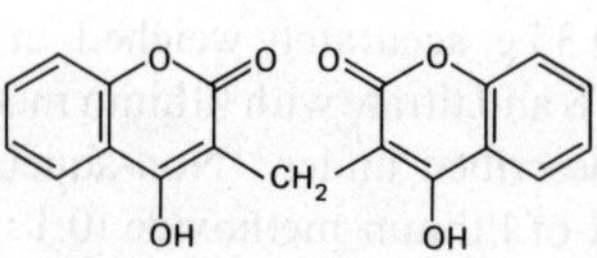

Chemical name. 3,3'-Methylenebis[4-hydroxycoumarin]; 3,3'-methylenebis[4-hydroxy-2H-1-benzopyran-2-one]; CAS Reg. No. 66-76-2.

Description. A white or creamy white, crystalline powder; odour, characteristic, faint.

Solubility. Practically insoluble in water, ethanol (~750 g/l) TS, and ether R; slightly soluble in chloroform R.

Category. Anticoagulant.

Storage. Dicoumarol should be kept in a well-closed container, protected from light.

REQUIREMENTS

General requirement. Dicoumarol contains not less than 98.5% and not more than 101.0% of $C_{19}H_{12}O_6$, calculated with reference to the dried substance.

Identity tests

• Either test A alone or tests B and C may be applied.

A. Carry out the examination as described under "Spectrophotometry in the infrared region" (vol. 1, p. 40). The infrared absorption spectrum is concordant with the spectrum obtained from dicoumarol RS or with the *reference spectrum* of dicoumarol.

B. Fuse 0.2 g with 0.2 g of potassium hydroxide R, cool, stir with 5 ml of water, filter and acidify the filtrate with hydrochloric acid (~250 g/l) TS; a white, crystalline precipitate is obtained (salicylic acid). Retain the filtrate for test C.

C. To 1 ml of the filtrate from test B add 5 ml of water and a mixture of 1 drop of ferric chloride (25 g/l) TS and 2 drops of hydrochloric acid (~70 g/l) TS; a violet colour is produced.

Sulfated ash. Not more than 2.5 mg/g.

Loss on drying. Dry to constant weight at 105 °C; it loses not more than 5.0 mg/g.

Acidity. Shake 0.5 g with 10 ml of carbon-dioxide-free water R for 1 minute and filter; titrate the filtrate with sodium hydroxide (0.1 mol/l) VS, methyl red/ethanol TS being used as indicator; not more than 0.1 ml is required to obtain the midpoint of the indicator (orange).

Assay. Dissolve about 0.35 g, accurately weighed, in 40 ml of 1-butylamine R, add 5 drops of azo violet TS and titrate with lithium methoxide (0.1 mol/l) VS to a deep-blue endpoint, as described under "Non-aqueous titration", Method B, (vol. 1, p. 132). Each ml of lithium methoxide (0.1 mol/l) VS is equivalent to 16.82 mg of $C_{19}H_{12}O_6$.

DIETHYLCARBAMAZINI DIHYDROGENOCITRAS

Diethylcarbamazine dihydrogen citrate

Molecular formula. $C_{10}H_{21}N_3O,C_6H_8O_7$ or $C_{16}H_{29}N_3O_8$

Relative molecular mass. 391.4

Graphic formula.

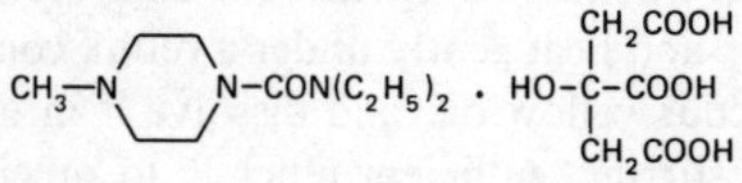

$$CH_3-N \underset{\smile}{\overset{\frown}{N}}-CON(C_2H_5)_2 \ . \ HO-\underset{\underset{CH_2COOH}{|}}{\overset{\overset{CH_2COOH}{|}}{C}}-COOH$$

Chemical name. N,N-Diethyl-4-methyl-1-piperazinecarboxamide citrate (1:1); N,N-diethyl-4-methyl-l-piperazinecarboxamide 2-hydroxy-1,2,3-propanetri-carboxylate (1:1); CAS Reg. No. 1642-54-2.

Description. A white, crystalline powder; odourless or almost odourless.

Solubility. Very soluble in water; soluble in 35 parts of ethanol (~750 g/l) TS; practically insoluble in chloroform R and ether R.

Category. Filaricide.

Storage. Diethylcarbamazine dihydrogen citrate should be kept in a tightly closed container, protected from light.

Additional information. Diethylcarbamazine dihydrogen citrate is hygroscopic; it has an acid and bitter taste. Even in the absence of light, Diethylcarbamazine dihydrogen citrate is gradually degraded on exposure to a humid atmosphere, the decomposition being faster at higher temperatures.

REQUIREMENTS

General requirement. Diethylcarbamazine dihydrogen citrate contains not less than 98.0% and not more than 101.0% of $C_{10}H_{21}N_3O,C_6H_8O_7$, calculated with reference to the anhydrous substance.

Identity tests

• Either tests A and D or tests B and C may be applied.
A. Dissolve 0.05 g in 25 ml of water. Add 1 ml of sodium hydroxide (~80 g/l) TS and 4 ml of carbon disulfide R, and shake for 2 minutes. Separate the aqueous layer. Centrifuge the lower layer if necessary, and filter through a dry filter,

collecting the filtrate in a small flask provided with a glass stopper. Carry out the examination of the filtered solution using carbon disulfide R as the blank as described under "Spectrophotometry in the infrared region" (vol. 1, p. 40). The infrared absorption spectrum is concordant with the spectrum obtained from diethylcarbamazine dihydrogen citrate RS treated similarly or with the *reference spectrum* of diethylcarbamazine base.

B. Dissolve 0.5 g in 10 ml of water, add 10 ml of sodium hydroxide (1 mol/l) VS, and extract with 4 successive quantities, each of 5 ml of chloroform R. Retain the aqueous layer for test C. Wash the combined chloroform extracts with water, filter through a plug of cotton wool, and evaporate the chloroform. Add 1 ml of ethyl iodide R to the residue, and heat gently under a reflux condenser for 5 minutes. Cool, separate the viscous yellow oil, and dissolve it in ethanol (~750 g/l) TS. Add, with continuous stirring, sufficient ether R to precipitate the quaternary ammonium salt, and filter. Dissolve the precipitate in ethanol (~750 g/l) TS, reprecipitate with ether R, and dry at 105 °C; melting temperature, about 152 °C (1-diethylcarbamoyl-4-methylpiperazine ethiodide).

C. The aqueous layer from test B yields reaction B described under "General identification tests" as characteristic of citrates (vol. 1, p. 113).

D. Melting temperature, after drying at 80 °C, about 137 °C.

Heavy metals. Use 1.0 g for the preparation of the test solution as described under "Limit test for heavy metals", Procedure 1 (vol. 1, p. 118); determine the heavy metals content according to Method A (vol. 1, p. 119); not more than 20 μg/g.

Sulfated ash. Not more than 1.0 mg/g.

Water. Determine as described under "Determination of water by the Karl Fischer method", Method A (vol. 1, p. 135), using about 1 g of the substance; the water content is not more than 10 mg/g.

pH value. pH of a 30 mg/ml solution, 3.5–4.5.

N-**Methylpiperazine.** Carry out the test as described under "Thin-layer chromatography" (vol. 1, p. 83), using silica gel R1 as the coating substance and a mixture of 6 volumes of ethanol (~750 g/l) TS, 3 volumes of glacial acetic acid R and 1 volume of water as the mobile phase. Apply separately to the plate 5 μl of each of 2 solutions in methanol R containing (A) 50 mg of the test substance per ml and (B) 0.050 mg of *N*-methylpiperazine R per ml. After removing the plate from the chromatographic chamber, allow it to dry in air, spray with a mixture of 3 volumes of platinic chloride (60 g/l) TS, 97 volumes of water and 100 volumes of potassium iodide (60 g/l) TS, and examine the chromatogram in daylight. The spot obtained with solution B is more intense than any spot, corresponding in position and appearance, obtained with solution A.

Assay. Dissolve about 0.35 g, accurately weighed, in 30 ml of glacial acetic acid R1, and titrate with perchloric acid (0.1 mol/l) VS as described under "Non-aqueous titration", Method A (vol. 1, p. 131). Each ml of perchloric acid (0.1 mol/l) VS is equivalent to 39.14 mg of $C_{10}H_{21}N_3O,C_6H_8O_7$.

DIGITOXINUM

Digitoxin

Molecular formula. $C_{41}H_{64}O_{13}$

Relative molecular mass. 765.0

Graphic formula.

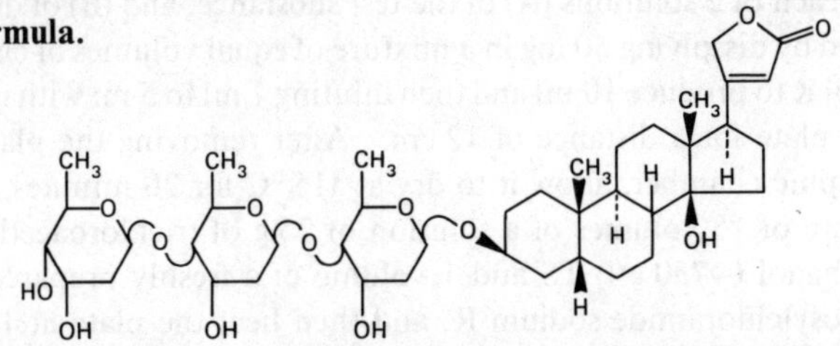

Chemical name. 3β-[(O-2,6-Dideoxy-β-D-ribo-hexopyranosyl-(1→4)-O-2,6-dideoxy-β-D-ribo-hexopyranosyl-(1→4)-2,6-dideoxy-β-D-ribo-hexopyranosyl)-oxy]-14-hydroxy-5β-card-20(22)-enolide; CAS Reg. No. 71-63-6.

Description. A white or almost white, microcrystalline powder; odourless.

Solubility. Practically insoluble in water; slightly soluble in ethanol (~750 g/l) TS; sparingly soluble in chloroform R.

Category. Cardiotonic.

Storage. Digitoxin should be kept in a well-closed container, protected from light.

Additional information. CAUTION: Digitoxin is extremely poisonous and should be handled with care.

REQUIREMENTS

General requirement. Digitoxin contains not less than 95.0% and not more than 105.0% of $C_{41}H_{64}O_{13}$, calculated with reference to the dried substance.

Identity tests

• Either tests A, B and D or tests B, C and D may be applied.

A. Carry out the examination as described under "Spectrophotometry in the infrared region" (vol. 1, p. 40). The infrared absorption spectrum is concordant with the spectrum obtained from digitoxin RS or with the *reference spectrum* of digitoxin.

B. Carry out the test as described under "Thin-layer chromatography" (vol. 1, p. 83), using kieselguhr R1 as the coating substance and a mixture of 10 volumes of formamide R and 90 volumes of acetone R to impregnate the plate, dipping it about 5 mm beneath the surface of the liquid. After the solvent has reached a height of at least 15 cm, remove the plate from the chromatographic chamber and allow to stand for at least 5 minutes. Use the impregnated plate within 2 hours, carrying out the chromatography in the same direction as the impregnation. As the mobile phase, use a mixture of 50 volumes of xylene R, 50 volumes of ethylmethylketone R and 4 volumes of formamide R. Apply separately to the plate 3 μl of each of 2 solutions (A) of the test substance, and (B) of digitoxin RS, each prepared by dissolving 50 mg in a mixture of equal volumes of chloroform R and methanol R to produce 10 ml and then diluting 1 ml to 5 ml with methanol R. Develop the plate for a distance of 12 cm. After removing the plate from the chromatographic chamber, allow it to dry at 115 °C for 20 minutes, cool, spray with a mixture of 15 volumes of a solution of 25 g of trichloroacetic acid R in 100 ml of ethanol (~750 g/l) TS and 1 volume of a freshly prepared 30 mg/ml solution of tosylchloramide sodium R, and then heat the plate at 115 °C for 5 minutes. Allow to cool, and examine the chromatogram in daylight and in ultraviolet light (365 nm). The principal spot obtained with solution A corresponds in position, appearance, and intensity with that obtained with solution B.

C. Dissolve 1 mg in 1 ml of ethanol (~750 g/l) TS by heating gently. Cool the solution and add 1 ml of dinitrobenzene/ethanol TS and 1 ml of potassium hydroxide (1 mol/l) VS; a violet colour develops and then fades.

D. Dissolve 1 mg in 2 ml of a solution prepared by mixing 0.5 ml of ferric chloride (25 g/l) TS and 100 ml of glacial acetic acid R; cautiously add 1 ml of sulfuric acid (~1760 g/l) TS to form a lower layer; a brown ring, but no red colour, is produced at the junction of the two liquids, and after some time the acetic acid layer acquires a blue colour (distinction from allied glycosides).

Specific optical rotation. Use a 10 mg/ml solution in chloroform R and calculate with reference to the dried substance; $[\alpha]_D^{20\,°C} = +16.5$ to $+18.5\,°$.

Sulfated ash. Not more than 1.0 mg/g.

Loss on drying. Dry to constant weight at 105 °C; it loses not more than 20 mg/g.

Gitoxin. Dissolve about 5 mg, accurately weighed, in 1 ml of methanol R and dilute to 25 ml with a mixture of equal volumes of hydrochloric acid (~250 g/l) TS and glycerol R. Allow to stand for 1 hour. The absorbance of a 1-cm layer of this solution at 352 nm, when measured against a solvent cell containing a mixture of equal volumes of hydrochloric acid (~250 g/l) TS and glycerol R, is not more than 0.28 (preferably use 2-cm cells for the measurement and calculate the absorbance of a 1-cm layer); the gitoxin content is about 50 mg/g.

Assay. Dissolve about 0.05 g, accurately weighed, in sufficient methanol R to produce 25 ml; dilute 5.0 ml of this solution to 100 ml with methanol R. Place 5.0 ml of the dilute solution to be tested in a 25-ml volumetric flask, add 15 ml of alkaline trinitrophenol TS, and dilute to 25 ml with methanol R. Set aside for 30 minutes, protected from light, and measure the absorbance in a 1-cm layer at the maximum at about 490 nm against a solvent cell containing a solution prepared by diluting 15 ml of alkaline trinitrophenol TS to 25 ml with methanol R. Calculate the amount of $C_{41}H_{64}O_{13}$ in the substance being tested by comparison with digitoxin RS, similarly and concurrently examined.

DIGOXINUM

Digoxin

Molecular formula. $C_{41}H_{64}O_{14}$

Relative molecular mass. 781.0

Graphic formula.

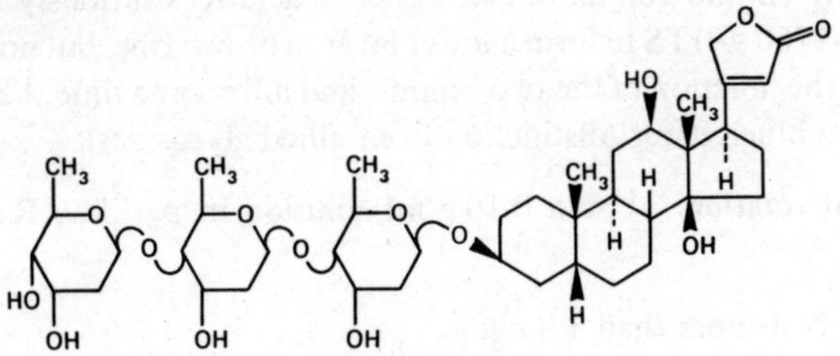

Chemical name. 3β-[(O-2,6-Dideoxy-β-D-*ribo*-hexopyranosyl)-(1→4)-O-2,6-dideoxy-β-D-*ribo*-hexopyranosyl-(1→4)-2,6-dideoxy-β-D-*ribo*-hexopyranosyl)-oxy]-12β,14-dihydroxy-5β-card-20(22)-enolide; CAS Reg. No. 20830-75-5.

Description. Colourless crystals or a white or almost white, crystalline powder; odourless.

Solubility. Practically insoluble in water and ether R; freely soluble in pyridine R; slightly soluble in ethanol (~750 g/l) TS and chloroform R.

Category. Cardiotonic.

Storage. Digoxin should be kept in a well-closed container, protected from light.

Additional information. CAUTION: Digoxin is extremely poisonous and should be handled with care.

REQUIREMENTS

General requirement. Digoxin contains not less than 95.0% and not more than 103.0% of $C_{41}H_{64}O_{14}$, calculated with reference to the dried substance.

Identity tests

• Either tests A, B and D or tests B, C and D may be applied.

A. Carry out the examination as described under "Spectrophotometry in the infrared region" (vol. 1, p. 40). The infrared absorption spectrum is concordant with the spectrum obtained from digoxin RS or with the *reference spectrum* of digoxin.

B. See the test described below under "Related substances". In daylight the principal spot obtained with solution A corresponds in position, appearance, and intensity with that obtained with solution B.

C. Dissolve 1 mg in 1 ml of ethanol (~750 g/l) TS by heating gently. Cool the solution, add 1 ml of dinitrobenzene/ethanol TS and 1 ml of potassium hydroxide (1 mol/l) VS; a violet colour develops and then fades.

D. Dissolve 1 mg in 2 ml of a solution prepared by mixing 0.5 ml of ferric chloride (25 g/l) TS and 100 ml of glacial acetic acid R; cautiously add 1 ml of sulfuric acid (~1760 g/l) TS to form a lower layer; a brown ring, but no red colour, is produced at the junction of the two liquids, and after some time the acetic acid layer acquires a blue colour (distinction from allied glycosides).

Specific optical rotation. Use a 0.10 g/ml solution in pyridine R; $[\alpha]_{546\,nm}^{20\,°C} = +13.6$ to $+14.2°$.

Sulfated ash. Not more than 1.0 mg/g.

Loss on drying. Dry to constant weight at ambient temperature under reduced pressure (not exceeding 0.6 kPa or about 5 mm of mercury); it loses not more than 10 mg/g.

Gitoxin. Dissolve about 5 mg, accurately weighed, in 1 ml of ethanol (~675 g/l) TS by heating gently, and dilute to 25 ml with a mixture of equal volumes of hydrochloric acid (~250 g/l) TS and glycerol R. Allow to stand for 1 hour. The absorbance of a 1-cm layer of this solution at 352 nm, when measured against a solvent cell containing a mixture of equal volumes of hydrochloric acid (~250 g/l) TS and glycerol R, is not more than 0.22 (preferably use 2-cm cells for the measurement and calculate the absorbance of a 1-cm layer); about 40 mg/g.

Related substances. Carry out the test as described under "Thin-layer chromatography" (vol. 1, p. 83), using kieselguhr R1 as the coating substance and a mixture of 10 volumes of formamide R and 90 volumes of acetone R to impregnate the plate, dipping it about 5 mm beneath the surface of the liquid. After the solvent has reached a height of at least 15 cm, remove the plate from the chromatographic chamber and allow to stand for at least 5 minutes. Use the impregnated plate within 2 hours, carrying out the chromatography in the same direction as the impregnation. As the mobile phase, use a mixture of 50 volumes of xylene R, 50 volumes of ethylmethylketone R, and 4 volumes of formamide R. Apply separately to the plate 1 μl of each of 3 solutions in a mixture of equal volumes of methanol R and chloroform R containing (A) 5.0 mg of the test substance per ml, (B) 5.0 mg of digoxin RS per ml and (C) 0.25 mg of digitoxin RS per ml. Develop the plate for a distance of 12 cm. After removal of the plate from the chromatographic chamber, allow it to dry at 115 °C for 20 minutes, cool, spray with a mixture of 15 volumes of a solution of 25 g of trichloroacetic acid R in 100 ml of ethanol (~750 g/l) TS and 1 volume of a freshly prepared 30 mg/ml solution of tosylchloramide sodium R, and then heat the plate at 115 °C for 5 minutes. Allow to cool, and examine the chromatogram in daylight and in ultraviolet light (365 nm). Any spot obtained with solution A in ultraviolet light, other than the principal spot, is not more intense than that obtained with solution C.

Assay. Dissolve about 0.05 g, accurately weighed, in sufficient methanol R to produce 25 ml; dilute 5.0 ml of this solution to 100 ml with methanol R. Place 5.0 ml of the dilute solution to be tested in a 25-ml volumetric flask, add 15 ml of alkaline trinitrophenol TS, and dilute to 25 ml with methanol R. Set aside for 30 minutes protected from light, and measure the absorbance in a 1-cm layer at the maximum of about 490 nm against a solvent cell containing a solution prepared by diluting 15 ml of alkaline trinitrophenol TS to 25 ml with methanol R. Calculate the amount of $C_{41}H_{64}O_{14}$ in the substance being tested by comparison with digoxin RS, similarly and concurrently examined.

EPINEPHRINI HYDROGENOTARTRAS

Epinephrine hydrogen tartrate

Molecular formula. $C_9H_{13}NO_3,C_4H_6O_6$ or $C_{13}H_{19}NO_9$

Relative molecular mass.   333.3

Graphic formula.

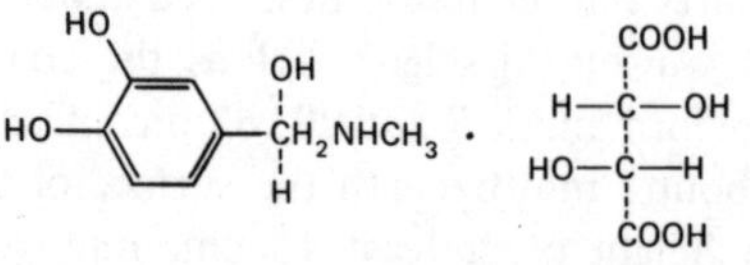

Chemical name.   (–)-(R)-3,4-Dihydroxy-α-[(methylamino)methyl]benzyl alcohol L-(+)-tartrate (1:1) (salt);   (–)-(R)-4-[1-hydroxy-2-(methylamino)ethyl]-1,2-ben-zenediol[R-(R*,R*)]-2,3-dihydroxybutanedioate (1:1) (salt); (–)-α-3,4-dihydroxy-phenyl-β-(methylamino)ethanol L-(+)-tartrate; CAS Reg. No. 51-42-3.

Other name.   Adrenalin tartrate.   (In certain countries the name Adrenalin is a trademark.   In those countries this name may be used only when applied to the product issued by the owners of the trademark.)

Description.   A white to greyish white, crystalline powder; odourless.

Solubility.   Soluble in 3 parts of water; slightly soluble in ethanol (~750 g/l) TS; practically insoluble in chloroform R and ether R.

Category.   Sympathomimetic.

Storage.   Epinephrine hydrogen tartrate should be kept in a tightly closed container, protected from light.

Additional information.   Epinephrine hydrogen tartrate gradually darkens in colour on exposure to air and light.   Even in the absence of light, Epinephrine hydrogen tartrate is gradually degraded on exposure to a humid atmosphere, the decomposition being faster at higher temperatures.

REQUIREMENTS

General requirement.   Epinephrine hydrogen tartrate contains not less than 98.0% and not more than 101.0% of $C_9H_{13}NO_3,C_4H_6O_6$, calculated with reference to the dried substance.

Identity tests

A. The absorption spectrum of a 0.10 mg/ml solution in hydrochloric acid (0.01 mol/l) VS, when observed between 230 nm and 350 nm exhibits a maximum at about 280 nm; the absorbance of a 1-cm layer at this wavelength is about 0.8.

B. Dissolve 10 mg in 10 ml of water and transfer 1 ml to a flask containing 10 ml of buffer phthalate, pH 3.4, TS; another buffer having the same pH may also be used. Add 1 ml of iodine (0.1 mol/l) VS, and allow to stand for 5 minutes. Add 2 ml of sodium thiosulfate (0.1 mol/l) VS, and allow to stand for 1 minute; a strong red colour is produced (distinction from levarterenol, which gives a clear solution with a pink tinge).

C. The filtrate obtained when carrying out the determination of specific optical rotation (see below) yields reaction B described under "General identification tests", as characteristic of tartrates (vol. 1, p. 115).

Specific optical rotation. Dissolve about 0.5 g in 20 ml of water containing about 0.1 g of sodium metabisulfite R, add a slight excess of ammonia ($\sim$100 g/l) TS, and allow to stand in the cold for 1 hour. Filter (keep the filtrate for identity test C, see above), wash the precipitate with 3 quantities, each of 2 ml of water, followed by 5 ml of ethanol ($\sim$750 g/l) TS and 5 ml of ether R. Dry the precipitate at ambient temperature under reduced pressure (not exceeding 0.6 kPa or about 5 mm of mercury) for 3 hours. Use a 20 mg/ml solution of epinephrine base in hydrochloric acid (0.5 mol/l) VS; $[\alpha]_D^{20\,°C} = -50$ to $-53°$.

Clarity and colour of solution. A solution of 1.0 g in 10 ml of water is clear and colourless.

Sulfated ash. Not more than 1.0 mg/g.

Loss on drying. Dry at ambient temperature under reduced pressure (not exceeding 0.6 kPa or about 5 mm of mercury) over silica gel, desiccant, R for 3 hours; it loses not more than 5.0 mg/g.

Adrenalone. The absorbance of a 1-cm layer of a 4.0 mg/ml solution in hydrochloric acid (0.1 mol/l) VS at 310 nm is not more than 0.2 (preferably use 2-cm cells for the measurement and calculate the absorbance of a 1-cm layer).

Levarterenol. Dissolve 10 mg in 1 ml of water, add 4 ml of buffer borate, pH 9.6, TS, or another buffer having the same pH, mix, add 1 ml of a freshly prepared solution of sodium 1,2-naphthoquinone-4-sulfonate (5 g/l) TS, mix, and allow to stand for 30 minutes. Add 0.2 ml of benzalkonium chloride TS1, mix, add 15 ml of toluene R, previously washed with buffer borate, pH 9.6, TS and filtered through a dry filter-paper, shake for 30 minutes and allow to separate, centrifuging if necessary. Any red or purple colour in the toluene-layer is not more intense than that produced by treating a solution of 0.40 mg of levarterenol hydrogen tartrate R and 9.0 mg of epinephrine hydrogen tartrate R in 1 ml of water in a similar manner, when compared as described under "Colour of liquids" (vol. 1, p. 50).

Assay. Dissolve about 0.3 g, accurately weighed, in 50 ml of glacial acetic acid R1, warming slightly if necessary, and titrate with perchloric acid (0.1 mol/l) VS, as described under "Non-aqueous titration", Method A (vol. 1, p. 131). Each ml of perchloric acid (0.1 mol/l) VS is equivalent to 33.33 mg of $C_9H_{13}NO_3,C_4H_6O_6$.

EPINEPHRINUM

Epinephrine

Molecular formula. $C_9H_{13}NO_3$

Relative molecular mass. 183.2

Graphic formula.

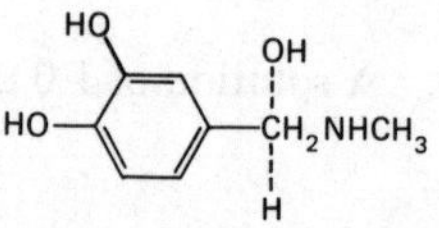

Chemical name. (–)-(R)-3,4-Dihydroxy-α-[(methylamino)methyl]benzyl alcohol; (–)-(R)-4-[1-hydroxy-2-(methylamino)ethyl]-1,2-benzenediol; (–)-α-3,4-dihydroxyphenyl-β-methylaminoethanol; CAS Reg. No. 51-43-4.

Other name. Adrenalin. (In certain countries the name Adrenalin is a trademark. In those countries this name may be used only when applied to the product issued by the owners of the trademark.)

Description. A white or almost white, microcrystalline powder; odourless.

Solubility. Very slightly soluble in water; practically insoluble in ethanol (~750 g/l) TS, ether R, chloroform R, and acetone R.

Category. Sympathomimetic.

Storage. Epinephrine should be kept in a hermetically closed container, protected from light.

Additional information. Epinephrine gradually darkens in colour on exposure to air and light. Even in the absence of light, Epinephrine is gradually degraded on exposure to a humid atmosphere, the decomposition being faster at higher temperatures.

REQUIREMENTS

General requirement. Epinephrine contains not less than 98.5% and not more than 101.0% of $C_9H_{13}NO_3$, calculated with reference to the dried substance.

Identity tests

A. The absorption spectrum of a 0.030 mg/ml solution in hydrochloric acid (0.01 mol/l) VS, when observed between 230 nm and 350 nm exhibits a maximum at about 280 nm; the absorbance of a 1-cm layer at this wavelength is about 0.45 (preferably use 2-cm cells for the measurement and calculate the absorbance of a 1-cm layer).

B. Dissolve 10 mg in 10 ml of hydrochloric acid (0.01 mol/l) VS and transfer 1 ml to a flask containing 10 ml of buffer phthalate, pH 3.4, TS; another buffer having the same pH may also be used. Add 1 ml of iodine (0.1 mol/l) VS, and allow to stand for 5 minutes. Add 2 ml of sodium thiosulfate (0.1 mol/l) VS, and allow to stand for 1 minute; a strong red colour is produced (distinction from levarterenol, which gives a clear solution with a pink tinge).

Specific optical rotation. Use a 40 mg/ml solution in hydrochloric acid (1 mol/l) VS; $[\alpha]_D^{20\,°C} = -50$ to $-53°$.

Sulfated ash. Not more than 1.0 mg/g.

Loss on drying. Dry at ambient temperature under reduced pressure (not exceeding 0.6 kPa or about 5 mm of mercury) over silica gel, desiccant, R for 18 hours; it loses not more than 10 mg/g.

pH value. pH of a 5.0 mg/ml solution in carbon-dioxide-free water R, above 7.5.

Adrenalone. The absorbance of a 1-cm layer of a 2.0 mg/ml solution in hydrochloric acid (0.1 mol/l) VS at 310 nm is not more than 0.2 (preferably use 2-cm cells for the measurement and calculate the absorbance of a 1-cm layer).

Levarterenol. Dissolve 5.0 mg in 1 ml of tartaric acid (5 g/l) TS, add 4 ml of buffer borate, pH 9.6, TS, or another buffer having the same pH, mix, add 1 ml of a freshly prepared solution of sodium 1,2-naphthoquinone-4-sulfonate (5 g/l) TS, mix, and allow to stand for 30 minutes. Add 0.2 ml of benzalkonium chloride TS1, mix, add 15 ml of toluene R, previously washed with buffer borate, pH 9.6,

TS and filtered through a dry filter-paper, shake for 30 minutes and allow to separate, centrifuging if necessary. Treat a solution of 0.40 mg of levarterenol hydrogen tartrate R and 9.0 mg of epinephrine hydrogen tartrate R in 1 ml of water in a similar manner. Any red or purple colour in the toluene layer is not more intense than that of the reference solution when compared as described under "Colour of liquids" (vol. 1, p. 50).

Assay. Dissolve about 0.35 g, accurately weighed, in 30 ml of glacial acetic acid R1, and titrate with perchloric acid (0.1 mol/l) VS, as described under "Non-aqueous titration", Method A (vol. 1, p. 131). Each ml of perchloric acid (0.1 mol/l) VS is equivalent to 18.32 mg of $C_9H_{13}NO_6$.

ERGOMETRINI HYDROGENOMALEAS

Ergometrine hydrogen maleate

Molecular formula. $C_{19}H_{23}N_3O_2,C_4H_4O_4$ or $C_{23}H_{27}N_3O_6$

Relative molecular mass. 441.5

Graphic formula.

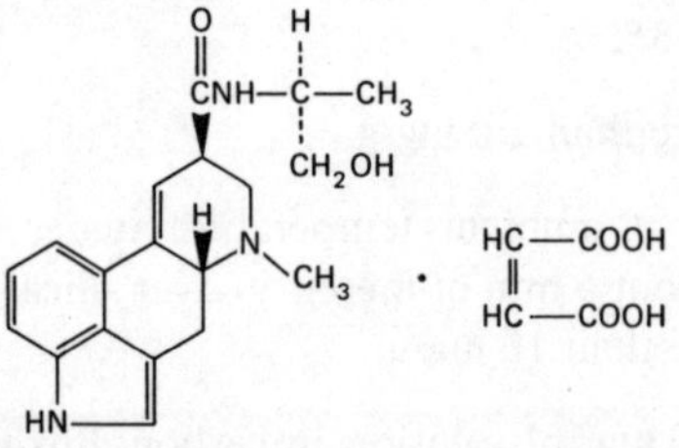

Chemical name. 9,10-Didehydro-N-[(S)-2-hydroxy-1-methylethyl]-6-methyl-ergoline-8β-carboxamide maleate (1:1) (salt); 9,10-didehydro-N-[(S)-2-hydroxy-1-methylethyl]-6-methylergoline-8β-carboxamide (Z)-2-butanedioate (1:1) salt; CAS Reg. No. 129-51-1.

Description. A white or faintly yellow, crystalline powder; odourless.

Solubility. Sparingly soluble in water and ethanol (~750 g/l) TS; practically insoluble in ether R and chloroform R.

Category. Oxytocic.

Storage. Ergometrine hydrogen maleate should be kept in a hermetically closed container, preferably in an inert atmosphere, such as nitrogen, protected from light and stored in a cool place.

Additional information. Ergometrine hydrogen maleate darkens in colour on exposure to light. Even in the absence of light, Ergometrine hydrogen maleate is gradually degraded on exposure to a humid atmosphere, the decomposition being faster at higher temperatures.

REQUIREMENTS

General requirement. Ergometrine hydrogen maleate contains not less than 98.0% and not more than 101.0% of $C_{19}H_{23}N_3O_2,C_4H_4O_4$, calculated with reference to the dried substance.

Identity tests

A. Dissolve 15 mg in 5 ml of water; a blue fluorescence is produced.

B. See the test described below under "Related alkaloids". The principal spot obtained with solution B corresponds in position, appearance, and intensity with that obtained with solution C.

C. Dissolve 2 mg in 20 ml of water; to 1 ml of this solution add 2 ml of 4-dimethylaminobenzaldehyde TS1 and allow to stand for about 5 minutes; a deep blue colour is produced.

D. Dissolve 2 mg in 1 ml of water, and add 1 drop of bromine TS1; the colour of the reagent is discharged.

Specific optical rotation. Use a 10 mg/ml solution and calculate with reference to the dried substance; $[\alpha]_D^{20\,°C} = +50$ to $+56°$.

Clarity and colour of solution. A solution of 0.10 g in 10 ml of carbon-dioxide-free water R is clear and not more intensely coloured than standard colour Yw3 when compared as described under "Colour of liquids" (vol. 1, p. 50).

Loss on drying. Dry to constant weight at 80 °C under reduced pressure (not exceeding 0.6 kPa or about 5 mm of mercury); it loses not more than 20 mg/g.

pH value. pH of a 10 mg/ml solution in carbon-dioxide-free water R, 3.0–5.0.

Related alkaloids. Carry out the test as described under "Thin-layer chromatography" (vol. 1, p. 83), using silica gel R1 as the coating substance and a mixture of 9 volumes of chloroform R and 1 volume of methanol R as the mobile phase. Place a sufficient volume of mobile phase to develop the chromatograms and a beaker containing 25 ml of ammonia (~260 g/l) TS into the chromatographic chamber, and equilibrate for 30 minutes. Apply separately to the plate 5 μl of each of 3 solutions in methanol R containing (A) 4.0 mg of the test substance per ml, and (B) 0.12 mg of the test substance per ml, and (C) 0.12 mg of ergometrine hydrogen maleate RS per ml. After removing the plate from the chromatographic chamber, allow it to dry in air until the solvents have evaporated, spray it with 4-dimethylaminobenzaldehyde TS2, and examine the chromatogram in daylight. Any spot obtained with solution A, other than the principal spot, is not more intense than that obtained with solution B.

Assay.   Dissolve about 0.20 g, accurately weighed, in 20 ml of glacial acetic acid R1 and 10 ml of acetic anhydride R, and titrate with perchloric acid (0.05 mol/l) VS, as described under "Non-aqueous titration", Method A (vol. 1, p. 131). Each ml of perchloric acid (0.05 mol/l) VS is equivalent to 22.07 mg of $C_{19}H_{23}N_3O_2,C_4H_4O_4$.

ERGOTAMINI TARTRAS

Ergotamine tartrate

Molecular formula. $(C_{33}H_{35}N_5O_5)_2,C_4H_6O_6$ or $C_{70}H_{76}N_{10}O_{16}$

Relative molecular mass.   1313

Graphic formula.

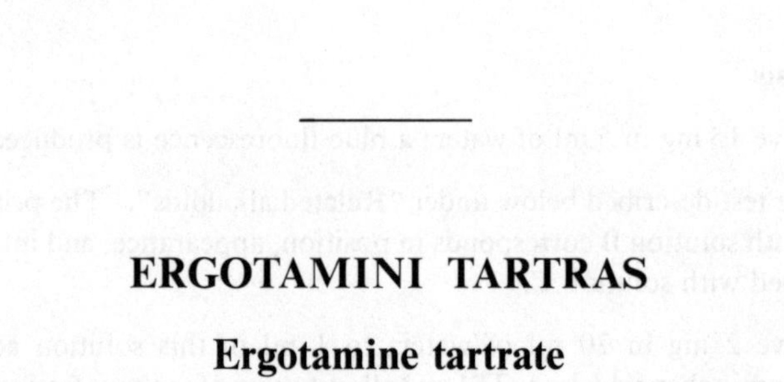

Chemical name.   Ergotamine L-(+)-tartrate (2:1) (salt); 12'-hydroxy-2'-methyl-5'α-(phenylmethyl)ergotaman-3',6',18-trione[R-(R*,R*)]-2,3-dihydroxybutane-dioate (2:1) (salt); CAS Reg. No. 379-79-3.

Description. Colourless crystals or a greyish white to yellowish white, crystalline powder; odourless.

Solubility. Slightly soluble in water and ethanol (~750 g/l) TS; practically insoluble in ether R, benzene R, and light petroleum R.

Category. Sympatholytic.

Storage. Ergotamine tartrate should be kept in a hermetically closed container, preferably in a inert atmosphere, such as nitrogen, protected from light and stored in a cool place.

Additional information. Even in the absence of light, Ergotamine tartrate is gradually degraded on exposure to a humid atmosphere, the decomposition being faster at higher temperatures.

REQUIREMENTS

General requirement. Ergotamine tartrate contains not less than 98.0% and not more than 101.0% of $(C_{33}H_{35}N_5O_5)_2,C_4H_6O_6$, calculated with reference to the dried substance.

Identity tests

A. See the test described below under "Related alkaloids". The principal spot obtained with solution B corresponds in position, appearance, and intensity with that obtained with solution C.

B. Dissolve 1 mg in a mixture of 5 ml of glacial acetic acid R and 5 ml of ethyl acetate R. To 1 ml of this solution add 1 ml of sulfuric acid (~1760 g/l) TS, with continuous shaking and cooling; a blue colour with a red tinge develops. Add 0.1 ml of ferric chloride (25 g/l) TS, previously diluted with an equal volume of water; the red tinge becomes less apparent and the blue colour more pronounced.

Specific optical rotation of ergotamine base

● Prepare and use the solution rapidly, in subdued light.

Place about 0.35 g, accurately weighed, in a separator, dissolve it in 25 ml of tartaric acid (10 g/l) TS, add 0.5 g of sodium hydrogen carbonate R, and mix gently. Add 10 ml of ethanol-free chloroform R, shake vigorously, allow to separate, and filter the chloroform-layer through a small filter-paper previously moistened with ethanol-free chloroform R into a 50-ml volumetric flask. Repeat the extraction of the aqueous layer with three 10-ml portions of ethanol-free chloroform R, passing the extracts through the same filter. Place the flask in a water-bath at 20°C for 10 minutes and adjust to 50 ml with the same solvent. Mix the solution and determine the optical rotation at 20°C, preferably using tubes that can be controlled thermostatically. Separately, measure 25.0 ml of the solution, evaporate on a water-bath, and dry to constant weight at 95°C under reduced pressure (not exceeding 0.6 kPa or about 5 mm of mercury). Calculate the specific optical rotation of the ergotamine base from the weight of the residue and the observed rotation; $[\alpha]_D^{20\,°C} = -150$ to $-160°$.

Clarity and colour of solution. Add 25 mg of tartaric acid R to 50 mg of the test substance and dissolve at 20°C in 10 ml of water; the solution is clear and not more intensely coloured than standard colour solution Yw2 when compared as described under "Colour of liquids" (vol.1, p. 50).

Loss on drying. Dry to constant weight at 95°C under reduced pressure (not exceeding 0.6 kPa or about 5 mm of mercury); it loses not more than 50 mg/g.

Related alkaloids. Carry out the test as described under "Thin-layer chromatography" (vol. 1, p. 83), using silica gel R1 as the coating substance and a mixture of 9 volumes of chloroform R and 1 volume of methanol R as the mobile phase. Place a sufficient volume of mobile phase to develop the chromatograms and a beaker containing 25 ml of ammonia (~260 g/l) TS into the chromatographic chamber, and equilibrate for 30 minutes. Apply separately to the plate 5 μl of each of 3 solutions in the mobile phase containing (A) 5.0 mg of the test substance per ml, (B) 0.25 mg of the test substance per ml, and (C) 0.25 mg of ergotamine tartrate RS per ml. After removing the plate from the chromatographic chamber, allow it to dry in air until the solvents have evaporated, spray it with 4-dimethylaminobenzaldehyde TS2, and examine the chromatogram in daylight. Any spot obtained with solution A, other than the principal spot, is not more intense than that obtained with solution B.

Assay. Dissolve about 0.3 g, accurately weighed, in 15 ml of a mixture of 6 volumes of acetic anhydride R and 100 volumes of glacial acetic acid R1. Titrate with perchloric acid (0.05 mol/l) VS as described under "Non-aqueous titrations", Method A (vol. 1, p. 131). Each ml of perchloric acid (0.05 mol/l) VS is equivalent to 32.83 mg of $(C_{33}H_{35}N_5O_5)_2,C_4H_6O_6$.

ETHAMBUTOLI HYDROCHLORIDUM

Ethambutol hydrochloride

Molecular formula. $C_{10}H_{24}N_2O_2,2HCl$

Relative molecular mass. 277.2

Graphic formula.

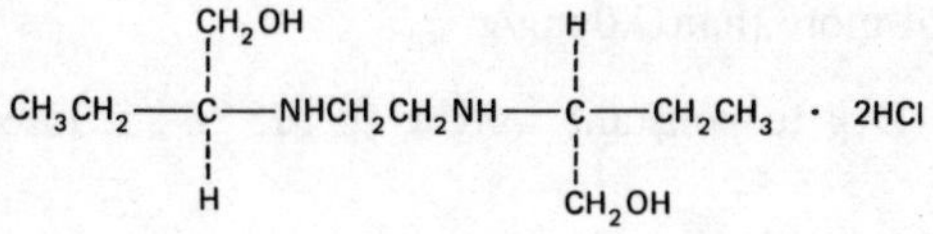

Chemical name. (+)-(S,S)-2,2'-(Ethylenediimino)di-1-butanol dihydrochloride; [S-(R*,R*)]-2,2'-(1,2-ethanediyldiimino)bis[1-butanol] dihydrochloride; CAS Reg. No. 1070-11-7.

Description. A white, crystalline powder; odourless.

Solubility. Soluble in 1 part of water and 850 parts of chloroform R; soluble in ethanol (~750 g/l) TS; practically insoluble in ether R.

Category. Antibacterial (tuberculostatic).

Storage. Ethambutol hydrochloride should be kept in a well-closed container.

REQUIREMENTS

General requirement. Ethambutol hydrochloride contains not less than 98.0% and not more than 100.5% of $C_{10}H_{24}N_2O_2,2HCl$, calculated with reference to the dried substance.

Identity tests

• Either tests A and C or tests B, C and D may be applied.

A. Carry out the examination as described under "Spectrophotometry in the infrared region" (vol. 1, p. 40). The infrared absorption spectrum is concordant with the spectrum obtained from ethambutol hydrochloride RS or with the *reference spectrum* of ethambutol hydrochloride.

B. See the test described below under "2(R-Aminobutanol)". The principal spot obtained with solution B corresponds in position, appearance, and intensity with that obtained with solution C.

C.   A 0.1 g/ml solution yields reaction B described under "General identification tests" as characteristic of chlorides (vol. 1, p. 113).

D.   Melting temperature, about 200 °C.

Specific optical rotation.   Use a 0.10 g/ml solution; $[\alpha]_D^{20\,°C} = +5.0$ to $+7.0°$.

Heavy metals.   Use 1.0 g for the preparation of the test solution as described under "Limit test for heavy metals", Procedure 3, (vol. 1, p. 118); determine the heavy metals content according to Method A (vol. 1, p. 119); not more than 20 μg/g.

Sulfated ash.   Not more than 2.0 mg/g.

Loss on drying.   Dry to constant weight at 105 °C; it loses not more than 5.0 mg/g.

pH value.   pH of a 0.10 g/ml solution, 3.0–4.5.

2(R-Aminobutanol).   Carry out the test as described under "Thin-layer chromatography" (vol. 1, p. 83), using silica gel R1 as the coating substance and a mixture of 11 volumes of ethyl acetate R, 7 volumes of glacial acetic acid R, 1 volume of hydrochloric acid ($\sim$420 g/l) TS, and 1 volume of water as the mobile phase. Apply separately to the plate 2 μl of each of 3 solutions in methanol R containing (A) 50 mg of the test substance per ml, (B) 0.50 mg of the test substance per ml, and (C) 0.50 mg of 2-aminobutanol R per ml.   After removing the plate from the chromatographic chamber, allow it to dry in air, heat at 105 °C for 5 minutes, cool, spray with triketohydrindene/cadmium TS, heat at 90 °C for 5 minutes, and examine the chromatogram in daylight.   The spot obtained with solution C is more intense than any spot, corresponding in position and appearance, obtained with solution A.

Assay.   Dissolve about 0.3 g, accurately weighed, in 100 ml of glacial acetic acid R1, add 10 ml of mercuric acetate/acetic acid TS and titrate with perchloric acid (0.1 mol/l) VS as described under "Non-aqueous titration", Method A (vol. 1, p. 131).   Each ml of perchloric acid (0.1 mol/l) VS is equivalent to 13.86 mg of $C_{10}H_{24}N_2O_2,2HCl$.

ETHINYLESTRADIOLUM

Ethinylestradiol

Molecular formula. $C_{20}H_{24}O_2$

Relative molecular mass. 296.4

Graphic formula.

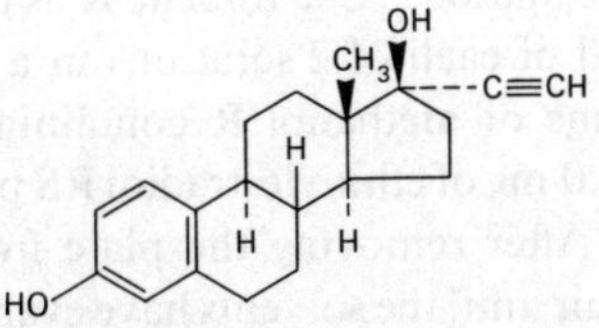

Chemical name. 19-Nor-17α-pregna-1,3,5(10)-trien-20-yne-3,17-diol; 17-ethy-nyl-estra-1,3,5,(10)-triene-3,17β-diol; CAS Reg. No. 57-63-6.

Description. A white to slightly yellowish white, crystalline powder; odour-less.

Solubility. Practically insoluble in water; freely soluble in ethanol (~750 g/l) TS; soluble in chloroform R, acetone R, and dioxan R.

Category. Estrogen.

Storage. Ethinylestradiol should be kept in a well-closed container, protected from light.

Additional information. Ethinylestradiol may exist in 2 polymorphic forms one of which melts at about 183°C, the other, metastable, at about 143°C.

REQUIREMENTS

General requirement. Ethinylestradiol contains not less than 97.0% and not more than 102.0% of $C_{20}H_{24}O_2$, calculated with reference to the dried substance.

Identity tests

• Either test A or test B may be applied.

A. Carry out the examination as described under "Spectrophotometry in the infrared region" (vol. 1, p. 40). The infrared absorption spectrum is concordant with the spectrum obtained from ethinylestradiol RS or with the *reference spectrum* of ethinylestradiol. If the spectrum obtained from the solid state of the test substance is not concordant with the spectrum obtained from the reference substance, compare the spectra of solutions in chloroform R containing 30 mg/ml, using a path length of 0.2 mm.

B.   Carry out the test as described under "Thin-layer chromatography" (vol. 1, p. 83), using kieselguhr R1 as the coating substance and a mixture of 1 volume of propylene glycol R and 9 volumes of acetone R to impregnate the plate, dipping it about 5 mm beneath the surface of the liquid. After the solvent has reached a height of at least 16 cm, remove the plate from the chromatographic chamber and allow it to stand at room temperature until the solvent has completely evaporated. Use the impregnated plate within 2 hours, carrying out the chromatography in the same direction as the impregnation. Use toluene R as the mobile phase. Apply separately to the plate 2 μl of each of 2 solutions in a mixture of 9 volumes of chloroform R and 1 volume of methanol R containing (A) 1.0 mg of the test substance per ml, and (B) 1.0 mg of ethinylestradiol RS per ml. Develop the plate for a distance of 15 cm. After removing the plate from the chromatographic chamber, allow it to dry in air until the solvents have evaporated, heat at 120 °C for 15 minutes, spray with 4-toluenesulfonic acid/ethanol TS, and then heat at 120 °C for 5–10 minutes. Allow to cool, and examine the chromatogram in daylight and in ultraviolet light (365 nm). The principal spot obtained with solution A corresponds in position, appearance, and intensity with that obtained with solution B.

Specific optical rotation. Use a 4.0 mg/ml solution in pyridine R and calculate with reference to the dried substance; $[\alpha]_D^{20\,°C} = -27.0$ to $-30.0°$.

Loss on drying. Dry to constant weight at 105 °C; it loses not more than 10 mg/g.

Estrone. Carry out the test as described under "Thin-layer chromatography" (vol. 1, p. 83), using silica gel R1 as the coating substance and a mixture of 92 volumes of dichloroethane R, 8 volumes of methanol R, and 0.5 volumes of water as the mobile phase. Apply separately to the plate 5 μl of each of 2 freshly prepared solutions in a mixture of 9 volumes of chloroform R and 1 volume of methanol R containing (A) 20 mg of the test substance per ml, and (B) 0.20 mg of estrone RS per ml. After removing the plate from the chromatographic chamber, allow it to dry in air until the odour of the solvent is no longer detectable; then heat at 110 °C for 10 minutes. Spray the hot plate with sulfuric acid/ethanol TS, heat again at 110 °C for 10 minutes, and examine the chromatogram in ultraviolet light (365 nm). The spot obtained with solution B is more intense than any spot, corresponding in position and appearance, obtained with solution A.

Assay. Dissolve about 0.05 g, accurately weighed, in sufficient dehydrated ethanol R to produce 100 ml, and dilute 10.0 ml of this solution to 50.0 ml with the same solvent. Measure the absorbance of a 1-cm layer of the diluted solution at the maximum at about 281 nm. Calculate the amount of $C_{20}H_{24}O_2$ in the substance being tested by comparison with ethinylestradiol RS, similarly and concurrently examined. In an adequately calibrated spectrophotometer the absorbance of the reference solution should be 0.72 ± 0.04.

ETHOSUXIMIDUM

Ethosuximide

Molecular formula. $C_7H_{11}NO_2$

Relative molecular mass. 141.2

Graphic formula.

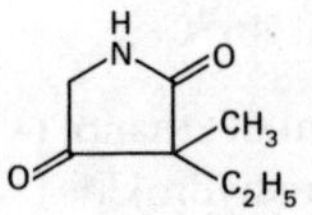

Chemical name. 2-Ethyl-2-methylsuccinimide; 3-ethyl-3-methyl-2,5-pyrroli-dinedione; CAS Reg. No. 77-67-8.

Description. A white or almost white powder or waxy solid; odourless or with a faint characteristic odour.

Solubility. Freely soluble in water; very soluble in ethanol (~750 g/l) TS, ether R, and chloroform R.

Category. Anticonvulsant.

Storage. Ethosuximide should be kept in a tightly closed container, protected from light.

Additional information. Even in the absence of light, Ethosuximide is gradually degraded on exposure to a humid atmosphere, the decomposition being faster at higher temperatures.

REQUIREMENTS

General requirement. Ethosuximide contains not less than 99.0% and not more than 100.5% of $C_7H_{11}NO_2$, calculated with reference to the anhydrous substance.

Identity tests

• Either test A alone or tests B and C may be applied.

A. Carry out the examination as described under "Spectrophotometry in the infrared region" (vol. 1, p. 40). The infrared absorption spectrum is concordant with the spectrum obtained from ethosuximide RS or with the *reference spectrum* of ethosuximide. If the spectrum obtained from the solid state of the test substance is not concordant with the spectrum obtained from the reference substance, dissolve a small amount of the substance in ethanol (~750 g/l) TS, evaporate to dryness on a water-bath, and prepare a potassium bromide disc as described in Method 3 (vol. 1, p. 41). Then compare the spectrum obtained from the disc with that of the reference substance.

B.   Heat 0.1 g with 0.2 g of resorcinol R and 2 drops of sulfuric acid (~1760 g/l) TS at 140 °C for 5 minutes, allow to cool, add 5 ml of water, make alkaline with sodium hydroxide (~80 g/l) TS, and pour a few drops into a large volume of water; a bright green fluorescence is obtained.

C.   Melting temperature, about 46 °C.

Cyanides.   Dissolve 1 g in 10 ml of ethanol (~750 g/l) TS, add 3 drops of ferrous sulfate (15 g/l) TS, 1 ml of sodium hydroxide (~80 g/l) TS and a few drops of ferric chloride (25 g/l) TS. Warm gently, and acidify with sulfuric acid (~100 g/l) TS; no blue precipitate or blue colour is produced within 15 minutes.

Sulfated ash.   Not more than 5.0 mg/g.

Water.   Determine as described under "Determination of water by the Karl Fischer method", Method A (vol. 1, p. 135), using about 1 g of the substance; the water content is not more than 5.0 mg/g.

Acidity.   Dissolve 5.0 g in 50 ml of water by warming on a water-bath for 5 minutes. Cool and titrate with sodium hydroxide (0.1 mol/l) VS, using bromocresol green/ethanol TS as indicator; not more than 0.7 ml is required to obtain the midpoint of the indicator (green).

Related substances.   Carry out the test as described under "Thin-layer chromatography" (vol. 1, p. 83), using silica gel R2 as the coating substance and a mixture of 9 volumes of chloroform R and 1 volume of acetone R as the mobile phase. Apply separately to the plate 10 μl of each of 2 solutions in ethanol (~750 g/l) TS containing (A) 50 mg of the test substance per ml and (B) 0.050 mg of the test substance per ml. After removing the plate from the chromatographic chamber allow it to dry in air, and examine the chromatogram in ultraviolet light (254 nm). Any spot obtained with solution A, other than the principal spot, is not more intense than that obtained with solution B.

Assay.   Dissolve about 0.28 g, accurately weighed, in 30 ml of dimethylformamide R, add 3 drops of azo violet TS and titrate with tetrabutylammonium hydroxide (0.1 mol/l) VS to a blue endpoint, as described under "Non-aqueous titration", Method B (vol. 1, p. 132). Each ml of tetrabutylammonium hydroxide (0.1 mol/l) VS is equivalent to 14.12 mg of $C_7H_{11}NO_2$.

FERROSI SULFAS

Ferrous sulfate

Ferrous sulfate, exsiccated
Ferrous sulfate heptahydrate

Molecular formula. $FeSO_4,nH_2O$ (exsiccated); $FeSO_4,7H_2O$ (heptahydrate).

Relative molecular mass. 151.9 (anhydrous); 278.0 (heptahydrate).

Chemical name. Iron(2+) sulfate (1:1); CAS Reg. No. 7720-78-7 (anhydrous). Iron(2+) sulfate (1:1) heptahydrate; CAS Reg. No. 7782-63-0 (heptahydrate).

Description. Exsiccated Ferrous sulfate is a greyish white powder; Ferrous sulfate heptahydrate has pale blue-green prisms or is a pale green, crystalline powder; both forms are odourless.

Solubility. Exsiccated Ferrous sulfate is slowly but almost completely soluble in carbon-dioxide-free water R; practically insoluble in ethanol (~750 g/l) TS. Ferrous sulfate heptahydrate is freely soluble in water; very soluble in boiling water; practically insoluble in ethanol (~750 g/l) TS.

Category. Haemopoietic (iron-deficiency anaemia).

Storage. Ferrous sulfate should be kept in a well-closed container.

Labelling. The designation on the container of Ferrous sulfate should state whether the substance is in the exsiccated form or is the heptahydrate.

Additional information. Exsiccated Ferrous sulfate is Ferrous sulfate deprived of part of its water of crystallization by drying at a temperature of 40°C. Ferrous sulfate heptahydrate is efflorescent in dry air. Even in the absence of light, Ferrous sulfate is gradually degraded on exposure to a humid atmosphere, the decomposition being faster at higher temperatures. The crystals rapidly oxidize becoming brown. Both forms have a metallic and astringent taste.

REQUIREMENTS

General requirement. Exsiccated Ferrous sulfate contains not less than 80.0% and not more than 90.0% of $FeSO_4$. Ferrous sulfate heptahydrate contains not less than 98.0% and not more than 105.0% of $FeSO_4,7H_2O$.

Identity tests

A. A 20 mg/ml solution yields the reactions described under "General identification tests" as characteristic of ferrous salts (vol. 1, p. 113).

B.   A 20 mg/ml solution yields reaction A described under "General identification tests" as characteristic of sulfates (vol. 1, p. 115).

Heavy metals.   Dissolve 1.0 g in 10 ml of hydrochloric acid (~250 g/l) TS, add
2 ml of hydrogen peroxide (~330 g/l) TS, and evaporate to 5 ml. Allow to cool,
dilute to 20 ml with hydrochloric acid (~250 g/l) TS, transfer the solution to a
separating funnel and shake for 3 minutes with 3 successive quantities, each of
20 ml, of a solution composed of 100 ml of freshly distilled methylisobutylketone
R shaken with 1 ml of hydrochloric acid (~250 g/l) TS. Allow the layers to
separate, evaporate the aqueous layer to half its volume, allow to cool and dilute to
50 ml with water. Neutralize 25 ml to litmus TS and determine the heavy metals
content as described under "Limit test for heavy metals", according to Method A
(vol. 1, p. 119), multiplying the result by a factor of 2; not more than 50 μg/g.

Alkaline salts.   Dissolve 1 g in 10 ml of water and oxidize by warming with a few
drops of nitric acid (~1000 g/l) TS, make alkaline with ammonia (~100 g/l) TS,
filter, evaporate the filtrate, ignite the residue and weigh; not more than
1.0 mg/g.

Arsenic.   Use a solution of 3.3 g in 35 ml of water and proceed as described under
"Limit test for arsenic" (vol. 1, p. 122); the arsenic content is not more than
3 μg/g.

Insoluble matter.   Dissolve 1.0 g in 10 ml of water, filter, wash the filter with
water and dry it at 105°C; the content of insoluble matter is not more than
5.0 mg/g.

pH value.   pH of a 0.05 g/ml solution, 3.0–4.0.

Assay.   For exsiccated Ferrous sulfate dissolve about 0.3 g, accurately weighed, in
a mixture of 30 ml of water and 20 ml of sulfuric acid (~100 g/l) TS and titrate with
ceric ammonium sulfate (0.1 mol/l) VS, using 2 drops of o-phenanthroline TS as
indicator. Each ml of ceric ammonium sulfate (0.1 mol/l) VS is equivalent to
15.19 mg of $FeSO_4$.

For Ferrous sulfate heptahydrate dissolve 2.5 g of sodium hydrogen carbonate
R in a mixture of 150 ml of water, 10.0 ml of sulfuric acid (~1760 g/l) TS, and
5.0 ml of phosphoric acid (~1440 g/l) TS. When the effervescence ceases, add
about 0.5 g of the test substance, accurately weighed, and when solution is
complete titrate with ceric ammonium sulfate (0.1 mol/1) VS, using 2 drops of
o-phenanthroline TS as indicator. Each ml of ceric ammonium sulfate (0.1 mol/l)
VS is equivalent to 27.80 mg of $FeSO_4,7H_2O$.

FLUPHENAZINI DECANOAS
Fluphenazine decanoate

Molecular formula. $C_{32}H_{44}F_3N_3O_2S$

Relative molecular mass. 591.8

Graphic formula.

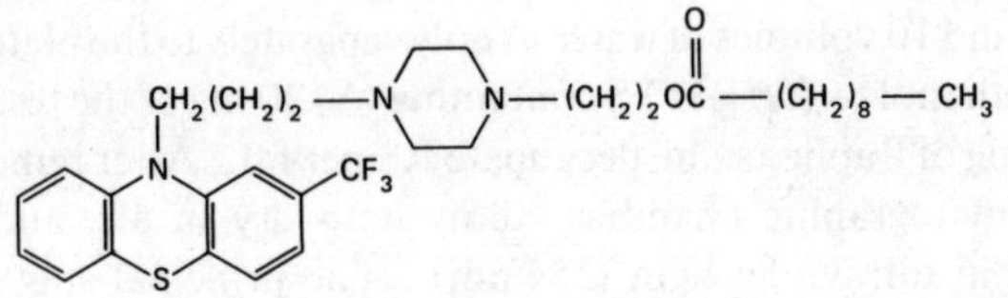

Chemical name. 4-[3-[2-(Trifluoromethyl)phenothiazin-10-yl]propyl]-1-piperazineethanol decanoate (ester); 4-[3-[2-(trifluoromethyl)-10H-phenothiazin-10-yl]propyl]-1-piperazineethanol decanoate (ester); CAS Reg. No. 5002-47-1.

Description. A pale yellow viscous liquid or a yellow, crystalline, oily solid; odour, faint, ester-like.

Miscibility. Immiscible with water; miscible with dehydrated ethanol R, chloroform R, and ether R.

Category. Neuroleptic.

Storage. Fluphenazine decanoate should be kept in a well-closed container, protected from light.

Additional information. Even in the absence of light, Fluphenazine decanoate is gradually degraded on exposure to a humid atmosphere, the decomposition being faster at higher temperatures.

REQUIREMENTS

General requirement. Fluphenazine decanoate contains not less than 98.5% and not more than 101.5% of $C_{32}H_{44}F_3N_3O_2S$, calculated with reference to the dried substance.

Identity tests

A. Carry out the examination as described under "Spectrophotometry in the infrared region" (vol. 1, p. 40). The infrared absorption spectrum is concordant

with the spectrum obtained from fluphenazine decanoate RS or with the *reference spectrum* of fluphenazine decanoate.

B.   Carry out the test as described under "Thin-layer chromatography" (vol. 1, p. 83), using silica gel R2 as the coating substance and a mixture of 5 volumes of *n*-tetradecane R and 95 volumes of hexane R to impregnate the plate, dipping it about 5 mm beneath the surface of the liquid. After the solvent has reached the top of the plate, remove the plate from the chromatographic chamber and allow to stand at room temperature until the solvents have completely evaporated. Use the impregnated plate immediately, carrying out the chromatography in the same direction as the impregnation. As the mobile phase, use a mixture of 90 volumes of methanol R and 10 volumes of water. Apply separately to the plate 1 μl of each of 2 solutions in ethanol (~750 g/l) TS containing (A) 20 mg of the test substance per ml and (B) 20 mg of fluphenazine decanoate RS per ml. After removing the plate from the chromatographic chamber, allow it to dry in air, and examine the chromatogram in ultraviolet light (254 nm). The principal spot obtained with solution A corresponds in position, appearance, and intensity with that obtained with solution B.

C.   Dissolve 5 mg in 2 ml of sulfuric acid (~1760 g/l) TS and allow to stand for 5 minutes; a reddish brown colour is produced.

Sulfated ash.   Not more than 2.0 mg/g.

Loss on drying.   Dry to constant weight at 60 °C under reduced pressure (not exceeding 0.6 kPa or about 5 mm of mercury); it loses not more than 10 mg/g.

Related substances.   Carry out the test as described under "Thin-layer chromatography" (vol. 1, p. 83), using silica gel R2 as the coating substance and a mixture of 80 volumes of acetone R, 30 volumes of cyclohexane R and 5 volumes of ammonia (~260 g/l) TS as the mobile phase. Apply separately to the plate 20 μl of each of 2 solutions in methanol R containing (A) 25 mg of the test substance per ml and (B) 0.25 mg of fluphenazine hydrochloride RS per ml. After removing the plate from the chromatographic chamber, allow it to dry in air, and examine the chromatogram in ultraviolet light (254 nm). Then spray the plate with sulfuric acid (~635 g/l) TS and examine the chromatogram in daylight. Using either method of visualization, any spot obtained with solution A, other than the principal spot, is not more intense than that obtained with solution B.

Assay.   Dissolve about 0.6 g, accurately weighed, in 30 ml of glacial acetic acid R1, and titrate with perchloric acid (0.1 mol/l) VS, as described under "Non-aqueous titration", Method A (vol. 1, p. 131). Each ml of perchloric acid (0.1 mol/l) VS is equivalent to 25.59 mg of $C_{32}H_{44}F_3N_3O_2S$.

FLUPHENAZINI ENANTAS

Fluphenazine enantate

Molecular formula. $C_{29}H_{38}F_3N_3O_2S$

Relative molecular mass. 549.7

Graphic formula.

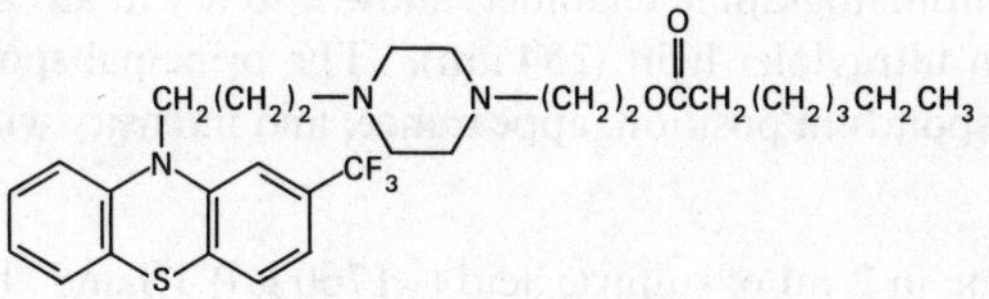

Chemical name. 4-[3-[2-(Trifluoromethyl)phenothiazin-10-yl]propyl]-1-piperazineethanol heptanoate (ester); 4-[3-[2-(trifluoromethyl)-10*H*-phenothiazin-10-yl]propyl]-1-piperazineethanol heptanoate (ester); CAS Reg. No. 2746-81-8.

Description. A pale yellow, viscous liquid or a yellow, crystalline, oily solid; odour, faint, ester-like.

Miscibility. Immiscible with water; miscible with dehydrated ethanol R, chloroform R, and ether R.

Category. Neuroleptic.

Storage. Fluphenazine enantate should be kept in a well-closed container, protected from light.

REQUIREMENTS

General requirement. Fluphenazine enantate contains not less than 98.5% and not more than 101.5% of $C_{29}H_{38}F_3N_3O_2S$, calculated with reference to the dried substance.

Identity tests

A. Carry out the examination as described under "Spectrophotometry in the infrared region" (vol. 1, p. 40). The infrared absorption spectrum is concordant with the spectrum obtained from fluphenazine enantate RS or with the *reference spectrum* of fluphenazine enantate.

B. Carry out the test as described under "Thin-layer chromatography" (vol. 1, p. 83), using silica gel R2 as the coating substance and a mixture of 5 volumes of n-tetradecane R and 95 volumes of hexane R to impregnate the plate, dipping it about 5 mm beneath the surface of the liquid. After the solvent has reached the top of the plate, remove the plate from the chromatographic chamber and allow it to stand at room temperature until the solvents have completely evaporated. Use the impregnated plate immediately, carrying out the chromatography in the same direction as the impregnation. As the mobile phase, use a mixture of 90 volumes of methanol R and 10 volumes of water. Apply separately to the plate 1 µl of each of 2 solutions in ethanol (~750 g/l) TS containing (A) 20 mg of the test substance per ml and (B) 20 mg of fluphenazine enantate RS per ml. After removing the plate from the chromatographic chamber, allow it to dry in air, and examine the chromatogram in ultraviolet light (254 nm). The principal spot obtained with solution A corresponds in position, appearance, and intensity with that obtained with solution B.

C.   Dissolve 5 mg in 2 ml of sulfuric acid (~1760 g/l) TS and allow to stand for 5 minutes; a reddish brown colour is produced.

Sulfated ash.   Not more than 2.0 mg/g.

Loss on drying.   Dry to constant weight at 60 °C under reduced pressure (not exceeding 0.6 kPa or about 5 mm of mercury); it loses not more than 10 mg/g.

Related substances.   Carry out the test as described under "Thin-layer chromatography" (vol. 1, p. 83), using silica gel R2 as the coating substance and a mixture of 80 volumes of acetone R, 30 volumes of cyclohexane R, and 5 volumes of ammonia (~260 g/l) TS as the mobile phase. Apply separately to the plate 20 µl of each of 2 solutions in methanol R containing (A) 25 mg of the test substance per ml and (B) 0.25 mg of fluphenazine hydrochloride RS per ml. After removing the plate from the chromatographic chamber, allow it to dry in air, and examine the chromatogram in ultraviolet light (254 nm). Then spray the plate with sulfuric acid (~635 g/l) TS and examine the chromatogram in daylight. Using either method of visualization, any spot obtained with solution A, other than the principal spot, is not more intense than that obtained with solution B.

Assay.   Dissolve about 0.55 g, accurately weighed, in 30 ml of glacial acetic acid R1, and titrate with perchloric acid (0.1 mol/l) VS, as described under "Non-aqueous titration", Method A (vol. 1, p. 131). Each ml of perchloric acid (0.1 mol/l) VS is equivalent to 27.49 mg of $C_{29}H_{38}F_3N_3O_2S$.

FLUPHENAZINI HYDROCHLORIDUM

Fluphenazine hydrochloride

Molecular formula. $C_{22}H_{26}F_3N_3OS,2HCl$

Relative molecular mass. 510.4

Graphic formula.

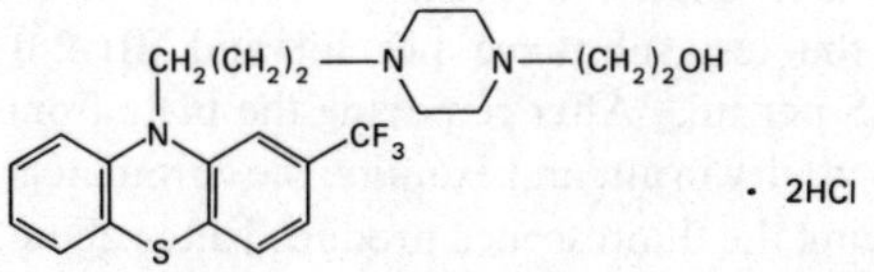

Chemical name. 4-[3-[2-(Trifluoromethyl)phenothiazin-10-yl]propyl]-1-piperazineethanol dihydrochloride; 4-[3-[2-(trifluoromethyl)-10H-phenothiazin-10-yl]propyl]-1-piperazineethanol dihydrochloride;CASReg.No.146-56-5.

Description. A white or almost white, crystalline powder; odourless.

Solubility. Soluble in 10 parts of water; sparingly soluble in ethanol (~750 g/l) TS; practically insoluble in ether R.

Category. Neuroleptic.

Storage. Fluphenazine hydrochloride should be kept in a well-closed container, protected from light.

Additional information. Even in the absence of light, Fluphenazine hydrochloride is gradually degraded on exposure to a humid atmosphere, the decomposition being faster at higher temperatures.

REQUIREMENTS

General requirement. Fluphenazine hydrochloride contains not less than 98.5% and not more than 101.5% of $C_{22}H_{26}F_3N_3OS,2HCl$, calculated with reference to the dried substance.

Identity tests

A. Carry out the examination as described under "Spectrophotometry in the infrared region" (vol. 1, p. 40). The infrared absorption spectrum is concordant with the spectrum obtained from fluphenazine hydrochloride RS or with the *reference spectrum* of fluphenazine hydrochloride.

B. Carry out the test in subdued light as described under "Thin-layer chromatography" (vol. 1, p. 83), using kieselguhr R1 as the coating substance and a mixture of 15 volumes of formamide R, 5 volumes of 2-phenoxyethanol R, and 180 volumes of acetone R to impregnate the plate, dipping it about 5 mm beneath the surface of the liquid. After the solvent has reached the top of the plate, remove the plate from the chromatographic chamber and allow to stand at room temperature until the solvents have completely evaporated. Use the impregnated plate immediately, carrying out the chromatography in the same direction as the impregnation. As the mobile phase, use a mixture of 2 volumes of diethylamine R and 100 volumes of light petroleum R1 saturated with 2-phenoxyethanol R. Apply separately to the plate 2 μl of each of 2 solutions in chloroform R containing (A) 2.0 mg of the test substance per ml and (B) 2.0 mg of fluphenazine hydrochloride RS per ml. After removing the plate from the chromatographic chamber, allow it to dry in air, and examine the chromatogram in ultraviolet light (365 nm), observing the fluorescence produced after about 2 minutes. Spray the plate with sulfuric acid/ethanol TS and examine the chromatogram in daylight. The principal spot obtained with solution A corresponds in position, appearance, and intensity with that obtained with solution B.

C. Dissolve 5 mg in 5 ml of sulfuric acid (~1760 g/l) TS; an orange colour is produced which becomes brownish red on warming.

D. Heat 0.5 ml of chromic acid TS in a small test-tube in a water-bath for 5 minutes; the solution wets the sides of the tube but there is no greasiness. Add about 3 mg of the test substance and again heat in a water-bath for 5 minutes; the solution no longer wets the sides of the tube.

E. A 0.05 g/ml solution yields reaction B described under "General identification tests" as characteristic of chlorides (vol. 1, p. 113).

Sulfated ash. Not more than 2.0 mg/g.

Loss on drying. Dry to constant weight at 105 °C; it loses not more than 10 mg/g.

Related substances. Carry out the test as described under "Thin-layer chromatography" (vol. 1, p. 83), using silica gel R2 as the coating substance and a mixture of 80 volumes of acetone R, 30 volumes of cyclohexane R and 5 volumes of ammonia (~260 g/l) TS as the mobile phase. Apply separately to the plate 10 μl of each of 2 solutions in sodium hydroxide/methanol TS containing (A) 10 mg of the test substance per ml and (B) 0.10 mg of the test substance per ml. After removing the plate from the chromatographic chamber, allow it to dry in air, and examine the chromatogram in ultraviolet light (254 nm). Any spot obtained with solution A, other than the principal spot, is not more intense than that obtained with solution B.

Assay. Dissolve about 0.5 g, accurately weighed, in 30 ml of glacial acetic acid R1, add 10 ml of mercuric acetate/acetic acid TS and titrate with perchloric acid (0.1 mol/l) VS, as described under "Non-aqueous titration", Method A (vol. 1, p. 131). Each ml of perchloric acid (0.1 mol/l) VS is equivalent to 25.52 mg of $C_{22}H_{26}F_3N_3OS,2HCl$.

FUROSEMIDUM

Furosemide

Molecular formula. $C_{12}H_{11}ClN_2O_5S$

Relative molecular mass. 330.8

Graphic formula.

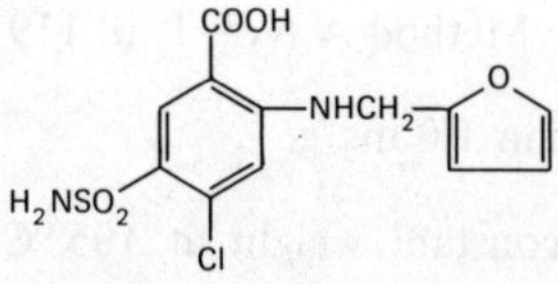

Chemical name. 4-Chloro-N-furfuryl-5-sulfamoylanthranilic acid; 5-(aminosulfonyl)-4-chloro-2-[(2-furanylmethyl)amino]benzoic acid; CAS Reg. No. 54-31-9.

Description. A white or almost white, crystalline powder; odourless.

Solubility. Practically insoluble in water; soluble in 75 parts of ethanol (~750 g/l) TS; slightly soluble in ether R; very slightly soluble in chloroform R.

Category. Diuretic.

Storage. Furosemide should be kept in a well-closed container, protected from light.

REQUIREMENTS

General requirement. Furosemide contains not less than 98.0% and not more than 101.0% of $C_{12}H_{11}ClN_2O_5S$, calculated with reference to the dried substance.

Identity tests

• Either test A alone or tests B and C may be applied.

A. Carry out the examination as described under "Spectrophotometry in the infrared region" (vol. 1, p. 40). The infrared absorption spectrum is concordant with the spectrum obtained from furosemide RS or with the *reference spectrum* of furosemide.

B. Dissolve 5 mg in 10 ml of methanol R. Transfer 1 ml of this solution to a flask, add 10 ml of hydrochloric acid (~70 g/l) TS and heat under a reflux condenser for 15 minutes. Cool and add 15 ml of sodium hydroxide (1 mol/l) VS and 5 ml of sodium nitrite (1 g/l) TS. Allow to stand for 3 minutes, then add 2 ml of

ammonium sulfamate (25 g/l) TS and mix.   Add 1 ml of N-(1-naphthyl)ethylene-
diamine hydrochloride (5 g/l) TS; a red-violet colour is produced.

C.   Dissolve 25 mg in 2.5 ml of ethanol (~750 g/l) TS and add, drop by drop, about
2 ml of 4-dimethylaminobenzaldehyde TS1; a transient green colour is produced,
which becomes deep red.

Heavy metals.   Use 1.0 g for the preparation of the test solution as described under
"Limit test for heavy metals", Procedure 3 (vol. 1, p. 118); determine the heavy
metals content according to Method A (vol. 1, p. 119); not more than 20 μg/g.

Sulfated ash.   Not more than 1.0 mg/g.

Loss on drying.   Dry to constant weight at 105 °C; it loses not more than
5.0 mg/g.

4-Chloro-5-sulfamoylanthranilic acid.   Dissolve 0.1 g in 25 ml of methanol R.
To 1 ml add 3 ml of dimethylformamide R, 12 ml of water, and 1 ml of
hydrochloric acid (1 mol/l) VS.   Cool, add 0.5 ml of sodium nitrite (10 g/l) TS,
shake, and allow to stand for 5 minutes.   Add 1 ml of ammonium sulfamate (25 g/l)
TS, shake, and allow to stand for 3 minutes.   Add 1 ml of N-(1-naphthyl)ethylene-
diamine hydrochloride (5 g/l) TS and sufficient water to produce 25 ml.   Measure
the absorbance of a 1-cm layer of the resulting solution at a maximum of about
530 nm, using as a blank a solution prepared by treating a mixture of 1 ml of
methanol R and 3 ml of dimethylformamide R in a similar manner; the
absorbance is not greater than 0.12 (0.3% of free primary aromatic amines
expressed as 4-chloro-5-sulfamoylanthranilic acid) (preferably use 2-cm cells for
the measurement and calculate the absorbance of a 1-cm layer).

Related substances.   Carry out the test as described under "Thin-layer chromatography" (vol. 1, p. 83), using silica gel R1 as the coating substance and a mixture
of 1 volume of toluene R, 1 volume of xylene R, 3 volumes of dioxan R, 3 volumes
of 2-propanol R and 2 volumes of ammonia (~260 g/l) TS as the mobile phase.
Apply separately to the plate 5 μl of each of 2 solutions in acetone R containing (A)
20 mg of the test substance per ml and (B) 0.30 mg of the test substance per ml.
After removing the plate from the chromatographic chamber, allow it to dry in air,
and examine the chromatogram in ultraviolet light (365 nm).   Any spot obtained
with solution A, other than the principal spot, is not more intense than that
obtained with solution B.

Assay.   Dissolve about 0.3 g, accurately weighed, in 40 ml of dimethylformamide
R, add 3 drops of bromothymol blue/dimethylformamide TS, and titrate with
sodium hydroxide (0.1 mol/l) VS to a blue endpoint.   Repeat the operation
without the substance being examined and make any necessary corrections.   Each
ml of sodium hydroxide (0.1 mol/l) VS is equivalent to 33.08 mg of
$C_{12}H_{11}ClN_2O_5S$.

GLUCOSUM

Glucose

Glucose, anhydrous
Glucose monohydrate

Molecular formula. $C_6H_{12}O_6$ (anhydrous); $C_6H_{12}O_6,H_2O$ (monohydrate).

Relative molecular mass. 180.2 (anhydrous); 198.2 (monohydrate).

Graphic formula.

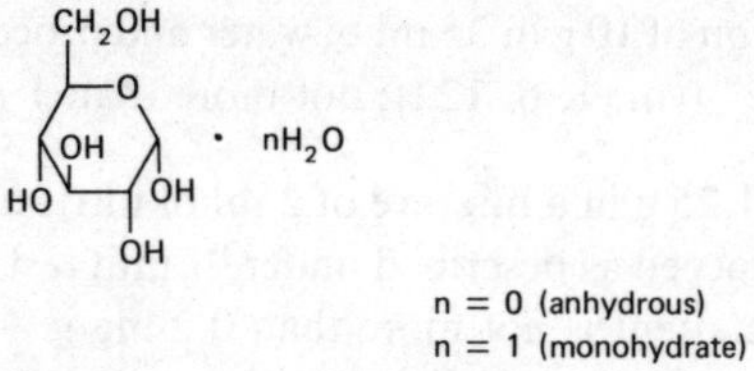

$$CH_2OH$$

$\cdot\ nH_2O$

$n = 0$ (anhydrous)
$n = 1$ (monohydrate)

Chemical name. α-D-Glucopyranose; CAS Reg. No. 492-62-6 (anhydrous). α-D-Glucopyranose monohydrate; CAS Reg. No. 14431-43-7 (monohydrate).

Other name. Dextrose.

Description. Colourless crystals or a white, crystalline or granular powder; odourless.

Solubility. Soluble in about 1 part of water; slightly soluble in ethanol ($\sim$750 g/l) TS; more soluble in boiling water and boiling ethanol ($\sim$750 g/l) TS.

Category. Nutrient; fluid replenisher.

Storage. Glucose should be kept in a well-closed container.

Labelling. The designation on the container of Glucose should state whether the substance is the monohydrate or is in the anhydrous form. If the material is not intended for parenteral use a designation "for oral use only" should be added.

Additional information. Glucose has a sweet taste.

REQUIREMENTS

General requirement. Glucose contains not less than 99.0% and not more than 101.5% of $C_6H_{12}O_6$, calculated with reference to the anhydrous substance.

Identity tests

A. When heated it melts, swells up and burns, evolving an odour of burnt sugar.

B.   Add a few drops of a 0.05 g/ml solution to 5 ml of hot potassio-cupric tartrate TS; a copious red precipitate is produced.

Specific optical rotation.   Dissolve 10.0 g in 50 ml of water, add 0.2 ml of ammonia (~100 g/l) TS, and sufficient water to produce 100 ml, and allow to stand for 30 minutes. Calculate the result with reference to the anhydrous substance; $[\alpha]_D^{20\,°C} = +52.5$ to $+53.0°$.

Heavy metals.   Use 1.0 g for the preparation of the test solution as described under "Limit test for heavy metals", Procedure 1 (vol. 1, p. 118); determine the heavy metals content according to Method A (vol. 1, p. 119); not more than 5 μg/g.

Arsenic.   Use a solution of 10 g in 35 ml of water and proceed as described under "Limit test for arsenic" (vol. 1, p. 122); not more than 1 μg/g.

Chlorides.   Dissolve 1.25 g in a mixture of 2 ml of nitric acid (~130 g/l) TS and 20 ml of water, and proceed as described under "Limit test for chlorides" (vol. 1, p. 116); the chloride content is not more than 0.2 mg/g.

Sulfates.   Dissolve 2.5 g in 20 ml of water and proceed as described under "Limit test for sulfates" (vol. 1, p. 116); the sulfate content is not more than 0.2 mg/g.

Less-soluble sugars and dextrins.   Boil 1 g with 30 ml of ethanol (~710 g/l) TS and cool; a clear solution is produced.

Soluble starch.   Dissolve 2.5 g in 25 ml of water, boil the solution for 1 minute, cool and add 0.1 ml of iodine (0.1 mol/l) VS; no blue colour is produced.

Sulfites.   Dissolve 2.5 g in 25 ml of water, add 0.1 ml of iodine (0.1 mol/l) VS and a few drops of starch TS; a blue colour is produced.

Clarity and colour of solution.   A solution of 5.0 g in 10 ml of water is clear and not more intensely coloured than standard colour solution Gn3 when compared as described under "Colour of liquids" (vol. 1, p. 50).

Sulfated ash.   Not more than 1.0 mg/g.

Water.   Determine as described under "Determination of water by the Karl Fischer method", Method A (vol. 1, p. 135). For the anhydrous form use about 1 g of the substance; the water content is not more than 10 mg/g. For the monohydrate use about 0.15 g of the substance; the water content is not less than 70 mg/g and not more than 95 mg/g.

Acidity.   Dissolve 5.0 g in 50 ml of carbon-dioxide-free water R and titrate with carbonate-free sodium hydroxide (0.02 mol/l) VS, using phenolphthalein/ethanol TS as indicator; not more than 0.5 ml is required to obtain the midpoint of the indicator (pink).

Assay. Dissolve about 0.10 g, accurately weighed, in 50 ml of water, add 25.0 ml of iodine (0.1 mol/l) VS and 10 ml of sodium carbonate (50 g/l) TS. Allow to stand for 20 minutes in the dark and add 15 ml of sulfuric acid (~100 g/l) TS. Titrate the excess of iodine with sodium thiosulfate (0.1 mol/l) VS, using starch TS as indicator. Repeat the operation without the substance being examined and make any necessary corrections. Each ml of iodine (0.1 mol/l) VS is equivalent to 9.008 mg of $C_6H_{12}O_6$.

GRISEOFULVINUM

Griseofulvin

Molecular formula. $C_{17}H_{17}ClO_6$

Relative molecular mass. 352.8

Graphic formula.

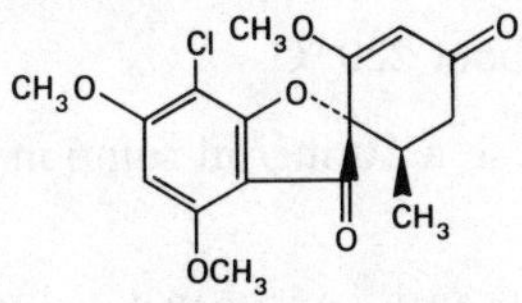

Chemical name. 7-Chloro-2′,4,6-trimethoxy-6′β-methylspiro[benzofuran-2(3H),1′-[2]cyclohexene]-3,4′-dione; (1′S-trans)-7-chloro-2′,4,6-trimethoxy-6′-methylspiro[benzofuran-2(3H),1′-[2]cyclohexene]-3,4′-dione; CAS Reg. No. 126-07-8.

Description. White to pale cream powder; almost odourless.

Solubility. Very slightly soluble in water; slightly soluble in ethanol (~750 g/l) TS; soluble in chloroform R; freely soluble in tetrachloroethane R.

Category. Antifungal.

Storage. Griseofulvin should be kept in a well-closed container.

Additional information. The particles of Griseofulvin are generally up to 5 μm in maximum dimension, although occasionally larger particles may be present that exceed 30 μm.

General requirement. Griseofulvin contains not less than 97.0% and not more than 102.0% of $C_{17}H_{17}ClO_6$, calculated with reference to the dried substance.

Identity tests

• Either tests A and D or tests B, C, and D may be applied.

A. Carry out the examination as described under "Spectrophotometry in the infrared region" (vol. 1, p. 40). The infrared absorption spectrum is concordant with the spectrum obtained from griseofulvin RS or with the *reference spectrum* of griseofulvin.

B. Carry out the test as described under "Thin-layer chromatography" (vol. 1, p. 83), using kieselguhr R1 as the coating substance and a mixture of 1 volume of ethylmethylketone R and 1 volume of xylene R as the mobile phase. Apply separately to the plate 10 μl of each of 2 solutions in chloroform R containing (A) 0.50 mg of the test substance per ml and (B) 0.50 mg of griseofulvin RS per ml. After removing the plate from the chromatographic chamber, allow it to dry in air, and examine the chromatogram in ultraviolet light (254 nm). The principal spot obtained with solution A corresponds in position, appearance, and intensity with that obtained with solution B.

C. Dissolve 5 mg in 1 ml of sulfuric acid (~1760 g/l) TS and add 5 mg of powdered potassium dichromate R; a wine-red colour is produced.

D. Melting temperature, about 220 °C.

Specific optical rotation. Use a 10 mg/ml solution in dimethylformamide R; $[\alpha]_D^{20\,°C} = +354$ to $+364°$.

Particle size. In a mortar grind 10 mg with 10 drops of hydroxyethylcellulose TS, add a further 3.50 ml of hydroxyethylcellulose TS and grind again. Transfer a drop of the suspension to a suitable counting chamber 0.10 mm deep, place a cover glass over it, and examine under a microscope 10 fields of vision of 0.04 mm^2 area each, using a magnification of 600×; not more than 30 crystals larger than 5 μm are visible in any field of vision.

Solution in dimethylformamide. A solution of 0.75 g in 10 ml of dimethylformamide R is clear and not more intensely coloured than standard colour solution Yw2 when compared as described under "Colour of liquids" (vol. 1, p. 50).

Matter soluble in light petroleum. Reflux 1.0 g with 40 ml of light petroleum R for 10 minutes, cool and filter. Wash the flask 3 times with 10 ml of light petroleum R, filter, evaporate the combined filtrates on a water-bath, and dry at 105 °C for 1 hour; the weight of the residue does not exceed 2.0 mg.

Sulfated ash. Not more than 2.0 mg/g.

Loss on drying. Dry to constant weight at 105 °C; it loses not more than 10 mg/g.

Acidity. Dissolve 0.25 g in 20 ml of neutralized ethanol TS and titrate with carbonate-free sodium hydroxide (0.02 mol/l) VS, phenolphthalein/ethanol TS being used as indicator; not more than 1.0 ml is required to obtain the midpoint of the indicator (pink).

Assay. Dissolve about 0.10 g, accurately weighed, in sufficient dehydrated ethanol R to produce 200 ml and dilute 2 ml of this solution to 100 ml with dehydrated ethanol R. Determine the absorbance of this solution in a 1-cm layer at the maximum at about 291 nm and calculate the content of $C_{17}H_{17}ClO_6$, using the absorptivity value of 68.6 ($E_{1\ cm}^{1\ \%}$ = 686).

HALOPERIDOLUM

Haloperidol

Molecular formula. $C_{21}H_{23}ClFNO_2$

Relative molecular mass. 375.9

Graphic formula.

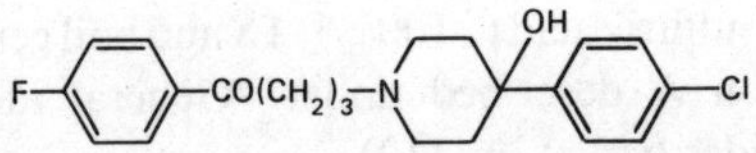

Chemical name. 4-[4-(*p*-Chlorophenyl)-4-hydroxypiperidino]-4′-fluorobutyro-phenone; 4-[4-(4-chlorophenyl)-4-hydroxy-1-piperidinyl]-1-(4-fluorophenyl)-1-butanone; CAS Reg. No. 52-86-8.

Description. A white to faintly yellowish, amorphous or microcrystalline powder; odourless.

Solubility. Practically insoluble in water; soluble in 50 parts of ethanol (~750 g/l) TS, in 20 parts of chloroform R, and in 200 parts of ether R.

Category. Neuroleptic.

Storage. Haloperidol should be kept in a well-closed container, protected from light.

REQUIREMENTS

General requirement. Haloperidol contains not less than 98.0% and not more than 101.0% of $C_{21}H_{23}ClFNO_2$, calculated with reference to the dried substance.

Identity tests

• Either tests A and C or tests B and C may be applied.

A. Carry out the examination as described under "Spectrophotometry in the infrared region" (vol. 1, p. 40). The infrared absorption spectrum is concordant with the spectrum obtained from haloperidol RS or with the *reference spectrum* of haloperidol.

B. The absorption spectrum of a 15 μg/ml solution in a mixture of 1 volume of hydrochloric acid (1 mol/l) VS and 99 volumes of methanol R, when observed between 230 nm and 350 nm, exhibits a maximum at about 245 nm; the absorbance of a 1-cm layer at this wavelength is between 0.49 and 0.53 (preferably use 2-cm cells for the measurement and calculate the absorbance of a 1-cm layer).

C. Carry out the combustion as described under "Oxyen flask method" (vol. 1, p. 125), using 20 mg of the test substance and a mixture of 3 ml of sodium hydroxide (~80 g/l) TS and 2 ml of water as the absorbing liquid. When the process is complete, dilute to 10 ml with water; the resulting solution complies with the following tests:

(a) Add 0.1 ml to a mixture of 0.1 ml of a freshly prepared sodium alizarinsulfonate (1 g/l) TS and 0.1 ml of zirconyl nitrate TS; the red colour of the solution changes to clear yellow.

(b) Acidify 5 ml with sulfuric acid (~100 g/l) TS and boil gently for 2 minutes; the solution yields reaction A described under "General identification tests" as characteristic of chlorides (vol. 1, p. 112).

Melting range. 147–152 °C.

Sulfated ash. Not more than 1.0 mg/g.

Loss on drying. Dry to constant weight at 60 °C under reduced pressure (not exceeding 0.6 kPa or about 5 mm of mercury); it loses not more than 5.0 mg/g.

Related substances. Carry out the test as described under "Thin-layer chromatography" (vol. 1, p. 83), using silica gel R5 as the coating substance (a precoated plate is preferable) and a mixture of 80 volumes of chloroform R, 10 volumes of glacial acetic acid R and 10 volumes of methanol R as the mobile phase. Apply separately to the plate 10 μl of each of 3 solutions in chloroform R containing (A) 10 mg of the test substance per ml, (B) 0.050 mg of the test substance per ml, and (C)

0.10 mg of the test substance per ml. After removing the plate from the chromatographic chamber, allow it to dry in air, spray with potassium iodobis-muthate TS2, and examine the chromatogram in daylight. Any spot obtained with solution A, other than the principal spot, is not more intense than that obtained with solution B. Not more than one of any such spots is more intense than the spot obtained with solution C.

Assay. Dissolve about 0.35 g, accurately weighed, in 30 ml of glacial acetic acid R1 and titrate with perchloric acid (0.1 mol/l) VS, determining the endpoint potentiometrically as described under "Non-aqueous titration", Method A (vol. 1, p. 131). Each ml of perchloric acid (0.1 mol/l) VS is equivalent to 37.59 mg of $C_{21}H_{23}ClFNO_2$.

HALOTHANUM

Halothane

Molecular formula. $C_2HBrClF_3$

Relative molecular mass. 197.4

Graphic formula.

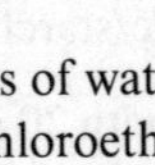

ClCHCF₃
|
Br

Chemical name. 2-Bromo-2-chloro-1,1,1-trifluoroethane; CAS Reg. No. 151-67-7.

Description. A colourless, mobile, heavy liquid; odour, characteristic, resembling that of chloroform.

Miscibility. Miscible with 400 parts of water; miscible with ethanol (~750 g/l) TS, chloroform R, ether R, and trichloroethylene R.

Category. General anaesthetic.

Storage. Halothane should be kept in a well-closed container, protected from light, and stored at a temperature not exceeding 25 °C.

Additional information. Halothane is a noninflammable liquid. Halothane contains not less than 0.08 mg/g and not more than 0.12 mg/g of thymol, as a stabilizer.

REQUIREMENTS

Identity tests

To a test-tube, transfer 2 ml of *tert.*-butanol R, 0.1 ml of the test liquid, 1 ml of copper edetate TS, 0.5 ml of ammonia (~260 g/l) TS and 2 ml of hydrogen peroxide (~60 g/l) TS; this constitutes solution 1. Similarly, prepare a blank without the test liquid; this constitutes solution 2. Place both tubes in a water-bath at 50 °C for 15 minutes, cool and add 0.3 ml of glacial acetic acid R.

A.   To 1 ml of each of solutions 1 and 2 add 0.5 ml of a mixture of equal volumes of sodium alizarinsulfonate (1 g/l) TS and zirconyl nitrate TS; a red colour is produced in solution 2 and a yellow colour in solution 1.

B.   To 1 ml of each of solutions 1 and 2 add 1 ml of a mixture of 1.02 g of potassium hydrogen phthalate R dissolved in 30 ml of sodium hydroxide (0.1 mol/l) VS and diluted to 100 ml with water (= buffer pH 5.2). Then add (a) 1 ml of phenol red/ethanol TS that has been previously diluted with an equal volume of water and (b) 0.1 ml of tosylchloramide sodium (15 g/l) TS; a yellow colour is produced in solution 2 and a bluish red colour in solution 1.

C.   To 2 ml of each of solutions 1 and 2 add 0.5 ml of sulfuric acid (~570 g/l) TS, 0.5 ml of acetone R and 0.2 ml of potassium bromate (50 g/l) TS. Shake, then place in a water-bath at 50 °C for 2 minutes. Cool, add 0.5 ml of a mixture of equal volumes of nitric acid (~1000 g/l) TS and water, and 0.1 ml of silver nitrate (40 g/l) TS; solution 2 remains clear and an opalescence is produced in solution 1, which changes to a white precipitate after a few minutes.

Mass density. ρ_{20} = 1.865–1.875 g/ml.

Free halides.   Shake 10 ml with 20 ml of carbon-dioxide-free water R for 3 minutes. To 5 ml of the aqueous layer add 5 ml of water, 1 drop of nitric acid (~1000 g/l) TS, and 0.2 ml of silver nitrate (40 g/l) TS; no opalescence is produced. (Keep the remaining aqueous layer for the test of free halogens).

Free halogens.   To 10 ml of the aqueous layer obtained from the test for free halides add 1 ml of potassium iodide/starch TS; no blue colour is produced.

Acidity or alkalinity.   Shake 20 ml with 20 ml of carbon-dioxide-free water R for 3 minutes. To the aqueous layer add a few drops of bromocresol purple/ethanol TS; not more than 0.1 ml of sodium hydroxide (0.01 mol/l) VS or 0.6 ml of hydrochloric acid (0.01 mol/l) VS is required to obtain the midpoint of the indicator (grey).

Thymol.   Use 3 dry 25-ml stoppered cylinders and place in the first one 0.5 ml of the test liquid, in the second one 0.5 ml of thymol TS2, and in the third one 0.5 ml of thymol TS3. To each of the 3 cylinders add 5 ml of carbon tetrachloride R and

5.0 ml of titanium dioxide/sulfuric acid TS. Shake the cylinders vigorously for 30 seconds and allow to stand until the layers have separated. When viewed transversally the yellowish-brown colour of the lower layer obtained in the cylinder containing the test liquid is intermediate in intensity between the colours of the corresponding layers in the other 2 cylinders (0.08–0.12 mg/g of thymol).

Related substances. Carry out the test as described under "Gas chromatography" (vol. 1, p. 94), using 3 solutions (1) trichlorotrifluoroethane TS serving as an internal standard, (2) the test liquid, and (3) the test liquid containing 0.05 μl of trichlorotrifluoroethane R per ml.

For the procedure use a glass column 2.75 m long and 5.0 mm in internal diameter, the first 1.8 m of which are packed with an adequate quantity of an adsorbent composed of 30 g of macrogol 400 R supported on 70 g of pink firebrick R, and the remainder with an adequate quantity of an adsorbent composed of 30 g of dinonyl phthalate R supported on 70 g of pink firebrick R. Maintain the column at 50 °C, use nitrogen R as the carrier gas and a flame ionization detector.

In the chromatogram obtained with solution 3, the peak area due to the trichlorotrifluoroethane is greater than the total area of any other peaks except that due to the halothane; in calculating the peak area due to the trichlorotrifluoroethane, allowance may be necessary for any impurities having the same retention time as revealed in the chromotogram obtained from solution 2.

HYDRARGYRI OXYCYANIDUM

Mercuric oxycyanide

Composition. Mercuric oxycyanide is a mixture of approximately 1 part of $Hg(CN)_2,HgO$ and 2 parts of $Hg(CN)_2$; CAS Reg. No. 73360-53-9.

Description. A white or almost white, crystalline powder; odourless.

Solubility. Soluble in 20 parts of water; sparingly soluble in ethanol (~750 g/l) TS.

Category. Antiseptic (for topical use).

Storage. Mercuric oxycyanide should be kept in a tightly closed container, protected from light.

Additional information. Mercuric oxycyanide is slowly discoloured by light. It might explode on triturating or mixing with other substances. The solution should not be heated on an open flame.

REQUIREMENTS

General requirement. Mercuric oxycyanide contains not less than 14.5% and not more than 17.2% of HgO, and not less than 82.5% and not more than 85.5% of $Hg(CN)_2$.

Identity tests

A. Immerse a small piece of copper plate in a 0.05 g/ml solution for some minutes, remove, wash with water, and rub the plate with paper; a bright silvery surface is produced.

B. To a 0.05 g/ml solution add potassium iodide (80 g/l) TS; a yellow solution is produced which on the addition of ammonia (~100 g/l) TS gives a reddish brown precipitate.

C. To 1 ml of a 0.05 g/ml solution add 0.05 g of ferrous sulfate R and sufficient sodium hydroxide (~80 g/l) TS to precipitate the iron as hydroxide. Boil the mixture and acidify with hydrochloric acid (~70 g/l) TS; a blue colour or precipitate is produced.

Chlorides. Dissolve 1.75 g in 20 ml of water, add 10 ml of sodium hydroxide (~80 g/l) TS and 25 ml of formaldehyde TS, and boil gently for 10 minutes. Cool, filter, wash the precipitate with water, combine the filtrate and washings, neutralize with nitric acid (~130 g/l) TS and add sufficient water to produce 100 ml. Proceed as described under "Limit test for chlorides" (vol. 1, p. 116), using 40 ml of this solution and 6 ml of nitric acid (~130 g/l) TS. To prepare the standard opalescence mix 10 ml of sodium hydroxide (~80 g/l) TS with 12.25 ml of hydrochloric acid ClTS, and boil the mixture gently for 10 minutes. Cool, filter, wash the filter with water, combine the filtrate and washings, neutralize with nitric acid (~130 g/l) TS, and add sufficient water to produce 100 ml. Proceed as described under "Limit test for chlorides", using 40 ml of this solution and 6 ml of nitric acid (~130 g/l) TS; the chloride content is not more than 0.35 mg/g.

Clarity of solution. A solution of 0.050 g in 10 ml of water is clear.

Sulfated ash. Carry out the ignition under a hood; not more than 2.5 mg/g.

Loss on drying. Dry to constant weight at 105 °C; it loses not more than 10 mg/g.

pH value. pH of a 0.05 g/ml solution in carbon-dioxide-free water R, 7.4–8.0.

Assay

For mercuric oxide. Dissolve about 0.5 g, accurately weighed, in 50 ml of water, add 1 g of sodium chloride R and titrate with hydrochloric acid (0.1 mol/l) VS using methyl orange/ethanol TS as indicator. Repeat the operation without the substance being examined and make any necessary corrections. Each ml of hydrochloric acid (0.1 mol/l) VS is equivalent to 10.83 mg of HgO. (Keep the solution for the assay for mercuric cyanide).

For mercuric cyanide. Use the solution obtained from the assay for mercuric oxide, add 3 g of potassium iodide R, and continue to titrate with hydrochloric acid (0.1 mol/l) VS. Each ml of hydrochloric acid (0.1 mol/l) VS is equivalent to 12.63 mg of $Hg(CN)_2$.

HYDROCHLOROTHIAZIDUM

Hydrochlorothiazide

Molecular formula. $C_7H_8ClN_3O_4S_2$

Relative molecular mass. 297.7

Graphic formula.

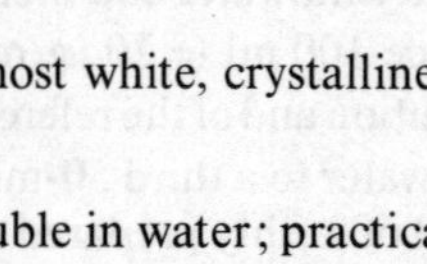

Chemical name. 6-Chloro-3,4-dihydro-2*H*-1,2,4-benzothiadiazine-7-sulfonamide 1,1-dioxide; CAS Reg. No. 58-93-5.

Description. A white or almost white, crystalline powder; odourless or almost odourless.

Solubility. Very slightly soluble in water; practically insoluble in chloroform R and ether R; soluble in 200 parts of ethanol (~750 g/l) TS and in 20 parts of acetone R.

Category. Diuretic.

Storage. Hydrochlorothiazide should be kept in a well-closed container.

REQUIREMENTS

General requirement. Hydrochlorothiazide contains not less than 98.0% and not more than 102.0% of $C_7H_8ClN_3O_4S_2$, calculated with reference to the dried substance.

Identity tests

A.   Carry out the examination as described under "Spectrophotometry in the infrared region" (vol. 1, p. 40).   The infrared absorption spectrum is concordant with the spectrum obtanied from hydrochlorothiazide RS or with the *reference spectrum* of hydrochlorothiazide.

B.   Mix 10 mg of the test substance and 10 mg of disodium chromotropate R, add 1 ml of water and, cautiously, 5 ml of sulfuric acid (~1760 g/l) TS; a purple colour is produced.

Heavy metals.   Use 1.0 g for the preparation of the test solution as described under "Limit test for heavy metals", Procedure 3 (vol. 1, p. 118); determine the heavy metals content according to Method A (vol. 1, p. 119); not more than 10 μg/g.

Free chlorides.   For the preparation of the test solution shake 0.3 g with 20 ml of water and 10 ml of nitric acid (~130 g/l) TS for 5 minutes, and filter.   Proceed with the filtrate as described under "Limit test for chlorides" (vol. 1, p. 116); the chloride content is not more than 0.8 mg/g.

Sulfated ash.   Not more than 1.0 mg/g.

Loss on drying.   Dry to constant weight at 105 °C; it loses not more than 10 mg/g.

Diazotizable substances.   For the test solution place about 0.10 g, accurately weighed, in a 50-ml volumetric flask, and dissolve in 10 ml of methanol R.   Dilute to volume with water and mix.

For the reference solution weigh 5.0 mg of 4-amino-6-chloro-1,3-benzenedisulfonamide R, transfer to a 10-ml volumetric flask, and dissolve in 1 ml of methanol R.   Dilute to volume with water and mix.   Dilute 4 ml of this solution with sufficient water to produce 100 ml (= 20 μg/ml).

Transfer 5 ml of the test solution and of the reference solution to separate 50-ml volumetric flasks, and 5 ml of water to a third 50-ml volumetric flask to serve as a blank.   To each flask add 1 ml of freshly prepared sodium nitrite (10 g/l) TS and 5 ml of hydrochloric acid (~70 g/l) TS, and allow to stand for 5 minutes.   Add 2 ml of ammonium sulfamate (25 g/l) TS, allow to stand for 5 minutes with frequent swirling, then add 2 ml of freshly prepared disodium chromotropate (10 g/l) TS and 10 ml of sodium acetate (150 g/l) TS.   Dilute with water to volume and mix.   Measure the absorbance at the maximum at about 500 nm, against the blank. The absorbance of the test solution does not exceed that of the reference solution (10 mg/g).

Assay. Dissolve about 0.3 g, accurately weighed, in 50 ml of pyridine R, add 5 drops of azo violet TS and titrate quickly with sodium methoxide (0.1 mol/l) VS to a deep blue endpoint, as described under "Non-aqueous titration", Method B (vol. 1, p. 132). Each ml of sodium methoxide (0.1 mol/l) VS is equivalent to 14.89 mg of $C_7H_8ClN_3O_4S_2$.

HYDROCORTISONI ACETAS

Hydrocortisone acetate

Molecular formula. $C_{23}H_{32}O_6$

Relative molecular mass. 404.5

Graphic formula.

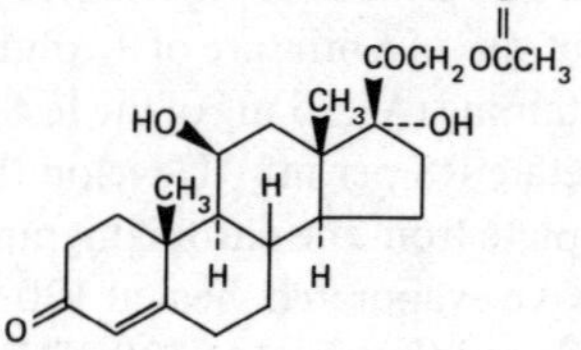

Chemical name. 21-(Acetyloxy)-11β,17-dihydroxypregn-4-ene-3,20-dione; 11β,17,21-trihydroxypregn-4-ene-3,20-dione 21-acetate; CAS Reg. No. 50-03-3.

Other name. Cortisol acetate.

Description. A white or almost white, crystalline powder; odourless.

Solubility. Practically insoluble in water; slightly soluble in ethanol (~750 g/l) TS and chloroform R; very slightly soluble in ether R.

Category. Adrenocortical steroid.

Storage. Hydrocortisone acetate should be kept in a well-closed container, protected from light.

Additional information. Hydrocortisone acetate melts at about 220 °C with decomposition.

REQUIREMENTS

General requirement. Hydrocortisone acetate contains not less than 97.0% and not more than 102.0% of $C_{23}H_{32}O_6$, calculated with reference to the dried substance.

Identity tests

• Either test A or test B may be applied.

A. Carry out the examination as described under "Spectrophotometry in the infrared region" (vol. 1, p. 40). The infrared absorption spectrum is concordant with the spectrum obtained from hydrocortisone acetate RS or with the *reference spectrum* of hydrocortisone acetate.

B. Carry out the test as described under "Thin-layer chromatography" (vol. 1, p. 83), using kieselguhr R1 as the coating substance and a mixture of 10 volumes of formamide R and 90 volumes of acetone R to impregnate the plate, dipping it about 5 mm beneath the surface of the liquid. After the solvent has reached a height of at least 16 cm, remove the plate from the chromatographic chamber and allow it to stand at room temperature until the solvent has completely evaporated. Use the impregnated plate within 2 hours and carry out the chromatography in the same direction as the impregnation. As the mobile phase, use a mixture of 75 volumes of toluene R and 25 volumes of chloroform R. Apply separately to the plate 2 μl of each of 2 solutions in a mixture of 9 volumes of chloroform R and 1 volume of methanol R containing (A) 2.5 mg of the test substance per ml and (B) 2.5 mg of hydrocortisone acetate RS per ml. Develop the plate for a distance of 15 cm. After removing the plate from the chromatographic chamber, allow it to dry in air until the solvents have evaporated, heat at 120 °C for 15 minutes, spray with sulfuric acid/ethanol TS, and then heat at 120 °C for 10 minutes. Allow to cool, and examine the chromatogram in daylight and in ultraviolet light (365 nm). The principal spot obtained with solution A corresponds in position, appearance, and intensity with that obtained with solution B.

Specific optical rotation. Use a 10 mg/ml solution in dioxan R; $[\alpha]_D^{20\,°C} = +157$ to $+168°$.

Loss on drying. Dry to constant weight at 105 °C; it loses not more than 10 mg/g.

Related substances. Carry out the test as described under "Thin-layer chromatography" (vol. 1, p. 83) using silica gel R2 as the coating substance and a mixture of 95 volumes of dichloroethane R, 5 volumes of methanol R and 0.2 volumes of water as the mobile phase. Apply separately to the plate 1 μl of each of 2 solutions in a mixture of 9 volumes of chloroform R and 1 volume of methanol R containing (A) 15 mg of the test substance per ml and (B) 0.30 mg of the test substance per ml. After removing the plate from the chromatographic chamber, allow it to dry in air until the solvents have evaporated; then heat at 105 °C for 10 minutes, allow to cool, and examine the chromatogram in ultraviolet light (254 nm). Any spot obtained with solution A, other than the principal spot, is not more intense than that obtained with solution B.

Assay. Dissolve about 20 mg, accurately weighed, in sufficient ethanol (~750 g/l) TS to produce 100 ml; dilute 5.0 ml of this solution to 100 ml with the same solvent. Measure the absorbance of a 1-cm layer of the diluted solution at the maximum at about 242 nm. Calculate the amount of $C_{23}H_{32}O_6$ in the substance being tested by comparison with hydrocortisone acetate RS, similarly and concurrently examined. In an adequately calibrated spectrophotometer the absorbance of the reference solution should be 0.40 ± 0.02 (preferably use 2-cm cells for the measurement and calculate the absorbance of a 1-cm layer).

HYDROCORTISONUM

Hydrocortisone

Molecular formula. $C_{21}H_{30}O_5$

Relative molecular mass.   362.5

Graphic formula.

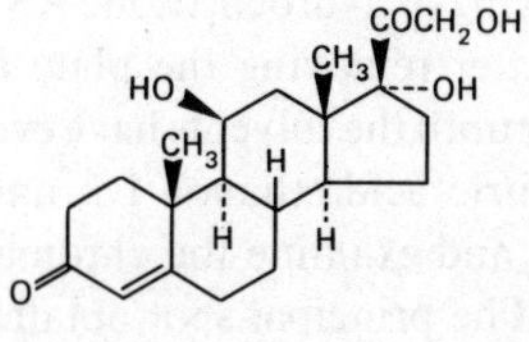

Chemical name. $11\beta,17,21$-Trihydroxypregn-4-ene-3,20-dione; CAS Reg. No. 50-23-7.

Other name.   Cortisol.

Description.   A white or almost white, crystalline powder; odourless.

Solubility.   Very slightly soluble in water and ether R; sparingly soluble in ethanol (~750 g/l) TS and acetone R; slightly soluble in chloroform R.

Category.   Adrenocortical steroid.

Storage. Hydrocortisone should be kept in a well-closed container, protected from light.

Additional information. Hydrocortisone melts at about 214 °C with decomposition.

REQUIREMENTS

General requirement. Hydrocortisone contains not less than 97.0% and not more than 102.0% of $C_{21}H_{30}O_5$, calculated with reference to the dried substance.

Identity tests

• Either test A or test B may be applied.

A. Carry out the examination as described under "Spectrophotometry in the infrared region" (vol. 1, p. 40). The infrared absorption spectrum is concordant with the spectrum obtained from hydrocortisone RS or with the *reference spectrum* of hydrocortisone.

B. Carry out the test as described under "Thin-layer chromatography" (vol. 1, p. 83), using kieselguhr R1 as the coating substance and a mixture of 10 volumes of formamide R and 90 volumes of acetone R to impregnate the plate, dipping it about 5 mm beneath the surface of the liquid. After the solvent has reached a height of at least 16 cm, remove the plate from the chromatographic chamber and allow it to stand at room temperature until the solvent has completely evaporated. Use the impregnated plate within 2 hours, carrying out the chromatography in the same direction as the impregnation. Use chloroform R as the mobile phase. Apply separately to the plate 2 μl of each of 2 solutions in a mixture of 9 volumes of chloroform R and 1 volume of methanol R containing (A) 2.5 mg of the test substance per ml, and (B) 2.5 mg of hydrocortisone RS per ml. Develop the plate for a distance of 15 cm. After removing the plate from the chromatographic chamber, allow it to dry in air until the solvents have evaporated, heat at 120 °C for 15 minutes, spray with sulfuric acid/ethanol TS, and then heat at 120 °C for 10 minutes. Allow to cool, and examine the chromatogram in daylight and in ultraviolet light (365 nm). The principal spot obtained with solution A corresponds in position, appearance, and intensity with that obtained with solution B.

Specific optical rotation. Use a 10 mg/ml solution in dioxan R; $[\alpha]_D^{20\,°C} = +150$ to +156 °.

Loss on drying. Dry to constant weight at 105 °C; it loses not more than 10 mg/g.

Related substances. Carry out the test as described under "Thin-layer chromatography" (vol. 1, p. 83), using silica gel R2 as the coating substance and a mixture of 77 volumes of dichloromethane R, 15 volumes of ether R, 8 volumes of methanol R and 1.2 volumes of water as the mobile phase. Apply separately to the plate 1 μl of each of 2 solutions in a mixture of 9 volumes of chloroform R and 1 volume of methanol R containing (A) 15 mg of the test substance per ml and (B) 0.30 mg of the test substance per ml. After removing the plate from the chromatographic chamber, allow it to dry in air until the solvents have evaporated, heat at 105 °C for 10 minutes, allow to cool, and examine the chromatogram in ultraviolet light (254 nm). Any spot obtained with solution A, other than the principal spot, is not more intense than that obtained with solution B.

Assay. Dissolve about 20 mg, accurately weighed, in sufficient ethanol (~750 g/l) TS to produce 100 ml; dilute 5.0 ml of this solution to 100 ml with the same solvent. Measure the absorbance of a 1-cm layer of the diluted solution at the maximum at about 242 nm. Calculate the amount of $C_{21}H_{30}O_5$ in the substance being tested by comparison with hydrocortisone RS, similarly and concurrently examined. In an adequately calibrated spectrophotometer the absorbance of the reference solution should be 0.44 ± 0.02 (preferably use 2-cm cells for the measurement and calculate the absorbance of a 1-cm layer).

IBUPROFENUM

Ibuprofen

Molecular formula. $C_{13}H_{18}O_2$

Relative molecular mass. 206.3

Graphic formula.

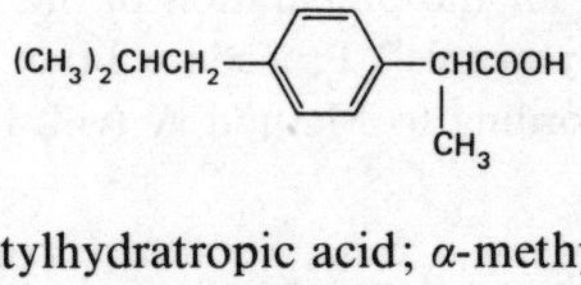

$(CH_3)_2CHCH_2$——⟨benzene ring⟩——CHCOOH
                                                    |
                                                   CH_3

Chemical name. *p*-Isobutylhydratropic acid; α-methyl-4-(2-methylpropyl)benzeneacetic acid; 2-(*p*-isobutylphenyl)propionic acid; CAS Reg. No. 15687-27-1.

Description. Colourless crystals or a white, crystalline powder; odour, characteristic.

Solubility. Practically insoluble in water; soluble in 1.5 parts of ethanol (~750 g/l) TS, in 1 part of chloroform R, in 2 parts of ether R, and in 1.5 parts of acetone R.

Category. Analgesic; anti-inflammatory.

Storage. Ibuprofen should be kept in a well-closed container.

REQUIREMENTS

General requirement. Ibuprofen contains not less than 98.5% and not more than 100.5% of $C_{13}H_{18}O_2$, calculated with reference to the dried substance.

Identity tests

- Either test A alone or tests B and C may be applied.

A. Carry out the examination as described under "Spectrophotometry in the infrared region" (vol. 1, p. 40). The infrared absorption spectrum is concordant with the spectrum obtained from ibuprofen RS or with the *reference spectrum* of ibuprofen.

B. The absorption spectrum of a 0.25 mg/ml solution in sodium hydroxide (0.1 mol/l) VS, when observed between 220 nm and 350 nm, is qualitatively similar to that of a 0.25 mg/ml solution of ibuprofen RS in sodium hydroxide (0.1 mol/l) VS (maxima occur at about 264 nm and 273 nm, and a shoulder at about 259 nm). The absorbances of the solutions at the respective maxima do not differ from each other by more than 3%. The absorbance of a 1-cm layer at the wavelengths of the main maxima at 264 nm and 273 nm are about 0.46 and 0.39, respectively (preferably use 2-cm cells for the measurement and calculate the absorbances of 1-cm layers).

C. Melting temperature, about 76 °C.

Heavy metals. Use 1.0 g for the preparation of the test solution as described under "Limit test for heavy metals", Procedure 3 (vol. 1, p. 118); determine the heavy metals content according to Method A (vol. 1, p. 119); not more than 10 μg/g.

Sulfated ash. Not more than 1.0 mg/g.

Loss on drying. Dry to constant weight at ambient temperature under reduced pressure (not exceeding 0.6 kPa or about 5 mm of mercury) over phosphorus pentoxide R; it loses not more than 5.0 mg/g.

Related substances

A. Carry out the test as described under "Gas chromatography" (vol. 1, p. 94), using a solution of the test substance prepared as follows: To 0.10 g add diazomethane TS until effervescence ceases and a persistent yellow colour is produced. Remove the solvent in a current of nitrogen, warming gently if necessary, and dissolve the residue in 2 ml of chloroform R. Use this solution in procedures A1 and A2.

In procedure A1 use a glass column 1.8 m long and 3.0 mm in internal diameter packed with an adsorbent composed of 1 g of macrogol 20M R and 9 g of acid-washed, silanized kieselguhr R3, and maintained at 135 °C. Use nitrogen R as the carrier gas and a flame ionization detector. In this system, determine only those impurities with a relative retention time of less than 2.5, taking the retention time of ibuprofen as 1.0. The ratio of the total area of the peaks due to these impurities to the area under the peak of ibuprofen does not exceed 0.010, and the corresponding ratio for the peak of any individual impurity does not exceed 0.003.

In procedure A2 use a glass column 1.8 m long and 3.0 mm in internal diameter packed with an adsorbent composed of 0.5 g of methyl silicone gum R, 0.2 g of cyanoethylmethyl silicone gum R and 9.3 g of acid-washed, silanized kieselguhr R4 and maintained at 170 °C. Use nitrogen R as the carrier gas and a flame ionization detector. In this system, determine only those impurities with a relative retention time of between 1.5 and 6.0, taking the retention time of ibuprofen as 1.0. The ratio of the total area of the peaks due to these impurities to the area under the peak of ibuprofen does not exceed 0.010.

The sum of the ratios found in procedures A1 and A2 does not exceed 0.015.

B. Carry out the test as described under "Thin-layer chromatography" (vol. 1, p. 83), using silica gel R1 as the coating substance and a mixture of 15 volumes of 1-hexane R, 5 volumes of ethyl acetate R and 1 volume of glacial acetic acid R as the mobile phase. Apply separately to the plate 5 μl of each of 2 solutions in chloroform R containing (A) 100 mg of the test substance per ml and (B) 1 mg of the test substance per ml. After removing the plate from the chromatographic chamber, allow it to dry in air, spray very lightly with a 10 mg/ml solution of potassium permanganate R in sulfuric acid ($\sim$100 g/l) TS, heat at 120 °C for 20 minutes, and examine the chromatogram in ultraviolet light (365 nm). Any spot obtained with solution A, other than the principal spot, is not more intense than that obtained with solution B.

Assay. Dissolve about 0.4 g, accurately weighed, in 100 ml of ethanol ($\sim$750 g/l) TS previously neutralized to phenolphthalein/ethanol TS, and titrate with carbonate-free sodium hydroxide (0.1 mol/l) VS, using phenolphthalein/ethanol TS as indicator. Repeat the operation without the substance being examined and make any necessary corrections. Each ml of carbonate-free sodium hydroxide (0.1 mol/l) VS is equivalent to 20.63 mg of $C_{13}H_{18}O_2$.

INDOMETACINUM

Indometacin

Molecular formula. $C_{19}H_{16}ClNO_4$

Relative molecular mass. 357.8

Graphic formula.

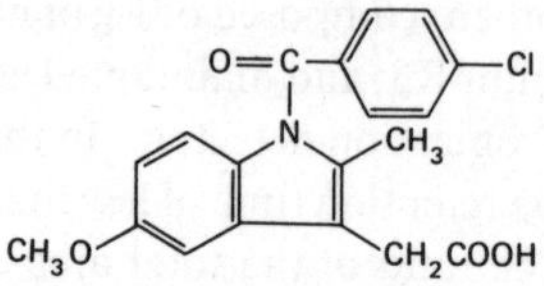

Chemical name. 1-(*p*-Chlorobenzoyl)-5-methoxy-2-methylindole-3-acetic acid; 1-(4-chlorobenzoyl)-5-methoxy-2-methyl-1*H*-indole-3-acetic acid; CAS Reg. No. 53-86-1.

Description. A white or a pale yellow, crystalline powder; odourless or almost odourless.

Solubility. Practically insoluble in water; sparingly soluble in ethanol (~750 g/l) TS, chloroform R, and ether R.

Category. Analgesic; anti-inflammatory.

Storage. Indometacin should be kept in a well-closed container, protected from light.

Additional information. Indometacin exhibits polymorphism. The polymorph specified in the monograph corresponds to the crystal form of indometacin RS.

REQUIREMENTS

General requirement. Indometacin contains not less than 98.0% and not more than 101.0% of $C_{19}H_{16}ClNO_4$, calculated with reference to the dried substance.

Identity tests

● Either test A alone or tests B and C may be applied.

A. Carry out the examination as described under "Spectrophotometry in the infrared region" (vol. 1, p. 40). The infrared absorption spectrum obtained from the solid state of the test substance is concordant with the spectrum obtained from indometacin RS or with the *reference spectrum* of indometacin (confirmation of polymorphic form).

B.   Dissolve 0.1 g in 100 ml of water containing 0.5 ml of sodium hydroxide (1 mol/l) VS.   To a 1 ml-portion add 1 ml of freshly prepared sodium nitrite (1 g/l) TS and allow to stand for 5 minutes.   Add 0.5 ml of sulfuric acid (~1760 g/l) TS; a deep yellow colour is produced.   To another 1-ml portion add 1 ml of sodium nitrite (1 g/l) TS, and allow to stand for 5 minutes.   Add 0.5 ml of hydrochloric acid (~420 g/l) TS; a green colour is produced.

C.   Melting temperature, about 160 °C.

Heavy metals.   Use 1.0 g for the preparation of the test solution as described under "Limit test for heavy metals", Procedure 3 (vol. 1, p. 118); determine the heavy metals content according to Method A (vol. 1, p. 119); not more than 20 μg/g.

Sulfated ash.   Not more than 2.0 mg/g.

Loss on drying.   Dry to constant weight at 105 °C under reduced pressure (not exceeding 0.6 kPa or about 5 mm of mercury); it loses not more than 5.0 mg/g.

Related substances.   Carry out the test as described under "Thin-layer chromatography" (vol. 1, p. 83), using silica gel R2 as the coating substance and preparing the slurry in sodium dihydrogen phosphate (45 g/l) TS.   As the mobile phase, use a mixture of 7 volumes of ether R and 3 volumes of light petroleum R.   Apply separately to the plate 10 μl of each of 2 solutions in methanol R containing (A) 20 mg of the test substance per ml and (B) 0.10 mg of the test substance per ml. After removing the plate from the chromatographic chamber, allow it to dry in air, and examine the chromatogram in ultraviolet light (254 nm).   Any spot obtained with solution A, other than the principal spot, is not more intense than that obtained with solution B.

Assay.   Dissolve about 0.33 g, accurately weighed, in 75 ml of acetone R through which nitrogen R free from carbon dioxide has previously been passed for 15 minutes.   Maintain a constant stream of nitrogen through the solution and titrate with carbonate-free sodium hydroxide (0.1 mol/l) VS using phenolphthalein/ethanol TS as indicator or determining the endpoint potentiometrically. Repeat the operation without the substance being examined and make any necessary corrections. Each ml of carbonate-free sodium hydroxide (0.1 mol/l) VS is equivalent to 35.78 mg of $C_{19}H_{16}ClNO_4$.

IODUM

Iodine

Molecular formula. I_2

Relative molecular mass. 253.8

Chemical name. Iodine; CAS Reg. No. 7553-56-2.

Description. Heavy, greyish black plates or granules, having a metallic lustre.

Solubility. Very slightly soluble in water; soluble in ethanol ($\sim$750 g/l) TS and chloroform R; freely soluble in carbon tetrachloride R, carbon disulfide R, and ether R.

Category. External antiseptic.

Storage. Iodine should be kept in a tightly closed container, preferably made of glass and provided with a glass stopper.

Additional information. Iodine volatilizes slowly at room temperature giving violet, irritant vapours.

REQUIREMENTS

General requirement. Iodine contains not less than 99.5% and not more than 100.5% of I.

Identity tests

A.   Dissolve 0.05 g in 10 ml of ethanol ($\sim$750 g/l) TS; the colour of the solution is reddish brown. Dissolve 0.05 g in 10 ml of carbon tetrachloride R; the colour of the solution is violet.

B.   To a saturated solution in water add starch TS; a blue colour is produced. Boil the mixture for a short time; the solution loses its colour, but on cooling the colour reappears.

Chlorides and bromides. Triturate 1.5 g with 10 ml of water, filter, wash the filter and dilute the filtrate to 15 ml with water. To the solution add 0.5 g of zinc R powder. When the solution has become decolourized, filter and wash the filter with sufficient water to adjust the volume of the filtrate to 20 ml. To 5 ml of the filtrate (keep the remaining filtrate for the test for cyanides) add 1.5 ml of ammonia ($\sim$260 g/l) TS and 3 ml of silver nitrate (40 g/l) TS, filter, wash the filter with sufficient water to adjust the volume of the filtrate to 10 ml, add 1.5 ml of nitric acid ($\sim$1000 g/l) TS and allow to stand for 1 minute. Any opalescence in the solution is not more intense than that obtained from a solution simultaneously prepared by mixing 10.75 ml of water, 0.25 ml of hydrochloric acid (0.01 mol/l) VS, 0.2 ml of nitric acid (~130 g/l) TS, and 0.3 ml of silver nitrate (40 g/l) TS; this indicates that the content of chlorides and bromides is not more than 0.25 mg/g.

Cyanides.   To 5 ml of the filtrate obtained in the test for chlorides and bromides add 0.2 ml of ferrous sulfate (15 g/l) TS and 1 ml of sodium hydroxide (~80 g/l) TS. Heat for a few minutes and acidify with hydrochloric acid (~70 g/l) TS; no blue or green colour is produced.

Non-volatile residue.   Place about 1 g, accurately weighed, in a porcelain dish and heat on a water-bath until the iodine has volatilized.   Dry the residue for 1 hour at 105 °C and weigh; not more than 1.0 mg/g.

Assay.   Dissolve about 0.5 g of finely powdered test substance, accurately weighed, in a solution of 1 g of potassium iodide R in 5 ml of water.   Dilute with water to about 50 ml, add 1 ml of hydrochloric acid (~70 g/l) TS and titrate with sodium thiosulfate (0.1 mol/l) VS, using starch TS as indicator.   Each ml of sodium thiosulfate (0.1 mol/l) VS is equivalent to 12.69 mg of I.

ISONIAZIDUM

Isoniazid

Molecular formula. $C_6H_7N_3O$

Relative molecular mass.   137.1

Graphic formula.

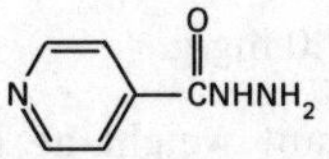

Chemical name.   4-Pyridinecarboxylic acid hydrazide; CAS Reg. No. 54-85-3.

Other name.   Isonicotinic acid hydrazide.

Description.   Colourless crystals or a white, crystalline powder; odourless.

Solubility.   Soluble in 8 parts of water and in 40 parts of ethanol (~750 g/l) TS; slightly soluble in chloroform R; very slightly soluble in ether R.

Category. Tuberculostatic.

Storage. Isoniazid should be kept in a well-closed container, protected from light.

REQUIREMENTS

General requirement. Isoniazid contains not less than 98.0% and not more than 101.0% of $C_6H_7N_3O$, calculated with reference to the dried substance.

Identity tests

• Either test A alone or tests B and C may be applied.

A. Carry out the examination as described under "Spectrophotometry in the infrared region" (vol. 1, p. 40). The infrared absorption spectrum is concordant with the spectrum obtained from isoniazid RS or with the *reference spectrum* of isoniazid.

B. Heat 0.05 g with about 1 g of anhydrous sodium carbonate R; pyridine, perceptible by its odour, is produced.

C. Dissolve 0.1 g in 2 ml of water and add 10 ml of a hot solution of vanillin (10 g/l) TS, scratch the inside of the test-tube and allow to stand; a yellow precipitate is obtained. Filter, recrystallize from 5 ml of ethanol (~600 g/l) TS, and dry at 105 °C; melting temperature, about 227 °C.

Melting range. 170–174 °C.

Heavy metals. Use 1.0 g for the preparation of the test solution as described under "Limit test for heavy metals", Procedure 1 (vol. 1, p. 118); determine the heavy metals content according to Method A (vol. 1, p. 119); not more than 20 $\mu g/g$.

Clarity and colour of solution. A solution of 0.50 g in 10 ml of water is clear and colourless.

Sulfated ash. Not more than 1.0 mg/g.

Loss on drying. Dry to constant weight at 105 °C; it loses not more than 10 mg/g.

pH value. pH of a 0.05 g/ml solution in carbon-dioxide-free water R, 6.0–8.0.

Free hydrazine. Carry out the test as described under "Thin-layer chromatography" (vol. 1, p. 83), using silica gel R1 as the coating substance and a mixture of 98 volumes of acetone R and 2 volumes of water as the mobile phase. Apply separately to the plate 10 μl of each of 2 solutions in a mixture of 1 volume of acetone R and 1 volume of water containing (A) 0.10 g of the test substance per ml, and (B) 20 μg of hydrazine hydrate R per ml. After removing the plate from the chromatographic chamber, allow it to dry in a current of air, spray with 4-dimethylaminobenzaldehyde TS3, and examine the chromatogram in daylight. The spot obtained with solution B is more intense than any spot, corresponding in position and appearance, obtained with solution A.

Assay. Dissolve about 0.25 g, accurately weighed, in sufficient water to produce 100 ml. To 25.0 ml of this solution add 100 ml of water, 20 ml of hydrochloric acid ($\sim$250 g/l) TS, 0.2 g of potassium bromide R, and 3 drops of methyl red/ethanol TS. Titrate with potassium bromate (0.0167 mol/l) VS, adding the titrant drop by drop and shaking till the red colour disappears. Repeat the operation without the substance being examined and make any necessary corrections. Each ml of potassium bromate (0.0167 mol/l) VS is equivalent to 3.429 mg of $C_6H_7N_3O$.

ISOPRENALINI HYDROCHLORIDUM

Isoprenaline hydrochloride

Molecular formula. $C_{11}H_{17}NO_3,HCl$

Relative molecular mass. 247.7

Graphic formula.

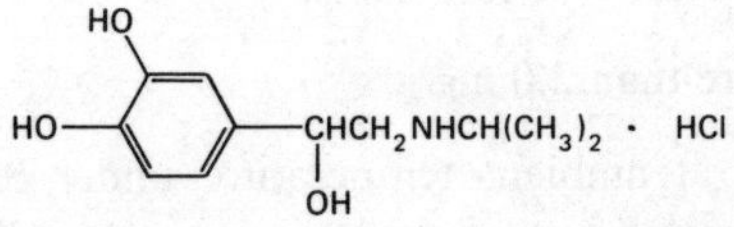

Chemical name. 3,4-Dihydroxy-α-[(isopropylamino)methyl]benzyl alcohol hydrochloride; 4-[1-hydroxy-2-[(1-methylethyl)amino]ethyl]-1,2-benzenediol hydrochloride; α-[(isopropylamino)methyl]protocatechuyl alcohol hydrochloride; CAS Reg. No. 51-30-9.

Description. A white or almost white, crystalline powder; odourless.

Solubility. Freely soluble in water; sparingly soluble in ethanol ($\sim$750 g/l) TS; practically insoluble in chloroform R and ether R.

Category. Bronchodilator.

Storage. Isoprenaline hydrochloride should be kept in a tightly closed container, protected from light.

Additional information. Isoprenaline hydrochloride gradually darkens in colour on exposure to air and light. Even in the absence of light, Isoprenaline hydrochloride is gradually degraded on exposure to a humid atmosphere, the decomposition being faster at higher temperatures.

REQUIREMENTS

General requirement. Isoprenaline hydrochloride contains not less than 97.5% and not more than 101.0% of $C_{11}H_{17}NO_3,HCl$, calculated with reference to the dried substance.

Identity tests

A.   The absorption spectrum of a 0.050 mg/ml solution, when observed between 240 nm and 350 nm, exhibits a maximum at about 280 nm; the absorbance of a 1-cm layer at this wavelength is about 0.50.

B.   Add 1 ml of a 1.0 mg/ml solution to each of two flasks, one containing 10 ml of buffer phthalate, pH 3.4, TS, the other containing 10 ml of buffer phosphate, pH 6.4, TS; other buffers having the same pH may also be used.   Add 1 ml of iodine (0.1 mol/l) VS, allow to stand for 5 minutes and add 2 ml of sodium thiosulfate (0.1 mol/l) VS.   In the solution of pH 3.4, a strong red colour is produced; in the solution of pH 6.4, a strong red-violet colour is produced (distinction from levarterenol).

C.   A 0.05 g/ml solution yields reaction B, described under "General identification test" as characteristic of chlorides (vol. 1, p. 113).

D.   Melting temperature, about 169 °C with decomposition.

Clarity and colour of solution. A solution of 0.50 g in 10 ml of carbon-dioxide-free water R is clear and colourless.

Sulfated ash. Not more than 2.0 mg/g.

Loss on drying. Dry at ambient temperature under reduced pressure (not exceeding 0.6 kPa or about 5 mm of mercury) over phosphorus pentoxide R for 4 hours; it loses not more than 10 mg/g.

pH value. pH of a 10 mg/ml solution, 4.5–6.0.

Isoprenalone. The absorbance of a 1-cm layer of a 1.0 mg/ml solution in sulfuric acid (0.005 mol/l) VS at 310 nm is not more than 0.2 (preferably use 2-cm cells for the measurement and calculate the absorbance of a 1-cm layer).

Assay. Dissolve about 0.5 g, accurately weighed, in 30 ml of glacial acetic acid R1 with the aid of the minimum of heat, add 10 ml of mercuric acetate/acetic acid TS, and titrate with perchloric acid (0.1 mol/l) VS as described under "Non-aqueous titration", Method A (vol. 1, p. 131).   Each ml of perchloric acid (0.1 mol/l) VS is equivalent to 24.77 mg of $C_{11}H_{17}NO_3,HCl$.

ISOPRENALINI SULFAS

Isoprenaline sulfate

Molecular formula. $(C_{11}H_{17}NO_3)_2,H_2SO_4,2H_2O$

Relative molecular mass. 556.6

Graphic formula.

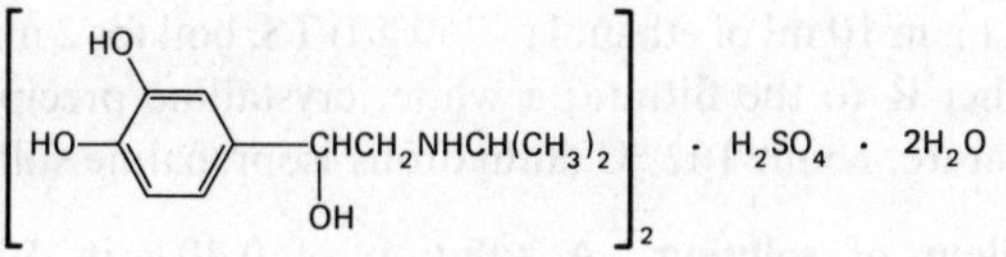

$$\left[HO-\underset{HO}{\bigcirc}-CHCH_2NHCH(CH_3)_2 \right]_2 \cdot H_2SO_4 \cdot 2H_2O$$
$$\underset{OH}{}$$

Chemical name. 3,4-Dihydroxy-α-[(isopropylamino)methyl]benzyl alcohol sulfate (2:1) (salt) dihydrate; 4-[1-hydroxy-2-[(1-methylethyl)amino]ethyl]-1,2-benzenediol sulfate (2:1) (salt) dihydrate; α-[(isopropylamino)methyl]protocatechuyl alcohol sulfate (2:1) (salt) dihydrate; CAS Reg. No. 6700-39-6.

Description. A white or almost white, crystalline powder; odourless.

Solubility. Freely soluble in water; very slightly soluble in ethanol ($\sim$750 g/l) TS; practically insoluble in chloroform R and ether R.

Category. Bronchodilator.

Storage. Isoprenaline sulfate should be kept in a tightly closed container, protected from light.

Additional information. Isoprenaline sulfate gradually darkens in colour on exposure to air and light. Even in the absence of light, Isoprenaline sulfate is gradually degraded on exposure to a humid atmosphere, the decomposition being faster at higher temperatures.

REQUIREMENTS

General requirement. Isoprenaline sulfate contains not less than 98.0% and not more than 101.0% of $(C_{11}H_{17}NO_3)_2,H_2SO_4$, calculated with reference to the anhydrous substance.

Identity tests

A. The absorption spectrum of a 0.050 mg/ml solution, when observed between 240 nm and 350 nm, exhibits a maximum at about 280 nm; the absorbance of a 1-cm layer at this wavelength is about 0.50.

B.   Add 1 ml of a 1.0 mg/ml solution to each of two flasks, one containing 10 ml of buffer phthalate, pH 3.4, TS, the other containing 10 ml of buffer phosphate, pH 6.4, TS; other buffers having the same pH may also be used.   Add 1 ml of iodine (0.1 mol/l) VS, allow to stand for 5 minutes and add 2 ml of sodium thiosulfate (0.1 mol/l) VS.   In the solution of pH 3.4, a strong red colour is produced; in the solution of pH 6.4, a strong red-violet colour is produced (distinction from levarterenol).

C.   A 0.05 g/ml solution yields reaction A, described under "General identification tests" as characteristic of sulfates (vol. 1, p. 115).

D.   Dissolve 0.1 g in 10 ml of ethanol (~750 g/l) TS, boil for 2 minutes and filter. Add 5 ml of ether R to the filtrate; a white, crystalline precipitate is formed; melting temperature, about 162 °C (anhydrous isoprenaline sulfate).

Clarity and colour of solution.   A solution of 0.40 g in 10 ml of carbon-dioxide-free water R is clear and colourless.

Sulfated ash.   Not more than 2.0 mg/g.

Water.   Determine as described under "Determination of water by the Karl Fischer method", Method A (vol. 1, p. 135), using about 0.15 g of the substance; not less than 50 mg/g and not more than 75 mg/g.

pH value.   pH of a 10 mg/ml solution, 4.0–5.5.

Isoprenalone.   The absorbance of a 1-cm layer of a 1.0 mg/ml solution in sulfuric acid (0.005 mol/l) VS at 310 nm is not more than 0.2 (preferably use 2-cm cells for the measurement and calculate the absorbance of a 1-cm layer).

Assay.   Dissolve about 0.45 g, accurately weighed, in 40 ml of glacial acetic acid R1 and 40 ml of acetonitrile R, and titrate with perchloric acid (0.1 mol/1) VS as described under "Non-aqueous titration", Method A (vol. 1, p. 131). Each ml of perchloric acid (0.1 mol/1) VS is equivalent to 52.06 mg of $(C_{11}H_{17}NO_3)_2,H_2SO_4$.

KALII CHLORIDUM

Potassium chloride

Potassium chloride (non-injectable)
Potassium chloride for parenteral use

Molecular formula. KCl

Relative molecular mass. 74.55

Chemical name. Potassium chloride; CAS Reg. No. 7447-40-7.

Description. Colourless crystals or a white, crystalline powder; odourless.

Solubility. Soluble in 3 parts of water; practically insoluble in ethanol ($\sim$750 g/l) TS.

Category. Ionic equilibration agent.

Storage. Potassium chloride should be kept in a well-closed container.

Labelling. The designation Potassium chloride for parenteral use indicates that the substance complies with the additional requirement given at the end of this monograph and may be used for parenteral administration or for other sterile applications.

REQUIREMENTS

General requirement. Potassium chloride contains not less than 99.0% and not more than 100.5% of KCl, calculated with reference to the dried substance.

Identity tests

A. To a 0.05 g/ml solution add 2 ml of sodium hydroxide ($\sim$80 g/l) TS; it yields the reaction described under "General identification tests" as characteristic of potassium (vol. 1, p. 114).

B. A 0.05 g/ml solution yields reaction A described under "General identification tests" as characteristic of chlorides (vol. 1, p. 112).

Heavy metals. Use 1.0 g for the preparation of the test solution as described under "Limit test for heavy metals", Procedure 1 (vol. 1, p. 118); determine the heavy metals content according to Method A (vol. 1, p. 119); not more than 10 μg/g.

Iron. Use 1.0 g; the solution complies with the "Limit test for iron" (vol. 1, p. 121); not more than 40 μg/g.

Calcium and magnesium.   To 20 ml of a 10 mg/ml solution add 2 ml of ammonia ($\sim$100 g/l) TS, 2 ml of ammonium oxalate (25 g/l) TS and 2 ml of disodium hydrogen phosphate (40 g/l) TS; no turbidity is produced within 5 minutes.

Barium.   Dissolve 0.5 g in 10 ml of carbon-dioxide-free and ammonia-free water R and add 1 ml of sulfuric acid ($\sim$100 g/l) TS; no turbidity is produced within 1 minute.

Arsenic.   Use a solution of 1.0 g in 35 ml of water and proceed as described under "Limit test for arsenic" (vol. 1, p. 122); the arsenic content is not more than 3 μg/g.

Bromides.   Dissolve 0.08 g in 10 ml of water, add 0.25 ml of sulfuric acid (0.5 mol/l) VS and 2 drops of tosylchloramide sodium (15 g/l) TS and mix; allow to stand for 2 minutes and extract with 5 ml of chloroform R.   Prepare a reference solution by treating a mixture of 1.0 ml of potassium bromide (0.119 g/l) TS and 9 ml of water in a similar manner.   Transfer the extracts to matched 10-ml stoppered test-tubes of transparent glass, add to each tube 3 ml of fuchsin TS, shake vigorously and allow to separate.   The colour of the chloroform layer of the test solution when viewed transversely against a white background is not more intense than that produced in the reference solution when compared as described under "Colour of liquids" (vol. 1, p. 50).

Iodides.   Moisten 5 g by adding, drop by drop, a recently prepared mixture composed of 25 ml of starch TS, 2 ml of sulfuric acid (0.5 mol/l) VS, 2 ml of sodium nitrite (10 g/l) TS, and 25 ml of water.   Examine the mixture in daylight; no particles show any trace of blue colour within 5 minutes.

Sulfates.   Dissolve 1.7 g in 20 ml of water and proceed as described under "Limit test for sulfates" (vol. 1, p. 116); the sulfate content is not more than 0.3 mg/g.

Clarity and colour of solution.   A solution of 1.0 g in 10 ml of water is clear and colourless.

Loss on drying.   Dry to constant weight at 130 °C; it loses not more than 10 mg/g.

Acidity or alkalinity.   Dissolve 5.0 g in 50 ml of carbon-dioxide-free water R, and add 0.1 ml of bromothymol blue/ethanol TS; not more than 0.2 ml of sodium hydroxide (0.02 mol/l) VS or 0.2 ml of hydrochloric acid (0.02 mol/l) VS is required to obtain the midpoint of the indicator (green).

Assay.   Dissolve about 1.0 g, accurately weighed, in sufficient water to produce 100 ml.   To 10.0 ml add 50 ml of water, 5 ml of nitric acid ($\sim$130 g/l) TS, 25.0 ml of silver nitrate (0.1 mol/l) VS, and 2 ml of dibutyl phthalate R, shake the flask and titrate with ammonium thiocyanate (0.1 mol/l) VS using 2.5 ml of ferric ammonium sulfate (45 g/l) TS as indicator.   Each ml of silver nitrate (0.1 mol/l) VS is equivalent to 7.455 mg of KCl.

Additional Requirement for Potassium Chloride for Parenteral Use

Sodium. Determine by atomic absorption spectrophotometry (vol. 1, p. 45) at a wavelength of 589 nm; use a standard solution of sodium chloride R, previously dried to constant weight, dissolved in 1000 ml of water to contain 508.4 mg of NaCl (0.2 mg of Na per ml); the sodium content is not more than 1.0 mg/g.

KALII IODIDUM
Potassium iodide

Molecular formula. KI

Relative molecular mass. 166.0

Chemical name. Potassium iodide; CAS Reg. No. 7681-11-0.

Description. Colourless crystals or a white, granular powder; odourless.

Solubility. Soluble in 0.7 part of water, in 17 parts of ethanol (~750 g/l) TS, in 2 parts of glycerol R, and in 75 parts of acetone R.

Category. Antifungal, expectorant.

Storage. Potassium iodide should be kept in a well-closed container, protected from light.

REQUIREMENTS

General requirement. Potassium iodide contains not less than 99.0% and not more than 101.0% of KI, calculated with reference to the dried substance.

Identity tests

A.   To a 0.05 g/ml solution add 2 ml of sodium hydroxide (~80 g/l) TS; it yields the reaction described under "General identification tests" as characteristic of potassium (vol. 1, p. 114).

B.   A 0.05 g/ml solution yields reaction B, described under "General identification tests" as characteristic of iodides (vol. 1, p. 113).

Heavy metals. Use 1.0 g for the preparation of the test solution as described under "Limit test for heavy metals", Procedure 1 (vol. 1, p. 118); determine the heavy metals content according to Method A (vol. 1, p. 119); not more than 10 μg/g.

Barium. Dissolve 0.5 g in 10 ml of carbon-dioxide-free and ammonia-free water R and add 1 ml of sulfuric acid (~100 g/l) TS; no turbidity is produced within 1 minute.

Iodates. Dissolve 0.5 g in 10 ml of carbon-dioxide-free water R, and add 2 drops of sulfuric acid (~100 g/l) TS, followed by 1 drop of starch TS; there is no immediate production of a blue colour.

Nitrates, nitrites and ammonia. To a solution of 1.0 g in 5 ml of water contained in a test-tube of about 40 ml capacity, add 5 ml of sodium hydroxide (~80 g/l) TS and about 0.2 g of aluminium R wire. Insert a small plug of purified cotton wool in the upper part of the test-tube, and place a piece of moistened red litmus paper R over the mouth of the tube. Heat the test-tube with its contents in a water-bath for 15 minutes; no blue coloration of the paper is discernible.

Sulfates. Dissolve 2.5 g in 20 ml of water and proceed as described under "Limit test for sulfates" (vol. 1, p. 116); the sulfate content is not more than 0.2 mg/g.

Thiosulfates. Dissolve 1.0 g in 10 ml of carbon-dioxide-free water R and add 0.1 ml of starch TS; not more than 0.1 ml of iodine (0.01 mol/l) VS is required to produce a blue colour.

Clarity and colour of solution. A solution of 1.0 g in 10 ml of water is clear and colourless.

Loss on drying. Dry to constant weight at 105 °C; it loses not more than 10 mg/g.

Alkalinity. Dissolve 1.0 g in 10 ml of carbon-dioxide-free water R, add 0.1 ml of sulfuric acid (0.05 mol/l) VS, and 1 drop of phenolphthalein/ethanol TS; no colour is produced.

Assay. Dissolve about 0.3 g, accurately weighed, in 10 ml of water. Add 10 ml of a mixture of 50 ml of starch TS and 1 drop of iodine/ethanol TS. Titrate with silver nitrate (0.1 mol/l) VS until a pale yellow colour is produced. Each ml of silver nitrate (0.1 mol/l) VS is equivalent to 16.60 mg of KI.

––––––––––––

LEVODOPUM

Levodopa

Molecular formula. $C_9H_{11}NO_4$

Relative molecular mass. 197.2

Graphic formula.

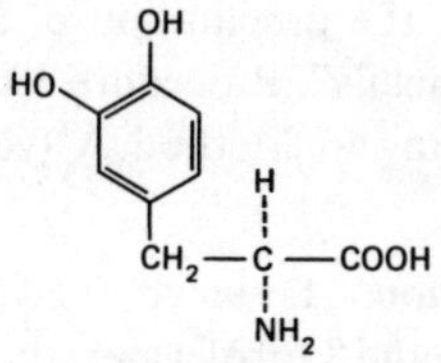

Chemical name. (−)-3-(3,4-Dihydroxyphenyl)-L-alanine; 3-hydroxy-L-tyrosine; CAS Reg. No. 59-92-7.

Description. A white or almost white, crystalline powder; odourless.

Solubility. Soluble in 300 parts of water; practically insoluble in ethanol (~750 g/l) TS, chloroform R, and ether R.

Category. Antiparkinsonism drug.

Storage. Levodopa should be kept in a tightly closed container, protected from light, and stored in a cool place.

REQUIREMENTS

General requirement. Levodopa contains not less than 98.5% and not more than 101.0% of $C_9H_{11}NO_4$, calculated with reference to the dried substance.

Identity tests

• Either test A alone or tests B and C may be applied.
A. Carry out the examination as described under "Spectrophotometry in the infrared region" (vol. 1, p. 40). The infrared absorption spectrum is concordant with the spectrum obtained from levodopa RS or with the *reference spectrum* of levodopa.

B. See the test described below under "Related substances". The principal spot obtained with solution B corresponds in position, appearance, and intensity with that obtained with solution C.

C.   To 5 mg add 1 ml of water, 1 ml of pyridine R and 5 mg of 4-nitrobenzoyl chloride R, mix and allow to stand for 3 minutes; a violet colour is produced which changes to pale yellow on boiling.   While shaking, add 0.1 ml of sodium carbonate (200 g/l) TS; the violet colour reappears.

Specific optical rotation.   Transfer about 0.5 g, accurately weighed, to a 25-ml volumetric flask, dissolve it in 10 ml of hydrochloric acid (1 mol/l) VS, add 5 g of methenamine R, swirl the contents to dissolve the methenamine, dilute with sufficient hydrochloric acid (1 mol/l) VS to produce 25 ml, mix, and allow to stand in the dark at 25 °C for 3 hours; $[\alpha]_D^{20\,°C} = -160$ to $-167\,°$.

Heavy metals.   Use 1.0 g for the preparation of the test solution as described under "Limit test for heavy metals", Procedure 3 (vol. 1, p. 118); determine the heavy metals content according to Method A (vol. 1, p. 119); not more than 10 μg/g.

Clarity and colour of solution.   Dissolve 0.50 g in a mixture of 2 ml of hydrochloric acid (~70 g/l) TS and 8 ml of water; the solution is clear and not more intensely coloured than standard colour solution Yw2 when compared as described under "Colour of liquids" (vol. 1, p. 50).

Sulfated ash.   Not more than 1.0 mg/g.

Loss on drying.   Dry to constant weight at 105 °C; it loses not more than 10 mg/g.

Related substances.   Carry out the test as described under "Thin-layer chromatography" (vol. 1, p. 83), using cellulose R2 as the coating substance and a mixture of 50 volumes of 1-butanol R, 25 volumes of glacial acetic acid R, and 25 volumes of water as the mobile phase.   Prepare a fresh solution of 0.10 g of the test substance dissolved in 5 ml of anhydrous formic acid R and dilute to 10 ml with methanol R; this constitutes solution A.   Dilute 0.5 ml of solution A to 100 ml with methanol R; this constitutes solution B.   Separately prepare a fresh solution of 0.10 g of levodopa RS dissolved in 5 ml of anhydrous formic acid R and dilute to 10 ml with methanol R.   Dilute 0.5 ml of this solution to 100 ml with methanol R; this constitutes solution C.   Dissolve 30 mg of tyrosine R in 1 ml of anhydrous formic acid R and dilute to 100 ml with methanol R.   Mix 1 ml of this solution with 1 ml of solution A; this constitutes solution D.   Apply separately to the plate 10 μl of each of solutions A, B, and C, and 20 μl of solution D.   Dry the plate in a stream of air before placing it in the chromatographic chamber.   Develop the plate, remove it from the chamber, allow it to dry in air, spray with a freshly prepared solution containing 2 volumes of ferric chloride (25 g/l) TS and 1 volume of potassium ferricyanide (50 g/l) TS, and examine the chromatogram immediately in ultraviolet light (365 nm).   Any spot obtained with solution A, other than the principal spot, is not more intense than that obtained with solution B. The test is valid only if the chromatogram obtained with solution D shows two distinctly separated spots.

Assay. Dissolve by heating about 0.18 g, accurately weighed, in 5 ml of anhydrous formic acid R, add 25 ml of glacial acetic acid R1 and 25 ml of dioxan R, and titrate with perchloric acid (0.1 mol/l) VS as described under "Non-aqueous titration", Method A (vol. 1, p. 131). Each ml of perchloric acid (0.1 mol/l) VS is equivalent to 19.72 mg of $C_9H_{11}NO_4$.

LIDOCAINI HYDROCHLORIDUM

Lidocaine hydrochloride

Molecular formula. $C_{14}H_{22}N_2O,HCl,H_2O$

Relative molecular mass. 288.8

Graphic formula.

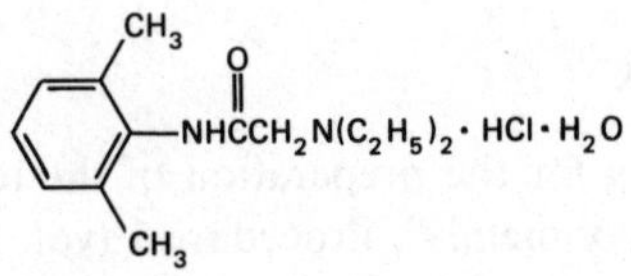

Chemical name. 2-(Diethylamino)-2',6'acetoxylidide monohydrochloride monohydrate; 2-(diethylamino)-N-(2,6-dimethylphenyl)acetamide mono-hydrochloride monohydrate; CAS Reg. No. 6108-05-0.

Description. A white, crystalline powder; odourless.

Solubility. Soluble in 0.7 part of water and in 1.5 parts of ethanol (~750 g/l) TS; soluble in chloroform R; practically insoluble in ether R.

Category. Local anaesthetic.

Storage. Lidocaine hydrochloride should be kept in a tightly closed container, protected from light.

Additional information. Lidocaine hydrochloride causes local numbness after being placed on the tongue. Even in the absence of light, Lidocaine hydrochloride is gradually degraded on exposure to a humid atmosphere, the decomposition being faster at higher temperatures.

REQUIREMENTS

General requirement. Lidocaine hydrochloride contains not less than 99.0% and not more than 101.0% of $C_{14}H_{22}N_2O,HCl$, calculated with reference to the anhydrous substance.

Identity tests

• Either tests A and C or tests B, C, and D may be applied.

A.   Carry out the examination as described under "Spectrophotometry in the infrared region" (vol. 1, p. 40).   The infrared absorption spectrum is concordant with the *reference spectrum* of lidocaine hydrochloride.

B.   Dissolve 0.15 g in 10 ml of water, make the solution alkaline with sodium hydroxide (~80 g/l) TS, filter, and wash the precipitate with water.   Dissolve the precipitate in 1 ml of ethanol (~750 g/l) TS, add 0.5 ml of cobaltous chloride TS, and shake for 2 minutes; a bluish green precipitate is produced.

C.   A 0.05 g/ml solution yields reaction B, described under "General identification tests" as characteristic of chlorides (vol. 1, p. 113).

D.   Dissolve 0.1 g in 10 ml of water and add 10 ml of trinitrophenol (7 g/l) TS. Filter, wash the precipitate with water and dry at 105 °C.   Melting temperature, about 230 °C (picrate).

Melting range.   74–79 °C.

Heavy metals.   Use 1.0 g for the preparation of the test solution as described under "Limit test for heavy metals", Procedure 1 (vol. 1, p. 118); determine the heavy metals content according to Method A (vol. 1, p. 119); not more than 10 μg/g.

Clarity and colour of solution.   A solution of 1.0 g in 10 ml of water is clear and colourless.

Sulfated ash.   Not more than 1.0 mg/g.

Water.   Determine as described under "Determination of water by the Karl Fischer method", Method A (vol. 1, p. 135), using about 0.2 g of the substance; the water content is not less than 50 mg/g and not more than 75 mg/g.

pH value.   pH of a 0.05 g/ml solution, 4.0–5.5.

Primary aromatic amines.   Dissolve 0.10 g in 4 ml of hydrochloric acid (~70 g/l) TS using a 100-ml volumetric flask.   Cool the solution in an ice-bath.   In a test-tube, dissolve 50 mg of sodium nitrite R in 10 ml of water and cool the solution.   To the flask in the ice-bath add half of the volume of the cooled sodium nitrite solution.   Allow to stand for 10 minutes, lift the flask from the ice-bath, and add 1 g of urea R.   Shake the flask frequently and when the evolution of gas has ceased (about 15 minutes), add 2.5 ml of sodium hydroxide (~80 g/l) TS in which 10 mg of thymol R has previously been dissolved. Add 5 ml of sodium hydroxide (~80 g/l) TS, allow to stand for 10 minutes, and dilute to volume. Prepare a blank as described above, but without the substance being examined. The test solution is not more intensely coloured than the blank solution when compared as described under "Colour of liquids" (vol. 1, p. 50).

Assay. Dissolve about 0.55 g, accurately weighed, in 30 ml of glacial acetic acid R1, add 10 ml of mercuric acetate/acetic acid TS, and titrate with perchloric acid (0.1 mol/l) VS, as described under "Non-aqueous titration", Method A (vol. 1, p. 131). Each ml of perchloric acid (0.1 mol/l) VS is equivalent to 27. 08 mg of $C_{14}H_{22}N_2O,HCl$.

LIDOCAINUM

Lidocaine

Molecular formula. $C_{14}H_{22}N_2O$

Relative molecular mass. 234.3

Graphic formula.

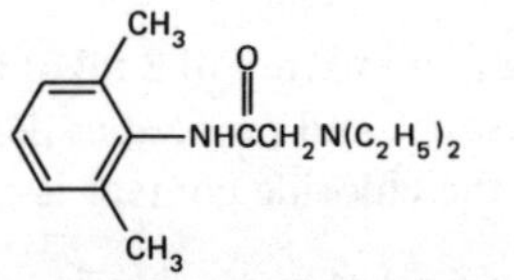

Chemical name. 2-(Diethylamino)-2′,6′-acetoxylidide; 2-(diethylamino)-N-(2,6-dimethylphenyl)acetamide; CAS Reg. No. 137-58-6.

Description. A white or slightly yellow, crystalline powder; odour, characteristic.

Solubility. Practically insoluble in water; very soluble in ethanol (~750 g/l) TS and chloroform R; freely soluble in benzene R and ether R.

Category. Local anaesthetic.

Storage. Lidocaine should be kept in a tightly closed container, protected from light.

Additional information. Lidocaine causes local numbness after being placed on the tongue.

REQUIREMENTS

General requirement.   Lidocaine contains not less than 99.0% and not more than 101.0% of $C_{14}H_{22}N_2O$, calculated with reference to the dried substance.

Identity tests

• Either test A alone or tests B and C may be applied.

A.   Carry out the examination as described under "Spectrophotometry in the infrared region" (vol. 1, p. 40).   The infrared absorption spectrum is concordant with the spectrum obtained from lidocaine RS or with the *reference spectrum* of lidocaine.

B.   Dissolve 0.1 g in 1 ml of ethanol (~750 g/l) TS, add 0.5 ml of cobaltous chloride TS, and shake for 2 minutes; a bluish green precipitate is produced.

C.   Dissolve 0.1 g in 15 ml of ethanol (~750 g/l) TS and add 10 ml of trinitrophenol (7 g/l) TS.   Filter, wash the precipitate with water, and dry at 105 °C.   Melting temperature, about 230 °C (picrate).

Melting range.   66–69 °C.

Heavy metals.   For the preparation of the test solution use 1.0 g dissolved in a mixture of 4 ml of hydrochloric acid (~70 g/l) TS and 21 ml of water, and proceed as described under "Limit test for heavy metals", Procedure 1 (vol. 1, p. 118); determine the heavy metals content according to Method A (vol. 1, p. 119); not more than 20 μg/g.

Chlorides.   Dissolve 0.50 g in a mixture of 2 ml of nitric acid (~130 g/l) TS and 20 ml of water, filter if necessary, and proceed as described under "Limit test for chlorides" (vol. 1, p. 116); the chloride content is not more than 0.5 mg/g.

Sulfates.   Dissolve 0.50 g in 5 ml of hydrochloric acid (~70 g/l) TS, and proceed as described under "Limit test for sulfates" (vol. 1, p. 116); the sulfate content is not more than 1 mg/g.

Sulfated ash.   Not more than 1.0 mg/g.

Loss on drying.   Dry to constant weight over phosphorus pentoxide R at ambient temperature; it loses not more than 5.0 mg/g.

Primary aromatic amines.   Dissolve 0.10 g in 4 ml of hydrochloric acid (~70 g/l) TS using a 100-ml volumetric flask.   Cool the solution in an ice-bath.   In a test-tube, dissolve 50 mg of sodium nitrite R in 10 ml of water and cool the solution.   To the flask in the ice-bath, add half of the volume of the cooled sodium nitrite solution.   Allow to stand for 10 minutes, lift the flask from the ice-bath, and add 1 g of urea R.   Shake the flask frequently and when the evolution of gas has ceased (about 15 minutes), add 2.5 ml of sodium hydroxide (~80 g/l) TS in which

10 mg of thymol R have previously been dissolved. Add 5 ml of sodium hydroxide (~80 g/l) TS, allow to stand for 10 minutes and dilute to volume. Prepare a blank as described above, but without the substance being examined. The test solution is not more intensely coloured than the blank solution when compared as described under "Colour of liquids" (vol. 1, p. 50).

Assay. Dissolve about 0.45 g, accurately weighed, in 30 ml of glacial acetic acid R1, and titrate with perchloric acid (0.1 mol/l) VS, as described under "Non-aqueous titration", Method A (vol. 1, p. 131). Each ml of perchloric acid (0.1 mol/l) VS is equivalent to 23.43 mg of $C_{14}H_{22}N_2O$.

LINDANUM
Lindane

Molecular formula. $C_6H_6Cl_6$

Relative molecular mass. 290.8

Graphic formula.

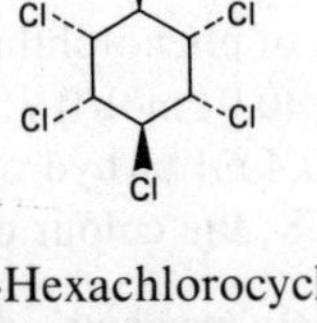

Chemical name. γ-1,2,3,4,5,6-Hexachlorocyclohexane; (1α,2α,3β,4α,5α,6β)-1,2,3,4,5,6-hexachlorocyclohexane; CAS Reg. No. 58-89-9.

Other names. Gamma benzene hexachloride; gammahexachlorcyclohexane.

Description. A white, crystalline powder; odour, slight.

Solubility. Practically insoluble in water; soluble in dehydrated ethanol R and ether R; freely soluble in chloroform R.

Category. Pediculicide; scabicide.

Storage. Lindane should be kept in a well-closed container.

REQUIREMENTS

General requirement. Lindane contains not less than 99.0% and not more than 100.5% of $C_6H_6Cl_6$, calculated with reference to the anhydrous substance.

Identity tests

A. Carry out the examination as described under "Spectrophotometry in the infrared region" (vol. 1, p. 40). The infrared absorption spectrum is concordant with the spectrum obtained from lindane RS or with the *reference spectrum* of lindane.

B. To 1 ml of a 5.0 mg/ml solution add 3 ml of ethanol (~750 g/l) TS and 1 ml of potassium hydroxide/ethanol TS1 and allow to stand for 10 minutes; the mixture yields reaction B, described under "General identification tests" as characteristic of chlorides (vol. 1, p. 113).

Congealing temperature. Not less than 112.0 °C.

Free chlorides. For the preparation of the test solution shake 1.2 g with 30 ml of water for 1 minute, and filter. To the filtrate add 10 ml of nitric acid (~130 g/l) TS and proceed as described under "Limit test for chlorides" (vol. 1, p. 116); the chloride content is not more than 0.2 mg/g.

Sulfated ash. Not more than 1.0 mg/g.

Water. Determine as described under "Determination of water by the Karl Fischer method", Method A (vol. 1, p. 135), using about 1 g of the substance; the water content is not more than 5.0 mg/g.

Acidity or alkalinity. Boil 1.5 g with 30 ml of water for 1 minute and filter. To 10 ml of the filtrate add 2 drops of phenolphthalein/ethanol TS and titrate with carbonate-free sodium hydroxide (0.01 mol/l) VS; not more than 0.2 ml is required to obtain a pink colour. Add 0.4 ml of hydrochloric acid (0.01 mol/l) VS and 5 drops of methyl red/ethanol TS; the colour changes to orange.

Assay. To about 0.4 g, accurately weighed, add 25 ml of ethanol (~750 g/l) TS and warm on a water-bath until dissolved. Cool, add 10 ml of potassium hydroxide/ethanol (1 mol/l) VS, swirl gently, and allow to stand for 10 minutes. Dilute to 150 ml with water, neutralize with nitric acid (~130 g/l) TS, add 10 ml in excess of the acid, followed by 50 ml of silver nitrate (0.1 mol/l) VS. Filter, wash the residue with water, and titrate the combined filtrate and washings with ammonium thiocyanate (0.1 mol/l) VS, using ferric ammonium sulfate (45 g/l) TS as indicator. Repeat the operation without the substance being examined and make any necessary corrections. Each ml of silver nitrate (0.1 mol/l) VS is equivalent to 9.693 mg of $C_6H_6Cl_6$.

———————

LITHII CARBONAS

Lithium carbonate

Molecular formula. Li_2CO_3

Relative molecular mass. 73.89

Chemical name. Dilithium carbonate; CAS Reg. No. 554-13-2.

Description. A white, crystalline powder; odourless.

Solubility. Soluble in 100 parts of water; less soluble in boiling water; very slightly soluble in ethanol ($\sim$750 g/l) TS.

Category. Antidepressant.

Storage. Lithium carbonate should be kept in a well-closed container.

Additional information. Lithium carbonate has a slightly alkaline taste.

REQUIREMENTS

General requirement. Lithium carbonate contains not less than 99.5% and not more than 100.5% of Li_2CO_3, calculated with reference to the dried substance.

Identity tests

A. Moisten a few crystals with hydrochloric acid ($\sim$420 g/l) TS and introduce them on a platinum wire into the flame of a Bunsen burner; a carmine-red colour is produced in the flame.

B. Dissolve 0.2 g in 5 ml of hydrochloric acid ($\sim$420 g/l) TS, boil, add 2 ml of sodium hydroxide ($\sim$80 g/l) TS, 5 ml of disodium hydrogen phosphate (40 g/l) TS and boil; a white precipitate is produced.

C. To a small amount add hydrochloric acid ($\sim$70 g/l) TS; it effervesces and the gas is colourless. Add a few drops of calcium hydroxide TS; immediately a white precipitate is formed.

Heavy metals. For the preparation of the test solution use 1.0 g dissolved in 10 ml of acetic acid ($\sim$60 g/l) TS, adjust the pH to 3–4, dilute to 40 ml with water and mix. Determine the heavy metals content as described under "Limit test for heavy metals", according to Method A (vol. 1, p. 119); not more than 20 μg/g.

Arsenic. Use a solution of 5.0 g dissolved in a mixture of 15 ml of brominated hydrochloric acid AsTS and 45 ml of water and remove the excess bromine with a few drops of stannous chloride AsTS; proceed with the solution as described under "Limit test for arsenic" (vol. 1, p. 122); the arsenic content is not more than 2 μg/g.

Calcium and magnesium. Dissolve 1.0 g in 30 ml of hydrochloric acid (1 mol/l) VS and neutralize with ammonia ($\sim$100 g/l) TS, filter if necessary, and divide into 2 equal portions. To one portion add 1 ml of ammonium oxalate (25 g/l) TS; no turbidity or precipitate is produced when the mixture is allowed to stand for 5 minutes (limit of calcium). To the second portion add 1 ml of disodium hydrogen phosphate (40 g/l) TS; no turbidity or precipitate is produced when the mixture is allowed to stand for 5 minutes (limit of magnesium).

Chlorides. Dissolve 0.35 g in a mixture of 3 ml of nitric acid ($\sim$130 g/l) TS and 30 ml of water, and proceed as described under "Limit test for chlorides" (vol. 1, p. 116); the chloride content is not more than 0.7 mg/g.

Sodium. Determine by atomic absorption spectrophotometry (vol. 1, p. 45) at a wavelength of 589 nm; use a standard solution prepared by dissolving sodium chloride R, previously dried to constant weight, in 1000 ml of water to give a solution containing 508.4 mg of NaCl (0.2 mg of Na per ml); the sodium content is not more than 2.0 mg/g.

Sulfates. Dissolve 0.5 g in 20 ml of water, add 3 ml of hydrochloric acid ($\sim$250 g/l) TS, and proceed as described under "Limit test for sulfates" (vol. 1, p. 116); the sulfate content is not more than 1 mg/g.

Loss on drying. Dry to constant weight at 105 °C; it loses not more than 5.0 mg/g.

Assay. Dissolve about 0.75 g, accurately weighed, in 100 ml of water, add 50 ml of hydrochloric acid (1 mol/l) VS, boil to remove carbon dioxide, cool, and titrate the excess acid with sodium hydroxide (1 mol/l) VS, using methyl orange/ethanol TS as indicator. Each ml of hydrochloric acid (1 mol/l) VS is equivalent to 36.95 mg of Li_2CO_3.

MANNITOLUM

Mannitol

Molecular formula. $C_6H_{14}O_6$

Relative molecular mass. 182.2

Graphic formula.

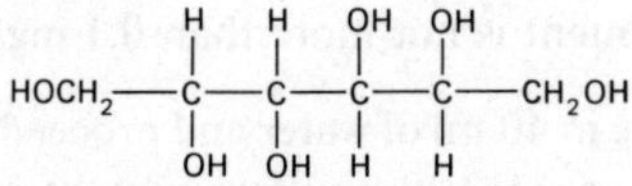

$$HOCH_2 - \overset{\overset{\displaystyle H}{|}}{\underset{\underset{\displaystyle OH}{|}}{C}} - \overset{\overset{\displaystyle H}{|}}{\underset{\underset{\displaystyle OH}{|}}{C}} - \overset{\overset{\displaystyle OH}{|}}{\underset{\underset{\displaystyle H}{|}}{C}} - \overset{\overset{\displaystyle OH}{|}}{\underset{\underset{\displaystyle H}{|}}{C}} - CH_2OH$$

Chemical name. D-Mannitol; CAS Reg. No. 69-65-8.

Description. A white, crystalline powder; odourless.

Solubility. Freely soluble in water; very slightly soluble in ethanol ($\sim$750 g/l) TS; practically insoluble in ether R.

Category. Diuretic.

Storage. Mannitol should be kept in a well-closed container.

Additional information. Mannitol has a sweet taste.

REQUIREMENTS

General requirement. Mannitol contains not less than 98.0% and not more than 102.0% of $C_6H_{14}O_6$, calculated with reference to the dried substance.

Identity tests

A. Transfer about 1.0 g, accurately weighed, to a 100-ml volumetric flask, and add 80 ml of ammonium molybdate (45 g/l) TS, previously filtered if necessary. Add sulfuric acid ($\sim$50 g/l) TS to volume and mix. Measure the optical rotation and calculate the specific rotation as described under "Determination of specific optical rotation" (vol. 1, pp. 29–31); $[\alpha]_D^{20\,°C} = +137$ to $+145°$.

B. To 0.5 g add 2.5 ml of acetyl chloride R, then add cautiously 0.5 ml of pyridine R. Warm the mixture until it becomes turbid, cool in ice, and collect the precipitate on a sintered-glass filter. Recrystallize the precipitate several times from ether R and dry at 60 °C for 1 hour; melting temperature, about 123 °C (mannitol hexaacetate).

Melting range. 165–169 °C.

Heavy metals. Use 1.0 g for the preparation of the test solution as described under "Limit test for heavy metals", Procedure 1 (vol. 1, p. 118); determine the heavy metals content according to method A (vol. 1, p. 119); not more than 10 μg/g.

Arsenic. Use a solution of 5.0 g in 35 ml of water and proceed as described under "Limit test for arsenic" (vol. 1, p. 122); the arsenic content is not more than 2 μg/g.

Chlorides. Dissolve 2.5 g in a mixture of 2 ml of nitric acid ($\sim$130 g/l) TS and 30 ml of water and proceed as described under "Limit test for chlorides" (vol. 1, p. 116); the chloride content is not more than 0.1 mg/g.

Sulfates. Dissolve 5.0 g in 40 ml of water and proceed as described under "Limit test for sulfates" (vol. 1, p. 116); the sulfate content is not more than 0.1 mg/g.

Clarity and colour of solution. A solution of 1.0 g in 10 ml of carbon-dioxide-free water R is clear and colourless.

Sulfated ash. Not more than 1.0 mg/g.

Loss on drying. Dry to constant weight at 105 °C; it loses not more than 5.0 mg/g.

Acidity. Dissolve 5.0 g in 50 ml of carbon-dioxide-free water R and titrate with carbonate-free sodium hydroxide (0.02 mol/l) VS, phenolphthalein/ethanol TS being used as indicator; not more than 0.3 ml is required to obtain the midpoint of the indicator (pink).

Sorbitol. Carry out the test as described under "Thin-layer chromatography" (vol. 1, p. 83), using silica gel R1 as the coating substance and a mixture of 85 volumes of 2-propanol R and 15 volumes of a 2 g/l solution of boric acid R as the mobile phase. Prepare a solution of 1.0 g of finely powdered test substance in 10 ml of ethanol ($\sim$750 g/l) TS, shake for 30 minutes and filter (solution A). Apply separately to the plate 1 μl of test solution A and 2 μl of a 1.0 mg/ml solution of sorbitol R in water (B).

Develop the plate at room temperature, the process taking up to 5 hours. After removing the plate from the chromatographic chamber, allow it to dry at 110 °C for 5 minutes, cool, and spray with a 1 g/l solution of potassium permanganate R in sulfuric acid (0.5 mol/l) VS. Heat the plate at 110 °C until brown spots appear and examine the chromatogram in daylight. The spot obtained with solution B is more intense than any spot, corresponding in position and appearance, obtained with solution A.

Assay. Dissolve about 0.4 g, accurately weighed, in sufficient water to produce 100 ml. Transfer 10 ml to a stoppered flask, add 20.0 ml of a 21.4 g/l solution of sodium metaperiodate R and 2 ml of sulfuric acid ($\sim$100 g/l) TS, and heat on a water-bath for 15 minutes. Cool, add 3 g of sodium hydrogen carbonate R,

25 ml of sodium arsenite (0.1 mol/l) VS, and 5 ml of a 200 g/l solution of potassium iodide R; allow to stand for 15 minutes, and titrate with iodine (0.1 mol/l) VS until the first trace of yellow colour appears. Repeat the procedure without the test substance and determine the difference in volume of iodine (0.1 mol/l) VS required for the titration. Each ml of iodine (0.1 mol/l) VS is equivalent to 1.822 mg of $C_6H_{14}O_6$.

METHYLDOPUM

Methyldopa

Molecular formula. $C_{10}H_{13}NO_4, 1\frac{1}{2}H_2O$

Relative molecular mass. 238.2

Graphic formula.

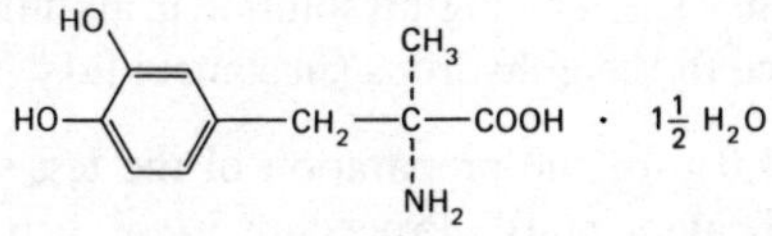

Chemical name. L-3-(3,4-Dihydroxyphenyl)-2-methylalanine sesquihydrate; 3-hydroxy-α-methyl-L-tyrosine sesquihydrate; CAS Reg. No. 41372-08-1.

Description. White to yellowish white, fine powder or lumps; odourless.

Solubility. Slightly soluble in water and ethanol (~750 g/l) TS; practically insoluble in ether R and chloroform R.

Category. Antihypertensive.

Storage. Methyldopa should be kept in a well-closed container, protected from light.

REQUIREMENTS

General requirement. Methyldopa contains not less than 98.0% and not more than 101.0% of $C_{10}H_{13}NO_4$, calculated with reference to the anhydrous substance.

Identity tests

• Either test A alone or tests B and C may be applied.

A.   Carry out the examination as described under "Spectrophotometry in the infrared region" (vol. 1, p. 40.).   The infrared absorption spectrum is concordant with the spectrum obtained from methyldopa RS or with the *reference spectrum* of methyldopa.

B.   Carry out the test as described under "Thin-layer chromatography" (vol. 1, p. 83), using cellulose R2 as the coating substance and a mixture of 50 volumes of 1-butanol R, 25 volumes of glacial acetic acid R and 25 volumes of water as the mobile phase.   Apply separately to the plate $5 \mu l$ of each of 2 solutions in hydrochloric acid (1 mol/l) VS containing (A) 10 mg of the test substance per ml and (B) 10 mg of methyldopa RS per ml.   After removing the plate from the chromatographic chamber, allow it to dry in a current of warm air, spray with a freshly prepared solution composed of 2 volumes of ferric chloride (25 g/l) TS and 1 volume of potassium ferricyanide (50 g/l) TS, and examine the chromatogram in daylight.   The principal spot obtained with solution A corresponds in position, appearance, and intensity with that obtained with solution B.

C.   To 5 mg add 1 ml of water, 1 ml of pyridine R, and 5 mg of 4-nitrobenzoyl chloride R and heat to boiling.   While shaking, add 0.1 ml of sodium carbonate (200 g/l) TS; an orange or amber colour is produced.

Specific optical rotation.   Use a 44 mg/ml solution in aluminium chloride TS and calculate with reference to the anhydrous substance; $[\alpha]_D^{20\,°C} = -25$ to $-28°$.

Heavy metals.   Use 1.0 g for the preparation of the test solution as described under "Limit test for heavy metals", Procedure 3 (vol. 1, p. 118); determine the heavy metals content according to Method A (vol. 1, p. 119); not more than $10 \mu g/g$.

Sulfated ash.   Not more than 1.0 mg/g.

Water.   Determine as described under "Determination of water by the Karl Fischer method", Method A (vol. 1, p. 135), using about 0.2 g of the substance; the water content is not less than 100 mg/g and not more than 130 mg/g.

Acidity.   Dissolve 1.0 g in 100 ml of carbon-dioxide-free water R with the aid of heat and titrate with sodium hydroxide (0.1 mol/l) VS, methyl red/ethanol TS being used as indicator; not more than 0.5 ml is required to obtain the midpoint of the indicator (orange).

3-*O*-Methyl derivative.   Carry out the test as described under "Thin-layer chromatography" (vol. 1, p. 83), using cellulose R2 as the coating substance and a mixture of 65 volumes of 1-butanol R, 15 volumes of glacial acetic acid R, and 25 volumes of water as the mobile phase.   Apply separately to the plate (A) 10 μl of a 10 mg/ml solution of the test substance dissolved in a mixture of 4 volumes of hydrochloric acid (~250 g/l) TS and 96 volumes of methanol R, (B) 10 μl of a 50 μg/ml solution of (–)-3-(4-hydroxy-3-methoxyphenyl)-2-methylalanine RS, and (C) 20 μl of a mixture of equal volumes of solutions A and B. After removing the plate from the chromatographic chamber, allow it to dry in a current of warm air, and spray with a mixture of 5 volumes of a 0.05 g/ml solution of sodium nitrite R and 45 volumes of a 3 mg/ml solution of 4-nitroaniline R dissolved in a mixture of 80 volumes of hydrochloric acid (~420 g/l) TS and 20 volumes of water. Dry in a current of warm air, spray with sodium carbonate (75 g/l) TS, and examine the chromatogram in daylight. The spot obtained with solution B is more intense than any spot, corresponding in position and appearance, obtained with solution A. The test is valid only if the chromatogram obtained with solution C shows two distinctly separated spots.

Assay. Dissolve about 0.20 g, accurately weighed, in 20 ml of glacial acetic acid R1, add 20 ml of dioxan R, and titrate with perchloric acid (0.1 mol/l) VS as described under "Non-aqueous titration", Method A (vol. 1, p. 131). Each ml of perchloric acid (0.1 mol/l) VS is equivalent to 21.12 mg of $C_{10}H_{13}NO_4$.

METHYLTESTOSTERONUM

Methyltestosterone

Molecular formula. $C_{20}H_{30}O_2$

Relative molecular mass. 302.5

Graphic formula.

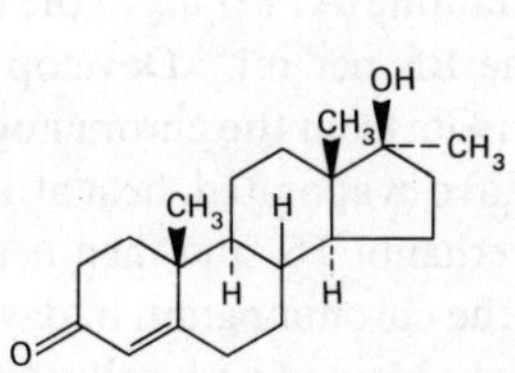

Chemical name. 17β-Hydroxy-17-methylandrost-4-en-3-one; CAS Reg. No. 58-18-4.

Description. Colourless or almost colourless crystals or a white or slightly yellowish white, crystalline powder; odourless.

Solubility.   Practically insoluble in water; freely soluble in ethanol (~750 g/l) TS and chloroform R; sparingly soluble in ether R.

Category.   Androgen.

Storage.   Methyltestosterone should be kept in a well-closed container, protected from light.

REQUIREMENTS

General requirement.   Methyltestosterone contains not less than 97.0% and not more than 102.0% of $C_{20}H_{30}O_2$, calculated with reference to the dried substance.

Identity tests

● Either test A alone or tests B and C may be applied.

A.   Carry out the examination as described under "Spectrophotometry in the infrared region" (vol. 1, p. 40).   The infrared absorption spectrum is concordant with the spectrum obtained from methyltestosterone RS or with the *reference spectrum* of methyltestosterone.

B.   Carry out the test as described under "Thin-layer chromatography" (vol. 1, p. 83), using kieselguhr R1 as the coating substance and a mixture of 10 volumes of propylene glycol R and 90 volumes of acetone R to impregnate the plate, dipping it about 5 mm beneath the surface of the liquid.   After the solvent has reached a height of at least 16 cm, remove the plate from the chromatographic chamber and allow it to stand at room temperature until the solvent has completely evaporated. Use the impregnated plate within 2 hours, carrying out the chromatography in the same direction as the impregnation.   As the mobile phase, use a mixture of 80 volumes of cyclohexane R and 20 volumes of toluene R.   Apply separately to the plate 2 μl of each of 2 solutions in a mixture of 9 volumes of chloroform R and 1 volume of methanol R containing (A) 1.0 mg of the test substance per ml and (B) 1.0 mg of methyltestosterone RS per ml.   Develop the plate for a distance of 15 cm.   After removing the plate from the chromatographic chamber, allow it to dry in air until the solvents have evaporated, heat at 120 °C for 15 minutes, spray with 4-toluenesulfonic acid/ethanol TS, and then heat at 120 °C for 10 minutes. Allow to cool, and examine the chromatogram in daylight and in ultraviolet light (365 nm).   The principal spot obtained with solution A corresponds in position, appearance, and intensity with that obtained with solution B.

C.   Melting temperature, about 165 °C.

Specific optical rotation.   Use a 10 mg/ml solution in ethanol (~750 g/l) TS; $[\alpha]_D^{20\,°C} = +78$ to $+85°$.

Solution in ethanol.   A solution of 0.50 g in 10 ml of ethanol (~750 g/l) TS is clear and not more intensely coloured than standard colour solution Yw2 when compared as described under "Colour of liquids" (vol. 1, p. 50).

Loss on drying.   Dry to constant weight at 105 °C; it loses not more than 10 mg/g.

Related substances.   Carry out the test as described under "Thin-layer chromatography" (vol. 1, p. 83), using silica gel R2 as the coating substance and a mixture of 90 volumes of chloroform R and 10 volumes of acetone R as the mobile phase. Apply separately to the plate 5 μl of each of 2 solutions in ethanol (~750 g/l) TS containing (A) 10 mg of the test substance per ml and (B) 0.10 mg of the test substance per ml.   After removing the plate from the chromatographic chamber, allow it to dry in air until the solvents have evaporated, and examine the chromatogram in ultraviolet light (254 nm).   Any spot obtained with solution A, other than the principal spot, is not more intense than that obtained with solution B.

Assay.   Dissolve about 20 mg, accurately weighed, in sufficient ethanol (~750 g/l) TS to produce 100 ml; dilute 5.0 ml of this solution to 100 ml with the same solvent.   Measure the absorbance of a 1-cm layer of the diluted solution at the maximum at about 242 nm.   Calculate the amount of $C_{20}H_{30}O_2$ in the substance being tested by comparison with methyltestosterone RS, similarly and concurrently examined.   In an adequately calibrated spectrophotometer the absorbance of the reference solution should be 0.54 ± 0.03.

METRONIDAZOLUM

Metronidazole

Molecular formula. $C_6H_9N_3O_3$

Relative molecular mass.   171.2

Graphic formula.

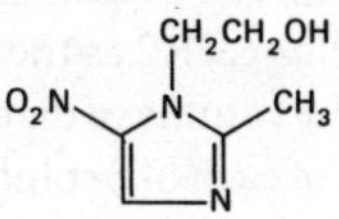

Chemical name.   2-Methyl-5-nitroimidazole-1-ethanol; 2-methyl-5-nitro-1H-imidazole-1-ethanol; CAS Reg. No. 443-48-1.

Description. A white or pale yellow, crystalline powder; odourless or almost odourless.

Solubility. Sparingly soluble in water; slightly soluble in ethanol (~750 g/l) TS, chloroform R, and ether R.

Category. Antitrichomonal; antiamoebic.

Storage. Metronidazole should be kept in a well-closed container, protected from light.

Additional information. Metronidazole is stable in air, but darkens on exposure to light.

REQUIREMENTS

General requirement. Metronidazole contains not less than 99.0% and not more than 101.0% of $C_6H_9N_3O_3$, calculated with reference to the dried substance.

Identity tests

A. Carry out the examination as described under "Spectrophotometry in the infrared region" (vol. 1, p. 40). The infrared absorption spectrum is concordant with the spectrum obtained from metronidazole RS or with the *reference spectrum* of metronidazole.

B. To 10 mg add 10 mg of zinc R powder, 1 ml of water, and 0.25 ml of hydrochloric acid (~250 g/l) TS and heat in a water-bath for 5 minutes; cool in ice, add 0.5 ml of sodium nitrite (100 g/l) TS, and remove the excess nitrite with sufficient sulfamic acid (50 g/l) TS. Add 0.5 ml of the resulting solution to a mixture of 0.5 ml of 2-naphthol TS1 and 2 ml of sodium hydroxide (~80 g/l) TS; an orange-red colour is produced.

Melting range. 159–163 °C.

Sulfated ash. Not more than 1.0 mg/g.

Loss on drying. Dry to constant weight at 105 °C; it loses not more than 5.0 mg/g.

Related substances. Carry out the test as described under "Thin-layer chromatography" (vol. 1, p. 83), using silica gel R2 as the coating substance and a mixture of 9 volumes of chloroform R and 1 volume of diethylamine R as the mobile phase. Apply separately to the plate 5 µl of each of 2 solutions in acetone R containing (A) 20 mg of the test substance per ml (warm slightly if necessary to dissolve the substance) and (B) 0.10 mg of the test substance per ml. After removing the plate from the chromatographic chamber, allow it to dry in air, and examine the chromatogram in ultraviolet light (254 nm). Any spot obtained with solution A, other than the principal spot, is not more intense than that obtained with solution B.

Assay. Dissolve about 0.35 g, accurately weighed, in 30 ml of glacial acetic acid R1, add 3 drops of 1-naphtholbenzein/acetic acid TS as indicator and titrate with perchloric acid (0.1 mol/l) VS, as described under "Non-aqueous titration", Method A (vol. 1, p. 131). Each ml of perchloric acid (0.1 mol/l) VS is equivalent to 17.12 mg of $C_6H_9N_3O_3$.

MORPHINI HYDROCHLORIDUM
Morphine hydrochloride

Molecular formula. $C_{17}H_{19}NO_3, HCl, 3H_2O$

Relative molcular mass. 375.9

Graphic formula.

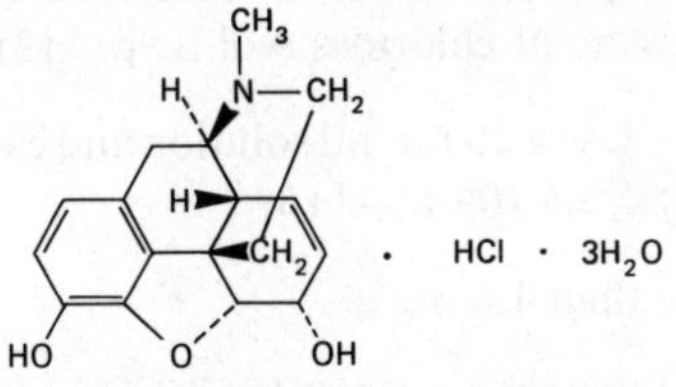

Chemical name. 7,8-Didehydro-4,5α-epoxy-17-methylmorphinan-3,6α-diol hydrochloride (1:1) (salt) trihydrate; CAS Reg. No. 6055-06-7.

Description. Colourless, needle-like crystals or a white, crystalline powder; odourless.

Solubility. Soluble in 25 parts of water; slightly soluble in ethanol (~750 g/l) TS; practically insoluble in chloroform R and ether R.

Category. Analgesic.

Storage. Morphine hydrochloride should be kept in a tightly closed container, protected from light.

Additional information. Even in the absence of light, Morphine hydrochloride is gradually degraded on exposure to a humid atmosphere, the decomposition being faster at higher temperatures.

REQUIREMENTS

General requirement. Morphine hydrochloride contains not less than 98.0% and not more than 101.0% of $C_{17}H_{19}NO_3$, HCl, calculated with reference to the dried substance.

Identity tests

A. To 5 ml of a 1 mg/ml solution add 3 drops of a freshly prepared potassium ferricyanide (10 g/l) TS and 1 drop of ferric chloride (25 g/l) TS; a bluish green colour is produced.

B. To 5 ml of a 1 mg/ml solution add 1 ml of hydrogen peroxide (~60 g/l) TS, 1 ml of ammonia (~100 g/l) TS, and 1 drop of copper(II) sulfate (80 g/l) TS; a transient red colour is produced.

C. To about 1 mg add 0.5 ml of sulfuric acid (~1760 g/l) TS containing 1 drop of formaldehyde TS; a purple colour is produced, which changes quickly to violet.

D. Dissolve a few mg in 5 ml of water, add 1 drop of hydrochloric acid (~70 g/l) TS and 1 ml of potassium iodobismuthate TS2; an orange or orange-red precipitate is produced immediately.

E. A 20 mg/ml solution yields reaction B, described under "General identification tests" as characteristic of chlorides (vol. 1, p. 113).

Specific optical rotation. Use a 20 mg/ml solution and calculate with reference to the dried substance; $[\alpha]_D^{20\,°C} = -109$ to $-115°$.

Sulfated ash. Not more than 1.0 mg/g.

Loss on drying. Dry to constant weight at 105 °C; it loses not less than 115 mg/g and not more than 150 mg/g.

Acidity. Dissolve 0.2 g in 10 ml of carbon-dioxide-free water R, and titrate with sodium hydroxide (0.02 mol/l) VS, using methyl red/ethanol TS as indicator; not more than 0.2 ml is required to obtain the midpoint of the indicator (orange).

Meconate. Dissolve 0.2 g in 5 ml of water, add 5 ml of hydrochloric acid (~70 g/l) TS and a few drops of ferric chloride (25 g/l) TS; no red colour is produced.

Related alkaloids. Transfer about 0.5 g, accurately weighed, to a separator, add 15 ml of water, 2 ml of sodium hydroxide (10 g/l) TS, and 10 ml of chloroform R. Shake, allow to separate and transfer the chloroform layer to another separator. Repeat the extraction with further quantities of chloroform R, each of 10 ml. Wash the combined chloroform solutions with 4 ml of sodium hydroxide (10 g/l) TS and then twice with water, using 5 ml each time. Separate the chloroform layer and evaporate it carefully to dryness on a water-bath. Add to the residue thus obtained 10 ml of sulfuric acid (0.01 mol/l) VS, heat until dissolved, cool, add 1 drop of methyl red/ethanol TS, and titrate the excess acid with sodium hydroxide (0.02 mol/l) VS; not less than 8.75 ml is required to obtain the midpoint of the indicator (orange).

Noscapine. Dissolve 0.05 g in 2 ml of sulfuric acid (~1760 g/l) TS and heat the solution on a water-bath; no violet colour is produced.

Assay. Dissolve about 0.3 g, accurately weighed, in 30 ml of glacial acetic acid R1, add 10 ml of mercuric acetate/acetic acid TS, and titrate with perchloric acid (0.1 mol/l) VS as described under "Non-aqueous titration", Method A (vol. 1, p. 131). Each ml of perchloric acid (0.1 mol/l) VS is equivalent to 32.18 mg of $C_{17}H_{19}NO_3, HCl$.

MORPHINI SULFAS

Morphine sulfate

Molecular formula. $(C_{17}H_{19}NO_3)_2, H_2SO_4, 5H_2O$

Relative molecular mass. 758.8

Graphic formula.

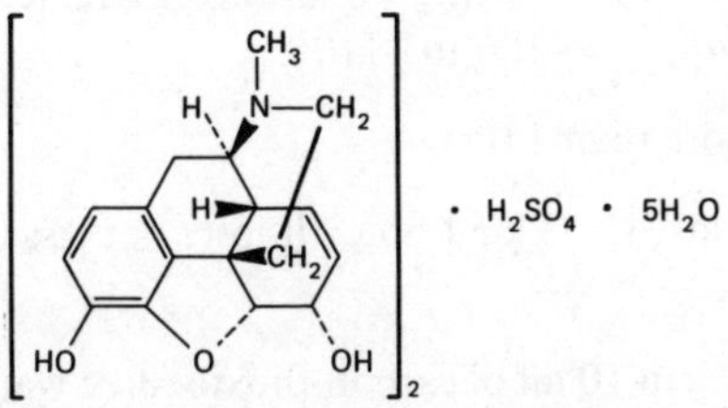

Chemical name. 7,8-Didehydro-4,5α-epoxy-17-methylmorphinan-3,6α-diol sulfate (2:1) (salt) pentahydrate; CAS Reg. No. 6211-15-0.

Description. White, feathery needles of a white, crystalline powder or cubical masses; odourless.

Solubility. Soluble in 20 parts of water; slightly soluble in ethanol (~750 g/l) TS; practically insoluble in chloroform R and ether R.

Category. Analgesic.

Storage. Morphine sulfate should be kept in a tightly closed container, protected from light.

Additional information. Morphine sulfate loses water of hydration on exposure to air and darkens in colour on prolonged exposure to light.

REQUIREMENTS

General requirement. Morphine sulfate contains not less than 98.0% and not more than 101.0% of $(C_{17}H_{19}NO_3)_2, H_2SO_4$, calculated with reference to the dried substance.

Identity tests

A. To 5 ml of a 1 mg/ml solution add 3 drops of a freshly prepared potassium ferricyanide (10 g/l) TS and 1 drop of ferric chloride (25 g/l) TS; a bluish green colour is produced.

B. To 5 ml of a 1 mg/ml solution add 1 ml of hydrogen peroxide (~60 g/l) TS, 1 ml of ammonia (~100 g/l) TS and 1 drop of copper(II) sulfate (80 g/l) TS; a transient red colour is produced.

C. To about 1 mg add 0.5 ml of sulfuric acid (~1760 g/l) TS containing 1 drop of formaldehyde TS; a purple colour is produced, which changes quickly to violet.

D. A 20 mg/ml solution yields reaction A described under "General identification tests" as characteristic of sulfates (vol. 1, p. 115).

Specific optical rotation. Use a 20 mg/ml solution and calculate with reference to the dried substance; $[\alpha]_D^{20\,°C} = -106$ to $-110°$.

Sulfated ash. Not more than 1.0 mg/g.

Loss on drying. Dry at 145 °C for 1 hour; it loses not less than 90 mg/g and not more than 120 mg/g.

Acidity. Dissolve 0.2 g in 10 ml of carbon-dioxide-free water R, and titrate with sodium hydroxide (0.02 mol/l) VS, using methyl red/ethanol TS as indicator; not more than 0.2 ml is required to obtain the midpoint of the indicator (orange).

Meconate. Dissolve 0.2 g in 5 ml of water, add 5 ml of hydrochloric acid (~70 g/l) TS and a few drops of ferric chloride (25 g/l) TS; no red colour is produced.

Related alkaloids. Transfer about 0.5 g, accurately weighed, to a separator, add 15 ml of water, 2 ml of sodium hydroxide (10 g/l) TS, and 10 ml of chloroform R. Shake, allow to separate, and transfer the chloroform layer to another separator. Repeat the extraction with further quantities of chloroform R, each of 10 ml.

Wash the combined chloroform solutions with 4 ml of sodium hydroxide (10 g/l) TS and twice with water, using 5 ml each time. Separate the chloroform layer and evaporate it carefully to dryness on a water-bath. Add to the residue thus obtained 10 ml of sulfuric acid (0.01 mol/l) VS, heat until dissolved, cool, add 1 drop of methyl red/ethanol TS, and titrate the excess acid with sodium hydroxide (0.02 mol/l) VS; not less than 8.75 ml is required to obtain the midpoint of the indicator (orange).

Noscapine. Dissolve 0.05 g in 2 ml of sulfuric acid (~1760 g/l) TS and heat the solution on a water-bath; no violet colour is produced.

Assay. Dissolve about 0.6 g, accurately weighed, in 30 ml of glacial acetic acid R1, and titrate with perchloric acid (0.1 mol/l) VS, determining the endpoint potentiometrically as described under "Non-aqueous titration", Method A (vol. 1, p. 131). Each ml of perchloric acid (0.1 mol/l) VS is equivalent to 66.88 mg of $(C_{17}H_{19}NO_3)_2, H_2SO_4$.

NATRII CHLORIDUM
Sodium chloride

Molecular formula. NaCl

Relative molecular mass. 58.44

Chemical name. Sodium chloride; CAS Reg. No. 7647-14-5.

Description. Colourless crystals or a white, crystalline powder; odourless.

Solubility. Freely soluble in water; slightly soluble in ethanol (~750 g/l) TS.

Category. Ionic equilibration agent.

Storage. Sodium chloride should be kept in a well-closed container.

Additional information. Sodium chloride has a saline taste.

REQUIREMENTS

General requirement. Sodium chloride contains not less than 99.0% and not more than 100.5% of NaCl, calculated with reference to the dried substance.

Identity tests

A. When tested for sodium as described under "General identification tests" (vol. 1, p. 115), yields the characteristic reactions. If reaction B is to be used, prepare a 20 mg/ml solution.

B. A 20 mg/ml solution yields reaction A described under "General identification tests" as characteristic of chlorides (vol. 1, p. 112).

Heavy metals. Use 1.0 g for the preparation of the test solution as described under "Limit test for heavy metals", Procedure 1 (vol. 1, p. 118); determine the heavy metals content according to Method A (vol. 1, p. 119); not more than 10 μg/g.

Arsenic. Use a solution of 2.5 g in 35 ml of water and proceed as described under "Limit test for arsenic" (vol. 1, p. 122); not more than 4 μg/g.

Barium. Dissolve 4 g in 20 ml of water, filter if necessary, divide the solution into 2 portions and place them in two separate matched tubes. To 1 portion add 2 ml of sulfuric acid (~100 g/l) TS and to the other, 2 ml of water; the solutions remain equally clear for not less than 30 minutes when viewed down the vertical axis of the tube in diffused light against a black background.

Calcium and magnesium. To 20 ml of a 10 mg/ml solution add 2 ml each of ammonia (~100 g/l) TS, ammonium oxalate (25 g/l) TS, and disodium hydrogen phosphate (40 g/l) TS; no turbidity is produced within 5 minutes.

Iodides and bromides. Digest 2 g of finely powdered test substance for 3 hours with 25 ml of warm ethanol (~750 g/l) TS, cool, and filter. Evaporate the filtrate to dryness, dissolve the residue in 5 ml of water, add 1 ml of chloroform R, and cautiously add, drop by drop, with constant agitation, 5 drops of chlorine TS, previously diluted with twice their volume of water; the chloroform does not acquire a violet, yellow or orange colour.

Iron and sodium ferrocyanides. To 0.5 g add 5 drops of sulfuric acid (~100 g/l) TS and carefully heat until dry. Dissolve the residue in 6 ml of water, add 1 ml of hydrochloric acid (~70 g/l) TS, 1 drop of hydrogen peroxide (~60 g/l) TS, and 2 ml of ammonium thiocyanate (~75 g/l) TS; this constitutes solution A. Prepare in a similar manner solution B using 0.40 ml of iron standard FeTS instead of the residue obtained from the test substance. Solution A is not more intensely coloured than solution B when compared as described under "Colour of liquids" (vol. 1, p. 50) (16 μg/g of total Fe).

Sulfates. Dissolve 1.7 g in 20 ml of water and proceed as described under "Limit test for sulfates" (vol. 1, p. 116); the sulfate content is not more than 0.3 mg/g.

Clarity and colour of solution. A solution of 1.0 g in 10 ml of carbon-dioxide-free water R is clear and colourless.

Loss on drying. Dry to constant weight at 130 °C; it loses not more than 10 mg/g.

Acidity or alkalinity. Dissolve 2 g in 20 ml of carbon-dioxide-free water R and add 2 drops of bromothymol blue/ethanol TS; not more than 0.1 ml of sodium hydroxide (0.02 mol/l) VS or 0.2 ml of hydrochloric acid (0.02 mol/l) VS is required to attain the midpoint of the indicator (green).

Assay. Dissolve about 0.25 g, accurately weighed, in 50 ml of water and titrate with silver nitrate (0.1 mol/l) VS, using potassium chromate (100 g/l) TS as indicator. Each ml of silver nitrate (0.1 mol/l) VS is equivalent to 5.844 mg of NaCl.

NATRII HYDROGENOCARBONAS

Sodium hydrogen carbonate

Molecular formula. $NaHCO_3$

Relative molecular mass. 84.01

Chemical name. Monosodium carbonate; CAS Reg, No. 144-55-8.

Other name. Sodium bicarbonate.

Description. A white, crystalline powder; odourless.

Solubility. Soluble in water; practically insoluble in ethanol (~750 g/l) TS.

Category. Systemic alkalinizing agent; antacid.

Storage. Sodium hydrogen carbonate should be kept in well-closed containers.

Additional information. Sodium hydrogen carbonate has a saline and slightly alkaline taste. It is stable in air, but slowly decomposes in moist air.

General requirement. Sodium hydrogen carbonate contains not less than 99.0% and not more than 101.0% of $NaHCO_3$, calculated with reference to the dried substance.

Identity tests

A. When tested for sodium as described under "General identification tests" (vol. 1, p. 115), yields the characteristic reactions. If reaction B is to be used, prepare a 20 mg/ml solution.

B. To a small amount add hydrochloric acid (~70 g/l) TS; it effervesces and the gas is colourless. Add a few drops of calcium hydroxide TS; immediately a white precipitate is formed.

C. To a 20 mg/ml solution add at room temperature a few drops of magnesium sulfate (50 g/l) TS; no precipitate is formed. Boil the mixture; a white precipitate is formed.

Heavy metals. Use 1.0 g for the preparation of the test solution as described under "Limit test for heavy metals", Procedure 1 (vol. 1, p. 118); determine the heavy metals content according to Method A (vol. 1, p. 119); not more than 10 μg/g.

Ammonium. Heat 1.0 g in a test-tube; the gas evolved does not turn moistened red litmus paper R blue.

Arsenic. Use a solution of 3.3 g in 35 ml of water and proceed as described under "Limit test for arsenic" (vol. 1, p. 122); the arsenic content is not more than 3 μg/g.

Calcium. Boil a 20 mg/ml solution for 5 minutes; the solution is clear or at most very slightly opalescent.

Carbonates. pH of a 50 mg/ml solution in carbon-dioxide-free water R, not more than 8.6.

Chlorides. Dissolve 1.7 g in a mixture of 2 ml of nitric acid (~130 g/l) TS and 40 ml of water, and proceed as described under "Limit test for chlorides" (vol. 1, p. 116); the chloride content is not more than 0.15 mg/g.

Sulfates. Dissolve 2.5 g in 40 ml of water, add 1 ml of hydrochloric acid (~250 g/l) TS, and proceed as described under "Limit test for sulfates" (vol. 1, p. 116); the sulfate content is not more than 0.2 mg/g.

Clarity and colour of solution. A solution of 0.50 g in 10 ml of carbon-dioxide-free water R is clear and colourless.

Loss on drying. Dry to constant weight over silica gel, desiccant, R at ambient temperature; it loses not more than 2.5 mg/g.

Assay. Dissolve about 0.5 g, accurately weighed, in 50 ml of water and titrate with hydrochloric acid (0.2 mol/l) VS, using 3 drops of methyl orange/ethanol TS as indicator. Each ml of hydrochloric acid (0.2 mol/l) VS is equivalent to 16.80 mg of $NaHCO_3$.

NATRII SALICYLAS
Sodium salicylate

Molecular formula. $C_7H_5NaO_3$

Relative molecular mass. 160.1

Graphic formula.

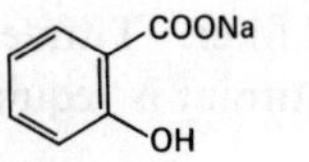

Chemical name. Sodium 2-hydroxybenzoate; CAS Reg. No. 54-21-7.

Description. Small, colourless crystals or shiny flakes, or a white, crystalline powder; odourless or almost odourless.

Solubility. Freely soluble in water and ethanol (~750 g/l) TS; practically insoluble in ether R and chloroform R.

Category. Analgesic; antiphlogistic.

Storage. Sodium salicylate should be kept in a well-closed container, protected from light.

Additional information. Sodium salicylate is discoloured on exposure to light.

REQUIREMENTS

General requirement. Sodium salicylate contains not less than 99.0% and not more than 101.0% of $C_7H_5NaO_3$, calculated with reference to the dried substance.

Identity tests

A. When tested for sodium as described under "General identification tests" (vol. 1, p. 115), yields the characteristic reactions. If reaction B is to be used, prepare a 20 mg/ml solution.

B. A 0.05 g/ml solution yields the reaction described under "General identification tests" as characteristic of salicylates (vol. 1, p. 114).

Heavy metals. For the preparation of the test solution use 2.0 g dissolved in 45 ml of water, add 5 ml of hydrochloric acid (~70 g/l) TS, and filter. Dilute 25 ml of the filtrate to 40 ml with water and mix; determine the heavy metals content as described under "Limit test for heavy metals", according to Method A (vol. 1, p. 119); not more than 20 μg/g.

Chlorides. Dissolve 1.25 g in a mixture of 5 ml of water and 5 ml of ethanol (~710 g/l) TS. Add 1 ml of nitric acid (~1000 g/l) TS, filter, and proceed with the filtrate as described under "Limit test for chlorides" (vol. 1, p. 116); the chloride content is not more than 0.2 mg/g.

Sulfates. Dissolve 0.85 g in 20 ml of water, add 1 ml of hydrochloric acid (~250 g/l) TS, and filter. Proceed with the filtrate as described under "Limit test for sulfates" (vol. 1, p. 116); the sulfate content is not more than 0.6 mg/g.

Sulfites and thiosulfates. Dissolve 1.0 g in 20 ml of water, add 1 ml of hydrochloric acid (~250 g/l) TS, and filter. Titrate the filtrate with iodine (0.1 mol/l) VS; not more than 0.15 ml of titrant is required to produce a yellow colour.

Clarity and colour of solution. A freshly prepared solution of 1.0 g in 10 ml of water is clear and not more intensely coloured than standard colour solution Rd1 when compared as described under "Colour of liquids" (vol. 1, p. 50).

Loss on drying. Dry to constant weight at 105 °C; it loses not more than 5.0 mg/g.

Acidity. Dissolve 2.0 g in 50 ml of carbon-dioxide-free water R and add 10 drops of phenol red/ethanol TS; the solution is yellow. Titrate with sodium hydroxide (0.1 mol/l) VS; not more than 0.2 ml is required to produce a red colour.

Assay. Dissolve about 0.3 g, accurately weighed, in 30 ml of glacial acetic acid R1, and titrate with perchloric acid (0.1 mol/l) VS as described under "Non-aqueous titration", Method A (vol. 1, p. 131). Each ml of perchloric acid (0.1 mol/l) VS is equivalent to 16.01 mg of $C_7H_5NaO_3$.

NEOSTIGMINI BROMIDUM
Neostigmine bromide

Molecular formula. $C_{12}H_{19}BrN_2O_2$

Relative molecular mass. 303.2

Graphic formula.

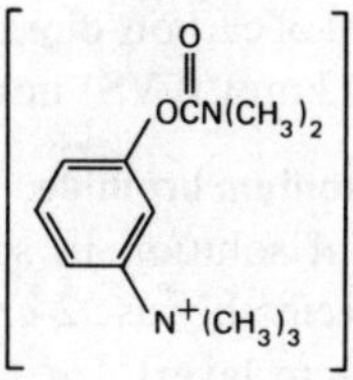

Chemical name. (*m*-Hydroxyphenyl)trimethylammonium bromide dimethyl-carbamate; 3-[[(dimethylamino)carbonyl]oxy]-*N,N,N*-trimethylbenzenaminium bromide; CAS Reg. No. 114-80-7.

Description. Colourless crystals or a white, crystalline powder; odourless.

Solubility. Very soluble in water; freely soluble in ethanol (~750 g/l) TS and chloroform R; practically insoluble in ether R.

Category. Cholinergic.

Storage. Neostigmine bromide should be kept in a tightly closed container, protected from light.

REQUIREMENTS

General requirement. Neostigmine bromide contains not less than 98.0% and not more than 101.0% of $C_{12}H_{19}BrN_2O_2$, calculated with reference to the dried substance.

Identity tests

A.   Heat 0.05 g with 0.4 g of potassium hydroxide R and 2 ml of ethanol (~750 g/l) TS on a water-bath for 3 minutes. Replace the evaporated ethanol, cool, and add 2 ml of water and 2 ml of diazobenzenedisulfonic acid TS; a red colour is produced.

B.   To a solution of 0.1 g in 5 ml of water add 15 ml of trinitrophenol (7 g/l) TS, wash the precipitate with water, and dry at 105 °C; melting temperature, about 185 °C (picrate).

C.   A 20 mg/ml solution yields reaction A described under "General identification tests" as characteristic of bromides (vol. 1, p. 112).

Sulfates.   Dissolve 2.5 g in 40 ml of water and proceed as described under "Limit test for sulfates" (vol. 1, p. 116); the sulfate content is not more than 0.2 mg/g.

Sulfated ash.   Not more than 1.5 mg/g.

Loss on drying.   Dry to constant weight at 105 °C; it loses not more than 20 mg/g.

Acidity.   Dissolve 0.2 g in 20 ml of carbon-dioxide-free water R and titrate to pH 7.0 with sodium hydroxide (0.02 mol/l) VS; not more than 0.1 ml is required.

3-Hydroxyphenyltrimethylammonium bromide.   The absorbance of a 1-cm layer of a freshly prepared 5.0 mg/ml solution in sodium carbonate (10 g/l) TS at 294 nm is not more than 0.2 (preferably use 2-cm cells for the measurement and calculate the absorbance of a 1-cm layer).

Assay.   Dissolve about 0.25 g, accurately weighed, in 20 ml of glacial acetic acid R1, add 5 ml of acetic anhydride R and 10 ml of mercuric acetate/acetic acid TS. Titrate with perchloric acid (0.1 mol/l) VS as described under "Non-aqueous titration", Method A (vol. 1, p. 131). Each ml of perchloric acid (0.1 mol/l) VS is equivalent to 30.32 mg of $C_{12}H_{19}BrN_2O_2$.

NICLOSAMIDUM

Niclosamide

Niclosamide, anhydrous
Niclosamide monohydrate

Molecular formula. $C_{13}H_8Cl_2N_2O_4$ (anhydrous); $C_{13}H_8Cl_2N_2O_4,H_2O$ (monohydrate)

Relative molecular mass.   327.1 (anhydrous); 345.1 (monohydrate)

Graphic formula.

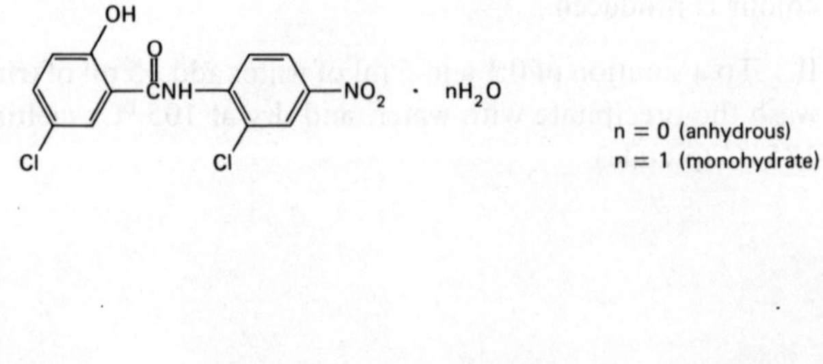

n = 0 (anhydrous)
n = 1 (monohydrate)

Chemical name. 2′,5-Dichloro-4′-nitrosalicylanilide; 5-chloro-*N*-(2-chloro-4-nitrophenyl)-2-hydroxybenzamide; CAS Reg. No. 50-65-7 (anhydrous). 2′,5-Dichloro-4′-nitrosalicylanilide monohydrate; 5-chloro-*N*-(2-chloro-4-nitrophenyl)-2-hydroxybenzamide monohydrate; CAS Reg. No. 73360-56-2 (monohydrate).

Description. A cream-coloured, crystalline powder; odourless.

Solubility. Practically insoluble in water; soluble in 150 parts of ethanol (~750 g/l) TS; slightly soluble in chloroform R, ether R, and acetone R.

Category. Taeniacide.

Storage. Niclosamide should be kept in a tightly closed container.

Labelling. The designation on the container of Niclosamide should state whether the substance is the monohydrate or is in the anhydrous form.

Additional information. Anhydrous Niclosamide is hygroscopic.

REQUIREMENTS

General requirement. Niclosamide contains not less than 98.0% and not more than 100.5% of $C_{13}H_8Cl_2N_2O_4$, calculated with reference to the dried substance.

Identity tests

• Either test A alone or tests B and C may be applied.

A. Carry out the examination as described under "Spectrophotometry in the infrared region" (vol. 1, p. 40). The infrared absorption spectrum is concordant with the *reference spectrum* of a relevant form of niclosamide.

B. Dissolve 1 mg in 2 ml of dimethylformamide R and add 2 drops of potassium hydroxide/ethanol TS1; a strong red colour is produced.

C. Dissolve 0.1 g in 1 ml of acetic anhydride R and boil for 10 minutes. Cool and add 10 ml of water. Collect the precipitate on a filter, wash with water, recrystallize from ethanol (~750 g/l) TS, and dry at 105 °C; melting temperature, about 178 °C (acetyl-derivative).

Sulfated ash. Not more than 1.0 mg/g.

Loss on drying. Dry to constant weight at 105 °C. Anhydrous Niclosamide loses not more than 5.0 mg/g. Niclosamide monohydrate loses not less than 40 mg/g and not more than 60 mg/g.

Acidity or alkalinity. Boil 0.8 g in 40 ml of water for 1 minute and filter. To 10 ml of the filtrate add 2 drops of phenolphthalein/ethanol TS and 0.2 ml of carbonate-free sodium hydroxide (0.01 mol/l) VS; a red colour is produced. Add 5 drops of methyl red/ethanol TS and 0.4 ml of hydrochloric acid (0.01 mol/l) VS; the colour of the solution changes from red to orange.

2-Chloro-4-nitroaniline. Boil 0.1 g with 20 ml of methanol R for 2 minutes, cool, add sufficient hydrochloric acid (1 mol/l) VS to produce 50 ml, and filter. To 10 ml of the filtrate add 1.0 ml of sodium nitrite (3 g/l) TS and allow to stand for 10 minutes; add 1 ml of ammonium sulfamate (25 g/l) TS, shake, allow to stand for 10 minutes, and add 1 ml of N-(1-naphthyl)ethylenediamine hydrochloride (5 g/l) TS. Treat similarly 10 μg of 2-chloro-4-nitroaniline R. The colour produced in the test solution is not more intense than that of the reference solution when compared as described under "Colour of liquids" (vol. 1, p. 50).

5-Chlorosalicylic acid. Boil 0.5 g with 10 ml of water for 2 minutes, cool, filter, and add to the filtrate a few drops of ferric chloride (25 g/l) TS; no red or violet colour is produced.

Assay. Dissolve about 0.3 g, accurately weighed, in 60 ml of dimethylformamide R and titrate with tetrabutylammonium hydroxide (0.1 mol/l) VS determining the endpoint potentiometrically as described under "Non-aqueous titration", Method B (vol. 1, p. 132). Each ml of tetrabutylammonium hydroxide (0.1 mol/l) VS is equivalent to 32.71 mg of $C_{13}H_8Cl_2N_2O_4$.

NICOTINAMIDUM

Nicotinamide

Molecular formula. $C_6H_6N_2O$

Relative molecular mass. 122.1

Graphic formula.

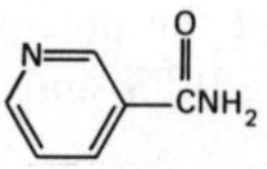

Chemical name. 3-Pyridinecarboxamide; 3-pyridinecarboxylic acid amide; CAS Reg. No. 98-92-0.

Description. Colourless crystals or a white, crystalline powder; odourless or almost odourless.

Solubility. Soluble in 1 part of water and 2 parts of ethanol (~750 g/l) TS; slightly soluble in ether R and chloroform R.

Category. Vitamin.

Storage. Nicotinamide should be kept in a well-closed container.

REQUIREMENTS

General requirement. Nicotinamide contains not less than 99.0% and not more than 101.0% of $C_6H_6N_2O$, calculated with reference to the dried substance.

Identity tests

• Either test A alone or tests B and C may be applied.

A. Carry out the examination as described under "Spectrophotometry in the infrared region" (vol. 1, p. 40). The infrared absorption spectrum is concordant with the spectrum obtained from nicotinamide RS or with the *reference spectrum* of nicotinamide.

B. Dissolve 10 mg in 10 ml of water. To 2 ml add 2 ml of thiocyanate reagent, obtained by adding, drop by drop, ammonium thiocyanate (0.1 mol/l) VS to bromine TS1 until the yellow coloration disappears. Then add 3 ml of aniline (25 g/l) TS and shake; a yellow colour is produced.

C. Boil gently 0.1 g with 1 ml of sodium hydroxide (~80 g/l) TS in a test-tube; ammonia, perceptible by its odour, is evolved.

Melting range. 128–131 °C.

Heavy metals. Use 1.0 g for the preparation of the test solution as described under "Limit test for heavy metals", Procedure 1 (vol. 1, p. 118); determine the heavy metals content according to Method A (vol. 1, p. 119); not more than 30 µg/g.

Clarity and colour of solution. A solution of 2.5 g in 10 ml of water is clear and not more intensely coloured than standard colour solution Yw2 when compared as described under "Colour of liquids" (vol. 1, p. 50).

Sulfated ash. Not more than 1.0 mg/g.

Loss on drying. Dry to constant weight at ambient temparature under reduced pressure (not exceeding 0.6 kPa or about 5 mm of mercury) over silica gel, desiccant, R or phosphorus pentoxide R; it loses not more than 5.0 mg/g.

pH value. pH of a 0.05 g/ml solution in carbon-dioxide-free water R, 6.0–8.0.

Related substances. Carry out the test as described under "Thin-layer chromatography" (vol. 1, p. 83), using silica gel R2 as the coating substance and a mixture of 48 volumes of chloroform R, 10 volumes of water and 45 volumes of dehydrated ethanol R as the mobile phase. Apply separately to the plate 5 μl of each of 2 solutions in a mixture of equal volumes of ethanol (~750 g/l) TS and water containing (A) 0.12 g of the test substance per ml and (B) 0.30 mg of the test substance per ml. After removing the plate from the chromatographic chamber, allow it to dry in air, and examine the chromatogram in ultraviolet light (254 nm). Any spot obtained with solution A, other than the principal spot, is not more intense than that obtained with solution B.

Assay. Dissolve about 0.25 g, accurately weighed, in 20 ml of glacial acetic acid R1, add 5 ml of acetic anhydride R, and titrate with perchloric acid (0.1 mol/l) VS as described under "Non-aqueous titration", Method A (vol. 1, p. 131). Each ml of perchloric acid (0.1 mol/l) VS is equivalent to 12.21 mg of $C_6H_6N_2O$.

NORETHISTERONI ACETAS
Norethisterone acetate

Molecular formula. $C_{22}H_{28}O_3$

Relative molecular mass. 340.5

Graphic formula.

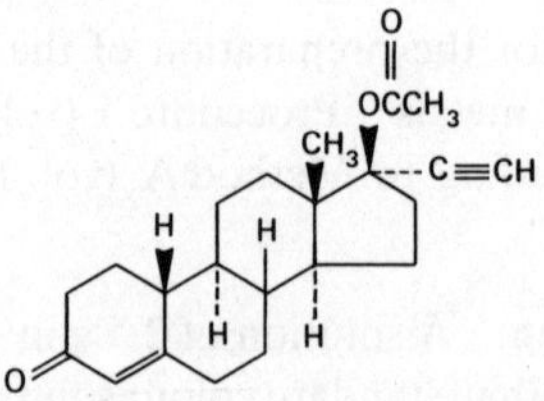

Chemical name. 17-Hydroxy-19-nor-17α-pregn-4-en-20-yn-3-one acetate; 17-(acetyloxy)-19-nor-17α-pregn-4-en-20-yn-3-one; 17α-ethynyl-17-hydroxyestr-4-en-3-one acetate; CAS Reg. No. 51-98-9.

Description. A white or creamy white, crystalline powder; odourless.

Solubility. Practically insoluble in water; soluble in 12.5 parts of ethanol (~750 g/l) TS and in 4 parts of acetone R; sparingly soluble in ether R.

Category. Progestational steroid.

Storage. Norethisterone acetate should be kept in a well-closed container, protected from light.

REQUIREMENTS

General requirement. Norethisterone acetate contains not less than 97.0% and not more than 103.0% of $C_{22}H_{28}O_3$, calculated with reference to the dried substance.

Identity tests

A. Carry out the examination as described under "Spectrophotometry in the infrared region" (vol. 1, p. 40). The infrared absorption spectrum is concordant with the spectrum obtained from norethisterone acetate RS or with the *reference spectrum* of norethisterone acetate.

B. See the test described under "Related substances". The principal spot obtained with solution B corresponds in position, appearance, and intensity with that obtained with solution C.

C. Heat 0.1 g with 2 ml of potassium hydroxide/ethanol (0.5 mol/l) VS in a water-bath for 5 minutes. Cool, add 2 ml of sulfuric acid (~700 g/l) TS and boil gently for 1 minute; ethyl acetate, perceptible by its odour (proceed with caution) is produced.

Specific optical rotation. Use a 20 mg/ml solution in dioxan R; $[\alpha]_D^{20\,°C} = -32$ to $-38°$.

Sulfated ash. Not more than 1.0 mg/g.

Loss on drying. Dry to constant weight at 105 °C; it loses not more than 5.0 mg/g.

Related substances. Carry out the test as described under "Thin-layer chromatography" (vol. 1, p. 83), using silica gel R1 as the coating substance and a mixture of equal volumes of toluene R and ethyl acetate R as the mobile phase. Apply separately to the plate 10 μl, in two portions of 5 μl, of each of 3 solutions in chloroform R containing (A) 10 mg of the test substance per ml, (B) 0.10 mg of the test substance per ml, and (C) 0.10 mg of norethisterone acetate RS per ml. After removing the plate from the chromatographic chamber, allow it to dry in air until the solvents have evaporated, and spray with sulfuric acid/ethanol TS. Heat the plate to 105 °C for 15 minutes, allow to cool, and examine the chromatogram in daylight. Any spot obtained with solution A, other than the principal spot, is not more intense than that obtained with solution B.

Assay. Dissolve about 10 mg, accurately weighed, in sufficient ethanol (~750 g/l) TS to produce 100 ml; dilute 10.0 ml of this solution to 100 ml with the same solvent. Measure the absorbance of a 1-cm layer of the diluted solution at the maximum at about 240 nm. Calculate the amount of $C_{22}H_{28}O_3$ in the substance being tested by comparison with norethisterone acetate RS, similarly and concurrently examined. In an adequately calibrated spectrophotometer the absorbance of the reference solution should be 0.51 ± 0.03.

NORETHISTERONUM

Norethisterone

Molecular formula. $C_{20}H_{26}O_2$

Relative molecular mass. 298.4

Graphic formula.

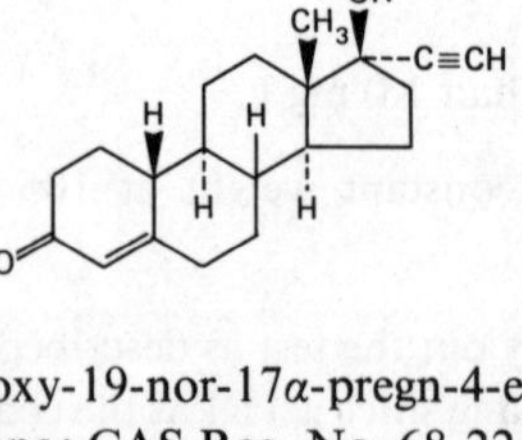

Chemical name. 17-Hydroxy-19-nor-17α-pregn-4-en-20-yn-3-one; 17α-ethynyl-17-hydroxyestr-4-en-3-one; CAS Reg. No. 68-22-4.

Description. A white or creamy white, crystalline powder; odourless.

Solubility. Practically insoluble in water; soluble in 150 parts of ethanol (~750 g/l) TS, in 80 parts of acetone R, and in 30 parts of chloroform R.

Category. Progestational steroid.

Storage. Norethisterone should be kept in a well-closed container, protected from light.

REQUIREMENTS

General requirement. Norethisterone contains not less than 97.0% and not more than 103.0% of $C_{20}H_{26}O_2$, calculated with reference to the dried substance.

Identity tests

A. Carry out the examination as described under "Spectrophotometry in the infrared region" (vol. 1, p. 40). The infrared absorption spectrum is concordant with the spectrum obtained from norethisterone RS or with the *reference spectrum* of norethisterone.

B. See the test described below under "Related substances". The principal spot obtained with solution B corresponds in position, appearance, and intensity with that obtained with solution C.

Specific optical rotation. Use a 10 mg/ml solution in chloroform R; $[\alpha]_D^{20\,°C} =$ −23 to −27 °.

Sulfated ash. Not more than 1.0 mg/g.

Loss on drying. Dry to constant weight at 105 °C; it loses not more than 5.0 mg/g.

Related substances. Carry out the test as described under "Thin-layer chromatography" (vol. 1, p. 83), using silica gel R1 as the coating substance and a mixture of 95 volumes of chloroform R and 5 volumes of methanol R as the mobile phase. Apply separately to the plate 10 μl in two portions of 5 μl, of each of 3 solutions in chloroform R containing (A) 10 mg of the test substance per ml, (B) 0.10 mg of the test substance per ml, and (C) 0.10 mg of norethisterone RS per ml. After removing the plate from the chromatographic chamber, allow it to dry in air until the solvents have evaporated, and spray with sulfuric acid/ethanol TS. Heat the plate to 105 °C for 15 minutes, allow to cool, and examine the chromatogram in daylight. Any spot obtained with solution A, other than the principal spot, is not more intense than that obtained with solution B.

Assay. Dissolve about 10 mg, accurately weighed, in sufficient ethanol (~750 g/l) TS to produce 100 ml; dilute 10.0 ml of this solution to 100 ml with the same solvent. Measure the absorbance of a 1-cm layer of the diluted solution at the maximum at about 240 nm. Calculate the amount of $C_{20}H_{26}O_2$ in the substance being tested by comparison with norethisterone RS, similarly and concurrently examined. In an adequately calibrated spectrophotometer the absorbance of the reference solution should be 0.58 ± 0.03.

PAPAVERINI HYDROCHLORIDUM

Papaverine hydrochloride

Molecular formula. $C_{20}H_{21}NO_4,HCl$

Relative molecular mass.   375.9

Graphic formula.

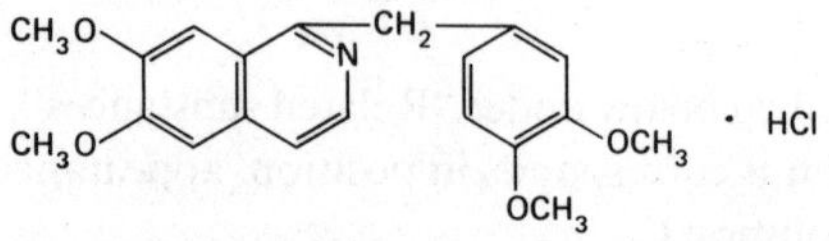

Chemical name.   6,7-Dimethoxy-1-veratrylisoquinoline hydrochloride; 1-[(3,4-dimethoxyphenyl)methyl]-6,7-dimethoxyisoquinoline hydrochloride; CAS Reg. No. 61-25-6.

Description.   Colourless crystals or a white, crystalline powder; odourless.

Solubility.   Sparingly soluble in water; soluble in 120 parts of ethanol ($\sim$750 g/l) TS; soluble in chloroform R; practically insoluble in ether R.

Category.   Spasmolytic.

Storage.   Papaverine hydrochloride should be kept in a well-closed container, protected from light.

REQUIREMENTS

General requirement.   Papaverine hydrochloride contains not less than 98.5% and not more than 101.0% of $C_{20}H_{21}NO_4,HCl$, calculated with reference to the dried substance.

Identity tests

• Either tests A and C or tests B, C, and D may be applied.

A.   Carry out the examination as described under "Spectrophotometry in the infrared region" (vol. 1, p. 40). The infrared absorption spectrum is concordant with the spectrum obtained from papaverine hydrochloride RS or with the *reference spectrum* of papaverine hydrochloride.

B.   Treat about 10 mg with 3 ml of acetic anhydride R, add cautiously 3 drops of sulfuric acid ($\sim$1760 g/l) TS and heat on a water-bath for 3–4 minutes; a yellow colour with a green fluorescence is produced.

C.   A 20 mg/ml solution yields reaction B described under "General identification tests" as characteristic of chlorides (vol. 1, p. 113).

D.   Dissolve 20 mg in 10 ml of water, add drop by drop ammonia (~100 g/l) TS, and set aside.   Filter, wash the precipitate with water, and dry at 105 °C; melting temperature, about 146 °C (papaverine base).

Clarity and colour of solution.   A solution of 0.20 g in 10 ml of carbon-dioxide-free water R is clear and not more intensely coloured than standard colour solution Gn2 when compared as described under "Colour of liquids" (vol. 1, p. 50).

Sulfated ash.   Not more than 1.0 mg/g.

Loss on drying.   Dry to constant weight at 105 °C; it loses not more than 10 mg/g.

pH value.   pH of a 20 mg/ml solution, 3.0–4.5.

Related substances.   Carry out the test as described under "Thin-layer chromatography" (vol. 1, p. 83), using silica gel R2 as the coating substance and a mixture of 7 volumes of toluene R, 2 volumes of ethyl acetate R, and 1 volume of diethylamine R as the mobile phase.   Apply separately to the plate 10 μl of each of 2 solutions in a mixture of 4 volumes of hydrochloric acid (0.01 mol/l) VS and 1 volume of ethanol (~750 g/l) TS containing (A) 0.050 g of the test substance per ml and (B) 0.50 mg of codeine R per ml.   After removing the plate from the chromatographic chamber, allow it to dry in a current of warm air until the odour of diethylamine is no longer perceptible, and examine the chromatogram in ultraviolet light (254 nm).   Any spot obtained with solution A, other than the principal spot, is not more intense than that obtained with solution B.

Assay.   Dissolve about 0.35 g, accurately weighed, in 30 ml of glacial acetic acid R1, add 10 ml of mercuric acetate/acetic acid TS and titrate with perchloric acid (0.1 mol/l) VS as described under "Non-aqueous titration", Method A (vol. 1, p. 131).   Each ml of perchloric acid (0.1 mol/l) VS is equivalent to 37.59 mg of $C_{20}H_{21}NO_4$,HCl.

PHENOBARBITALUM
Phenobarbital

Molecular formula. $C_{12}H_{12}N_2O_3$

Relative molecular mass.   232.2

Graphic formula.

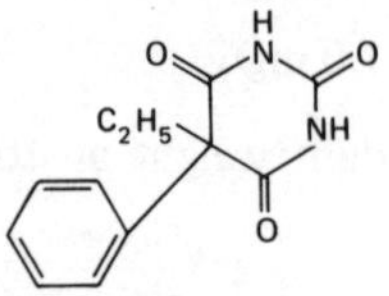

Chemical name.   5-Ethyl-5-phenylbarbituric acid; 5-ethyl-5-phenyl-2,4,6-(1H,3H,5H)-pyrimidinetrione; CAS Reg. No. 50-06-6.

Description.   Colourless crystals or a white, crystalline powder; odourless.

Solubility.   Soluble in about 1100 parts of water, in about 10 parts of ethanol (~750 g/l) TS, in about 15 parts of ether R, and in about 40 parts of chloroform R.

Category.   Hypnotic; sedative; anticonvulsant.

Storage.   Phenobarbital should be kept in a well-closed container.

Additional information.   Phenobarbital may exhibit polymorphism.

REQUIREMENTS

General requirement.   Phenobarbital contains not less than 98.0% and not more than 101.0% of $C_{12}H_{12}N_2O_3$, calculated with reference to the dried substance.

Identity tests

• Either test A alone or all 3 tests B, C, and D may be applied.

A.   Carry out the examination as described under "Spectrophotometry in the infrared region" (vol. 1, p. 40). The infrared absorption spectrum is concordant with the *reference spectrum* of phenobarbital.

B.   Dissolve 20 mg in 5 ml of ethanol (~750 g/l) TS, add 1 drop of cobaltous chloride TS and 1 drop of ammonia (~100 g/l) TS; a violet colour is produced.

C. Shake for 3 minutes 0.1 g with 4 ml of sodium hydroxide (0.1 mol/l) VS and 1 ml of water. Filter and to 2 ml of the filtrate add 4 drops of mercuric chloride (65 g/l) TS; a white precipitate is formed, which dissolves on the addition of 5 ml of ammonia (~100 g/l) TS.

D. Dissolve 0.1 g in 2 ml of sulfuric acid (~1760 g/l) TS, add about 10 mg of sodium nitrite R, and warm on a water-bath for 10 minutes; an orange-yellow colour with a brownish sheen is produced.

Melting range. 174–178 °C.

Solution in alkali. Dissolve 1.0 g in 4.0 ml of sodium hydroxide (~80 g/l) TS and add 6.0 ml of water; the solution is clear and colourless.

Sulfated ash. Not more than 1.0 mg/g.

Loss on drying. Dry to constant weight at 105 °C; it loses not more than 10 mg/g.

Acidity. Boil 1.0 g with 50 ml of water for 2 minutes, adjust the volume to 50 ml, and filter. To 10 ml of the filtrate add 0.15 ml of methyl red/ethanol TS; not more than 0.1 ml of sodium hydroxide (0.1 mol/l) VS is required to obtain the midpoint of the indicator (orange).

Phenylbarbituric acid. Boil 1.0 g with 5 ml of ethanol (~750 g/l) TS for 3 minutes under a reflux condenser; a clear solution is produced.

Neutral and basic impurities. Dissolve 1.0 g in a mixture of 5 ml of sodium hydroxide (~80 g/l) TS and 10 ml of water and shake for 1 minute with 25 ml of ether R. Wash the ethereal layer 3 times, each time with 5 ml of water, evaporate the ether, and dry the residue at 105 °C for 1 hour; the residue weighs not more than 3.0 mg.

Related substances. Carry out the test as described under "Thin-layer chromatography" (vol. 1, p. 83), using silica gel R2 as the coating substance and a mixture of 80 volumes of chloroform R, 15 volumes of ethanol (~750 g/l) TS, and 1 volume of ammonia (~260 g/l) TS as the mobile phase. Apply separately to the plate 10 μl of each of 2 solutions in ethanol (~750 g/l) TS containing (A) 10 mg of the test substance per ml and (B) 0.20 mg of the test substance per ml. After removing the plate from the chromatographic chamber, allow it to dry in air, and examine the chromatogram in ultraviolet light (254 nm). Any spot obtained with solution A, other than the principal spot, is not more intense than that obtained with solution B.

Assay. Dissolve about 0.20 g, accurately weighed, in 30 ml of dimethylformamide R, add 2 drops of thymolphthalein/dimethylformamide TS and titrate with sodium methoxide (0.1 mol/l) VS to a blue endpoint, as described under "Non-aqueous titration", Method B (vol. 1, p. 132). Each ml of sodium methoxide (0.1 mol/l) VS is equivalent to 23.22 mg of $C_{12}H_{12}N_2O_3$.

PHENOBARBITALUM NATRICUM
Phenobarbital sodium

Molecular formula. $C_{12}H_{11}N_2NaO_3$

Relative molecular mass. 254.2

Graphic formula.

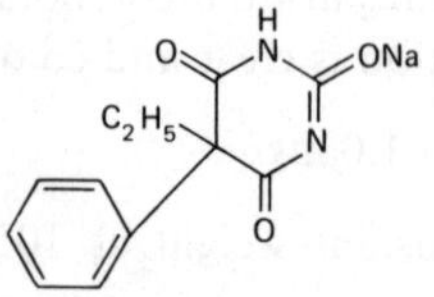

Chemical name. Sodium 5-ethyl-5-phenylbarbiturate; 5-ethyl-5-phenyl-2,4,6-(1H,3H,5H)-pyrimidinetrione monosodium salt; CAS Reg. No. 57-30-7.

Description. White, crystalline granules or a white, crystalline powder; odourless.

Solubility. Freely soluble in water; soluble in ethanol (~750 g/l) TS; practically insoluble in ether R and chloroform R.

Category. Hypnotic; sedative; anticonvulsant.

Storage. Phenobarbital sodium should be kept in a tightly closed container, protected from light.

Additional information. Phenobarbital sodium is hygroscopic. Even in the absence of light, Phenobarbital sodium is gradually degraded on exposure to a humid atmosphere, the decomposition being faster at higher temperatures.

REQUIREMENTS

General requirement. Phenobarbital sodium contains not less than 98.0% and not more than 101.0% of $C_{12}H_{11}N_2NaO_3$, calculated with reference to the dried substance.

Identity tests

• Either tests A and D or tests B, C, and D may be applied.
A. Carry out the examination as described under "Spectrophotometry in the infrared region" (vol. 1, p. 40). The infrared absorption spectrum is concordant with the *reference spectrum* of phenobarbital sodium.

B. Dissolve 0.2 g in 10 ml of water and add 2 ml of hydrochloric acid (~70 g/l) TS; a white, crystalline precipitate is produced. Wash the precipitate with water until free from chlorides, and dry at 105 °C; melting temperature, about 175 °C (phenobarbital). Keep the precipitate for test C.

C. Dissolve 20 mg of the precipitate obtained from test B in 5 ml of ethanol (~750 g/l) TS, add 1 drop of cobaltous chloride TS and 1 drop of ammonia (~100 g/l) TS; a violet colour is produced.

D. When tested for sodium as described under "General identification tests" (vol. 1, p. 115), yields the characteristic reactions. If reaction B is to be used, prepare a 20 mg/ml solution.

Clarity and colour of solution. A solution of 1.0 g in 10 ml of carbon-dioxide-free water R remains clear and colourless during 15 minutes.

Loss on drying. Dry to constant weight at 140 °C; it loses not more than 70 mg/g.

pH value. pH of a 0.10 g/ml solution in carbon-dioxide-free water R, 9.0–10.8.

Neutral and basic impurities. Dissolve 1.0 g in a mixture of 5 ml of sodium hydroxide (~80 g/l) TS and 10 ml of water, and shake for 1 minute with 25 ml of ether R. Wash the ethereal layer 3 times, each time with 5 ml of water, evaporate the ether, and dry the residue at 105 °C for 1 hour; the residue weighs not more than 3.0 mg.

Related substances. Carry out the test as described under "Thin-layer chromatography" (vol. 1, p. 40), using silica gel R2 as the coating substance and a mixture of 80 volumes of chloroform R, 15 volumes of ethanol (~ 750 g/l) TS and 5 volumes of ammonia (~260 g/l) TS as the mobile phase. Apply separately to the plate 10 μl of each of 2 solutions in ethanol (~ 750 g/l) TS containing (A) 10 mg of the test substance per ml and (B) 0.20 mg of the test substance per ml. After removing the plate from the chromatographic chamber, allow it to dry in air, and examine the chromatogram in ultraviolet light (254 nm). Any spot obtained with solution A, other than the principal spot, is not more intense than that obtained with solution B.

Assay. Dissolve about 0.5 g, accurately weighed, in 15 ml of water, add 5 ml of hydrochloric acid (2 mol/l) VS, and extract with 50 ml of ether R and then with successive quantities, each of 25 ml of ether R, until complete extraction has been effected. Wash the combined extracts twice with water, using 5 ml each time. Add the ether extract to the main ether extract, evaporate to low bulk, add 2 ml of dehydrated ethanol R, evaporate to dryness, and dry the residue to constant weight at 105 °C. Each g of residue is equivalent to 1.095 g of $C_{12}H_{11}N_2NaO_3$.

PHENOXYMETHYLPENICILLINUM

Phenoxymethylpenicillin

Molecular formula. $C_{16}H_{18}N_2O_5S$

Relative molecular mass. 350.4

Graphic formula.

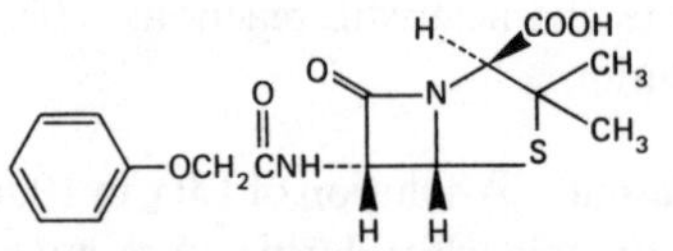

Chemical name. (2S,5R,6R)-3,3-Dimethyl-7-oxo-6-(2-phenoxyacetamido)-4-thia-1-azabicyclo[3.2.0]heptane-2-carboxylic acid; [2S-(2α,5α,6β)]-3,3-dimethyl-7-oxo-6-[(phenoxyacetyl)amino]-4-thia-1-azabicyclo[3.2.0]heptane-2-carboxylic acid: CAS Reg. No. 87-08-1.

Description. A white, fine crystalline powder.

Solubility. Soluble in 1700 parts of water and in 7 parts of ethanol (~750 g/l) TS.

Category. Antibiotic.

Storage. Phenoxymethylpenicillin should be kept in a tightly closed container, protected from light.

Additional information. Even in the absence of light, Phenoxymethylpenicillin is gradually degraded on exposure to a humid atmosphere, the decomposition being faster at higher temperatures.

REQUIREMENTS

General requirement. Phenoxymethylpenicillin contains not less than 95.0% and not more than 102.0% of $C_{16}H_{18}N_2O_5S$, calculated with reference to the anydrous substance.

Identity tests

• Either tests A and B or tests B and C may be applied.
A. Carry out the examination as described under "Spectrophotometry in the infrared region" (vol. 1, p. 40). The infrared absorption spectrum is concordant with the spectrum obtained from phenoxymethylpenicillin RS or with the *reference spectrum* of phenoxymethylpenicillin.

B. To 2 mg in a test-tube add 1 drop of water followed by 2 ml of sulfuric acid (~1760 g/l) TS and mix; the solution is colourless. Immerse the test-tube for 1 minute in a water-bath; the solution remains colourless.

C. Place 2 mg in a test-tube, add 1 drop of water and 2 ml of formaldehyde/sulfuric acid TS and mix; the solution is red. Immerse the test-tube for 1 minute in a water-bath; a red-brown colour is produced.

Specific optical rotation. Use a 10 mg/ml solution in 1-butanol R and calculate with reference to the anhydrous substance; $[\alpha]_D^{20\,°C} = +186$ to $+200\,°$.

Water. Determine as described under "Determination of water by the Karl Fischer method", Method B (vol. 1, p. 135), using about 0.3 g of the substance; not more than 15 mg/g.

pH value. pH of a 5.0 mg/ml suspension in water, 2.4–4.0.

p-**Hydroxyphenoxymethylpenicillin.** Dissolve about 0.1 g, accurately weighed, in sufficient sodium hydroxide (0.1 mol/l) VS to produce 100 ml. Measure the absorbance of a 1-cm layer at the maximum at about 306 nm; not more than 0.36 (preferably use 2-cm cells for the measurement and calculate the absorbance of a 1-cm layer).

Ultraviolet absorbance range. Dilute 20 ml of the solution obtained in the test for *p*-hydroxyphenoxymethylpenicillin to 100 ml with sodium hydroxide (0.1 mol/l) VS. Measure the absorbance of a 1-cm layer at the maximum at about 274 nm; not less than 0.56 and not more than 0.62.

Assay. Dissolve about 50 mg, accurately weighed, in a mixture of 0.6 ml of sodium hydrogen carbonate (40 g/l) TS and 10 ml of water and dilute with sufficient water to produce 1000 ml. Transfer two 2.0-ml aliquots of this solution into separate stoppered tubes. To one tube add 10.0 ml of imidazole/mercuric chloride TS, mix, stopper the tube, and place it in a water-bath at 60 °C for exactly 25 minutes. Cool the tube rapidly to 20 °C (solution A). To the second tube add 10.0 ml of water and mix (solution B).

Without delay measure the absorbance of a 1-cm layer at the maximum at about 325 nm against a solvent cell containing a mixture of 2.0 ml of water and 10.0 ml of imidazole/mercuric chloride TS for solution A and water for solution B.

From the difference between the absorbance of solution A and that of solution B, calculate the amount of $C_{16}H_{18}N_2O_5S$ in the substance being examined by comparison with phenoxymethylpenicillin potassium RS similarly and concurrently examined, but omitting the addition of sodium hydrogen carbonate (40 g/l) TS; each mg of phenoxymethylpenicillin potassium RS ($C_{16}H_{17}KN_2O_5S$) is equivalent to 0.902 mg of phenoxymethylpenicillin ($C_{16}H_{18}N_2O_5S$). In an adequately calibrated spectrophotometer the absorbance of the reference solution should be 0.63 ± 0.03.

PHENOXYMETHYLPENICILLINUM CALCICUM

Phenoxymethylpenicillin calcium

Molecular formula. $(C_{16}H_{17}N_2O_5S)_2Ca,2H_2O$ or $C_{32}H_{34}CaN_4O_{10}S_2,2H_2O$

Relative molecular mass. 774.9

Graphic formula.

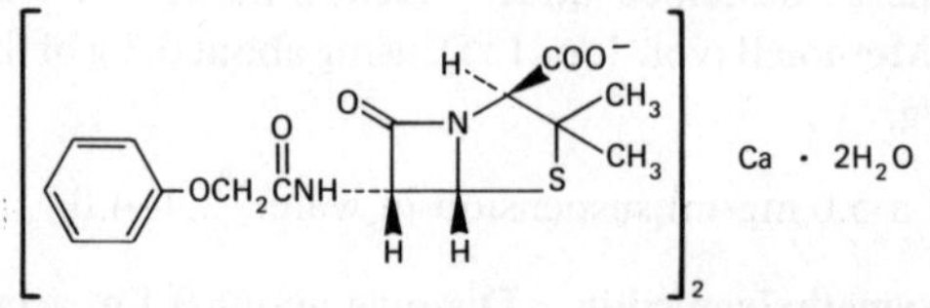

Chemical name. Calcium bis[(2S.5R.6R)-3,3-dimethyl-7-oxo-6-(2-phenoxy-acetamido)-4-thia-1-azabicyclo[3.2.0]heptane-2-carboxylate] dihydrate; calcium bis[[2S-(2α,5α,6β)]3,3-dimethyl-7-oxo-6-[(phenoxyacetyl)amino]-4-thia-1-azabi-cyclo[3.2.0]heptane-2-carboxylate] dihydrate; CAS Reg. No. 73368-74-8.

Description. A white, fine crystalline powder; odourless or with a faint characteristic odour.

Solubility. Slowly soluble in 120 parts of water.

Category. Antibiotic.

Storage. Phenoxymethylpenicillin calcium should be kept in a well-closed container.

Additional information. Even in the absence of light, Phenoxymethylpenicillin calcium is gradually degraded on exposure to a humid atmosphere, the decomposition being faster at higher temperatures.

REQUIREMENTS

General requirement. Phenoxymethylpenicillin calcium contains not less than 95.0% and not more than 102.0% of $(C_{16}H_{17}N_2O_5S)_2Ca$, calculated with reference to the anhydrous substance.

Identity tests

• Either tests A and D or tests B, C, and D may be applied.
A. Carry out the examination as described under "Spectrophotometry in the infrared region" (vol. 1, p. 40). The infrared absorption spectrum is concordant

with the spectrum obtained from phenoxymethylpenicillin calcium RS or with the *reference spectrum* of phenoxymethylpenicillin calcium.

B.   To 2 mg in a test-tube add 1 drop of water followed by 2 ml of sulfuric acid (~1760 g/l) TS and mix; the solution is colourless. Immerse the test-tube for 1 minute in a water-bath; the solution remains colourless.

C.   Place 2 mg in a test-tube, add 1 drop of water and 2 ml of formaldehyde/ sulfuric acid TS and mix; the solution is red. Immerse the test-tube for 1 minute in a water-bath; a red-brown colour is produced.

D.   Ignite a small quantity, dissolve the residue in hydrochloric acid (~70 g/l) TS, and make the solution alkaline by the addition of ammonia (~100 g/l) TS; the solution yields the reactions described under "General identification tests" as characteristic of calcium (vol. 1, p. 112).

Water.   Determine as described under "Determination of water by the Karl Fischer method", Method A (vol. 1, p. 135), using about 0.2 g of the substance; not more than 50 mg/g.

pH value.   pH of a 5.0 mg/ml solution in carbon-dioxide-free water R, 5.0–7.5.

p-**Hydroxyphenoxymethylpenicillin.**   Dissolve about 0.11 g, accurately weighed, in sufficient sodium hydroxide (0.1 mol/l) VS to produce 100 ml. Measure the absorbance of a 1-cm layer at the maximum at about 306 nm; not more than 0.36 (use preferably 2-cm cells for the measurement and calculate the absorbance of a 1-cm layer).

Ultraviolet absorbance range.   Dilute 20 ml of the solution obtained in the test for *p*-hydroxyphenoxymethylpenicillin to 100 ml with sodium hydroxide (0.1 mol/l) VS. Measure the absorbance of a 1-cm layer at the maximum at about 274 nm; not less than 0.56 and not more than 0.62.

Assay.   Dissolve about 50 mg, accurately weighed, in sufficient water to produce 1000 ml. Transfer two 2.0-ml aliquots of this solution into separate stoppered tubes. To one tube add 10.0 ml of imidazole/mercuric chloride TS, mix, stopper the tube, and place it in a water-bath at 60 °C for exactly 25 minutes. Cool the tube rapidly to 20 °C (solution A). To the second tube add 10.0 ml of water and mix (solution B).

   Without delay measure the absorbance of a 1-cm layer at the maximum at about 325 nm against a solvent cell containing a mixture of 2.0 ml of water and 10.0 ml of imidazole/mercuric chloride TS for solution A and water for solution B.

   From the difference between the absorbance of solution A and that of solution B, calculate the amount of $(C_{16}H_{17}N_2O_5S)_2Ca$ in the substance being tested by comparison with phenoxymethylpenicillin potassium RS, similarly and concurrently examined, taking into account that each mg of phenoxymethylpenicillin potassium RS ($C_{16}H_{17}KN_2O_5S$) is equivalent to 0.951 mg of phenoxymethylpenicillin calcium ($C_{16}H_{17}N_2O_5S)_2Ca$. In an adequately calibrated spectrophotometer the absorbance of the reference solution should be 0.63 ± 0.03.

PHENOXYMETHYLPENICILLINUM KALICUM
Phenoxymethylpenicillin potassium

Molecular formula. $C_{16}H_{17}KN_2O_5S$

Relative molecular mass. 388.5

Graphic formula.

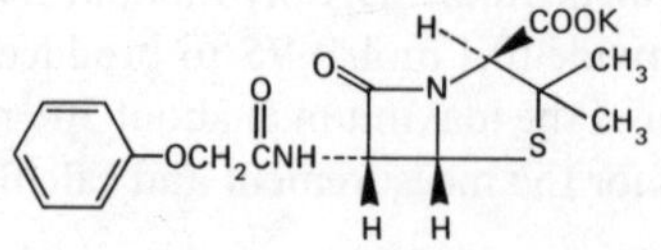

Chemical name. Potassium (2*S*,5*R*,6*R*)-3,3-dimethyl-7-oxo-6-(2-phenoxy-acetamido)-4-thia-1-azabicyclo[3.2.0]heptane-2-carboxylate; potassium [2*S*-(2α,5α,6β)]-3,3-dimethyl-7-oxo-6-[(phenoxyacetyl)amino]-4-thia-1-azabicyclo-[3.2.0]heptane-2-carboxylate; CAS Reg. No. 132-98-9.

Description. A white or almost white, crystalline powder; odourless or with a faint characteristic odour.

Solubility. Soluble in about 1.5 parts of water; practically insoluble in chloroform R and ether R.

Category. Antibiotic.

Storage. Phenoxymethylpenicillin potassium should be kept in a tightly closed container; protected from light.

Additional information. Even in the absence of light, Phenoxymethylpenicillin potassium is gradually degraded on exposure to a humid atmosphere, the decomposition being faster at higher temperatures.

REQUIREMENTS

General requirement. Phenoxymethylpenicillin potassium contains not less than 95.0% and not more than 102.0% of $C_{16}H_{17}KN_2O_5S$, calculated with reference to the dried substance.

Identity tests

• Either tests A and D or tests B, C, and D may be applied.

A. Carry out the examination as described under "Spectrophotometry in the infrared region" (vol. 1, p. 40). The infrared absorption spectrum is concordant with the spectrum obtained from phenoxymethylpenicillin potassium RS or with the *reference spectrum* of phenoxymethylpenicillin potassium.

B. To 2 mg in a test-tube add 1 drop of water followed by 2 ml of sulfuric acid (~1760 g/l) TS and mix; the solution is colourless. Immerse the test-tube for 1 minute in a water-bath; the solution remains colourless.

C. Place 2 mg in a test-tube, add 1 drop of water and 2 ml of formaldehyde/ sulfuric acid TS and mix; the solution is red. Immerse the test-tube for 1 minute in a water-bath; a red-brown colour is produced.

D. Ignite a small quantity, dissolve the residue in water and filter. To the filtrate, add 2 ml of sodium hydroxide (~80 g/l) TS; it yields the reaction described under "General identification tests" as characteristic of potassium (vol. 1, p. 114).

Specific optical rotation. Use a 10 mg/ml solution and calculate with reference to the dried substance; $[\alpha]_D^{20\,°C} = +215$ to $+235\,°$.

Clarity of solution. A solution of 0.2 g in 10 ml of water is not more than slightly opalescent.

Loss on drying. Dry to constant weight at 105 °C; it loses not more than 15 mg/g.

pH value. pH of a 5.0 mg/ml solution in carbon-dioxide-free water R, 5.0–7.5.

p-**Hydroxyphenoxymethylpenicillin.** Dissolve about 0.11 g, accurately weighed, in sufficient sodium hydroxide (0.1 mol/l) VS to produce 100 ml. Measure the absorbance of a 1-cm layer at the maximum at about 306 nm; not more than 0.36 (preferably use 2-cm cells for the measurement and calculate the absorbance of a 1-cm layer).

Ultraviolet absorbance range. Dilute 20 ml of the solution obtained in the test for *p*-hydroxyphenoxymethylpenicillin to 100 ml with sodium hydroxide (0.1 mol/l) VS. Measure the absorbance of a 1-cm layer at the maximum at about 274 nm; not less than 0.56 and not more than 0.62.

Assay. Dissolve about 50 mg, accurately weighed, in sufficient water to produce 1000 ml. Transfer two 2.0-ml aliquots of this solution into separate stoppered tubes. To one tube add 10.0 ml of imidazole/mercuric chloride TS, mix, stopper the tube and place it in a water-bath at 60 °C for exactly 25 minutes. Cool the tube rapidly to 20 °C (solution A). To the second tube add 10.0 ml of water and mix (solution B).

Without delay measure the absorbance of a 1-cm layer at the maximum at about 325 nm against a solvent cell containing a mixture of 2.0 ml of water and 10.0 ml of imidazole/mercuric chloride TS for solution A and water for solution B.

From the difference between the absorbance of solution A and that of solution B, calculate the amount of $C_{16}H_{17}KN_2O_5S$ in the substance being tested by comparison with phenoxymethylpenicillin potassium RS, similarly and concurrently examined. In an adequately calibrated spectrophotometer the absorbance of the reference solution should be 0.63 ± 0.03.

PHENYTOINUM

Phenytoin

Molecular formula. $C_{15}H_{12}N_2O_2$

Relative molecular mass. 252.3

Graphic formula.

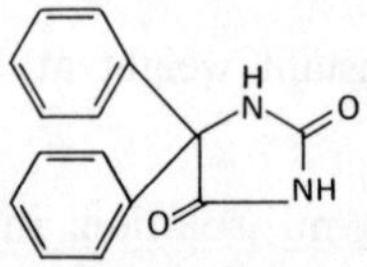

Chemical name. 5,5-Diphenylhydantoin; 5,5-diphenyl-2,4-imidazolidine-dione; CAS Reg. No. 57-41-0.

Description. A white, crystalline powder; odourless.

Solubility. Practically insoluble in water; sparingly soluble in ethanol (~750 g/l) TS; slightly soluble in ether R and chloroform R.

Category. Anticonvulsant.

Storage. Phenytoin should be kept in a tightly closed container, protected from light.

REQUIREMENTS

General requirement. Phenytoin contains not less than 98.0% and not more than 101.0% of $C_{15}H_{12}N_2O_2$, calculated with reference to the dried substance.

Identity tests

• Either test A alone or all 3 tests B, C, and D may be applied.

A. Carry out the examination as described under "Spectrophotometry in the infrared region" (vol. 1, p. 40). The infrared absorption spectrum is concordant with the spectrum obtained from phenytoin RS or with the *reference spectrum* of phenytoin.

B. Dissolve 20 mg in 2 ml of ammonia (~100 g/l) TS and add 5 ml of silver nitrate (40 g/l) TS; a white precipitate is produced.

C. Dissolve 5 mg in 1 ml of boiling ethanol (~750 g/l) TS, add 2 ml of water, 2 drops of pyridine R, and 2 drops of copper(II) sulfate (80 g/l) TS; allow to cool; a blue-violet, crystalline precipitate is produced.

D. Melting temperature, about 295 °C.

Heavy metals. Use 1.0 g for the preparation of the test solution, as described under "Limit test for heavy metals", Procedure 3 (vol. 1, p. 118); determine the heavy metals content according to Method A (vol. 1, p. 119); not more than 10 μg/g.

Sulfated ash. Not more than 1.0 mg/g.

Loss on drying. Dry to constant weight at 105 °C; it loses not more than 10 mg/g.

Acidity or alkalinity. Shake 2 g for 1 minute with 40 ml of carbon-dioxide-free water R, and filter. To 10 ml of the filtrate add 2 drops of phenolphthalein/ethanol TS; no colour is produced. Add 0.15 ml of carbonate-free sodium hydroxide (0.01 mol/l) VS; a pink colour is produced. Add 0.3 ml of hydrochloric acid (0.01 mol/l) VS and 5 drops of methyl red/ethanol TS; a red or orange colour is produced.

Assay. Dissolve about 0.5 g, accurately weighed, in 50 ml of dimethylformamide R, add 2 drops of thymol blue/dimethylformamide TS and titrate with sodium methoxide (0.1 mol/l) VS to a blue endpoint, as described under "Non-aqueous titration", Method B (vol. 1, p. 132). Each ml of sodium methoxide (0.1 mol/l) VS is equivalent to 25.23 mg of $C_{15}H_{12}N_2O_2$.

PHENYTOINUM NATRICUM
Phenytoin sodium

Molecular formula. $C_{15}H_{11}N_2NaO_2$

Relative molecular mass. 274.3

Graphic formula.

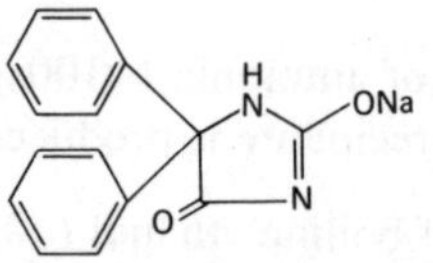

Chemical name. 5,5-Diphenylhydantoin monosodium salt; 5,5-diphenyl-2,4-imidazolidinedione monosodium salt; CAS Reg. No. 630-93-3.

Description. A white powder; odourless.

Solubility. Soluble in water, giving a slightly turbid solution owing to partial hydrolysis; soluble in ethanol (~750 g/l) TS; practically insoluble in ether R and chloroform R.

Category. Anticonvulsant.

Storage. Phenytoin sodium should be kept in a tightly closed container.

Additional information. Phenytoin sodium is somewhat hygroscopic and on exposure to air gradually absorbs carbon dioxide.

REQUIREMENTS

General requirement. Phenytoin sodium contains not less than 98.5% and not more than 101.0% of $C_{15}H_{11}N_2NaO_2$, calculated with reference to the dried substance.

Identity tests

• Either tests A and D or tests B, C, D, and E may be applied.
A. Shake 0.1 g with 20 ml of water, acidify with hydrochloric acid (~70 g/l) TS, and extract with chloroform R; wash the chloroform extract with water and

evaporate to dryness. Carry out the examination with the residue as described under "Spectrophotometry in the infrared region" (vol. 1, p. 40). The infrared absorption spectrum is concordant with the spectrum obtained from phenytoin RS or with the *reference spectrum* of phenytoin.

B. Dissolve 0.1 g in a mixture of 1 ml of pyridine R and 9 ml of water, add 1 ml of copper(II) sulfate/pyridine TS, and allow to stand for 10 minutes; a blue precipitate is produced.

C. Dissolve 10 mg in 1 ml of water, add 1 drop of ammonia (~100 g/l) TS and heat until boiling begins. Add 1 drop of copper(II) sulfate/ammonia TS and shake; a pink, crystalline precipitate is formed.

D. When tested for sodium as described under "General identification tests" (vol. 1, p. 115), yields the characteristic reactions. If reaction B is to be used, prepare a 20 mg/ml solution.

E. Shake 0.1 g with 20 ml of water, acidify with hydrochloric acid (~70 g/l) TS, and extract with chloroform R; wash the chloroform extract with water and evaporate to dryness. Melting temperature of the residue, about 295 °C (phenytoin).

Heavy metals. To 1.0 g add 24 ml of water and 6 ml of hydrochloric acid (~70 g/l) TS; heat the mixture until boiling begins. Filter, cool, and filter again through a suitable sintered glass filter. Dilute to 40 ml with water, mix, and determine the content of heavy metals as described under "Limit test for heavy metals", according to Method A (vol. 1, p. 119); not more than 10 μg/g.

Solution in alkali. To 20 mg add 8.0 ml of carbon-dioxide-free water R and then add gradually 2.0 ml of carbonate-free sodium hydroxide (0.1 mol/l) VS; the solution is clear and not more intensely coloured than standard colour solution Yw2 when compared as described under "Colour of liquids" (vol. 1, p. 50).

Loss on drying. Dry to constant weight at 105 °C; it loses not more than 30 mg/g.

Assay. Dissolve about 0.55 g, accurately weighed, in 30 ml of glacial acetic acid R1, add 3 drops of 1-naphtholbenzein/acetic acid TS as indicator and titrate with perchloric acid (0.1 mol/l) VS, as described under "Non-aqueous titration", Method A (vol. 1, p. 131). Each ml of perchloric acid (0.1 mol/l) VS is equivalent to 27.43 mg of $C_{15}H_{11}N_2NaO_2$.

PHYSOSTIGMINI SALICYLAS
Physostigmine salicylate

Molecular formula. $C_{15}H_{21}N_3O_2,C_7H_6O_3$ or $C_{22}H_{27}N_3O_5$

Relative molecular mass. 413.5

Graphic formula.

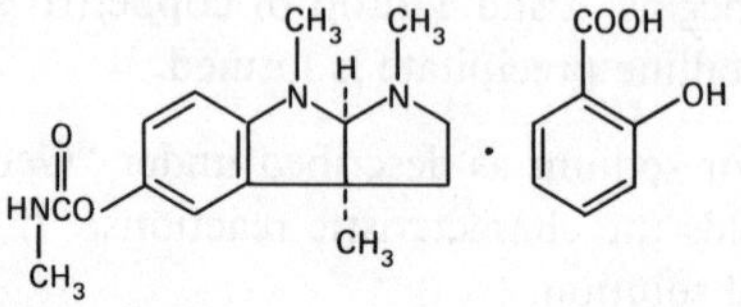

Chemical name. Physostigmine monosalicylate; (3aS-cis)-1,2,3,3a,8,8a-hexa-hydro-1,3a,8-trimethylpyrrolo[2,3-b]indol-5-ol, methylcarbamate (ester), mono-(2-hydroxybenzoate); CAS Reg. No. 57-64-7.

Other name. Eserine salicylate.

Description. Colourless crystals; odourless.

Solubility. Sparingly soluble in water; soluble in ethanol (~750 g/l) TS; freely soluble in chloroform R; slightly soluble in ether R.

Category. Anticholinesterase; miotic.

Storage. Physostigmine salicylate should be kept in a tightly closed container, protected from light, and preferably in quantities not exceeding 1 g.

Additional information. Physostigmine salicylate is very poisonous. It acquires a red tint when exposed to air or light. All tests should be performed on freshly prepared solutions.

REQUIREMENTS

General requirement. Physostigmine salicylate contains not less than 98.0% and not more than 101.0% of $C_{15}H_{21}N_3O_2,C_7H_6O_3$, calculated with reference to the dried substance.

Identity tests

A. To a 10 mg/ml solution add a few drops of sodium hydroxide (~80 g/l) TS; a white precipitate is produced, which gradually turns pink. It dissolves in an excess of the reagent to give a red solution.

B. Warm 10 mg with a few drops of ammonia (~100 g/l) TS; an orange solution is produced. Evaporate this solution and dissolve the residue in ethanol (~750 g/l) TS. To the resulting blue solution add a few drops of acetic acid (~300 g/l) TS; the colour is intensified. Dilute with water; a red fluorescence appears.

C. To a 10 mg/ml solution add a few drops of ferric chloride (25 g/l) TS; a violet colour, which remains after the addition of ethanol (~750 g/l) TS, appears.

D. Melting temperature, about 186 °C.

Specific optical rotation. Use a 10 mg/ml solution; $[\alpha]_D^{20\,°C} = -90$ to $-94\,°$.

Clarity and colour of solution. A solution of 0.10 g in 10 ml of water is clear and colourless.

Sulfated ash. Not more than 1.0 mg/g.

Loss on drying. Dry to constant weight at 105 °C; it loses not more than 10 mg/g.

pH value. pH of a 10 mg/ml solution, 4.6–5.2.

Eseridine. To 5 ml of a 10 mg/ml solution add 5 drops of hydrochloric acid (~70 g/l) TS, 1.5 ml of potassium iodate (0.01 mol/l) VS and 1 ml of chloroform R. Shake for 1 minute; no violet colour develops in the chloroform layer.

Assay. Dissolve about 0.35 g, accurately weighed, in 30 ml of a mixture of equal volumes of chloroform R and glacial acetic acid R1. Titrate with perchloric acid (0.1 mol/l) VS, determining the endpoint potentiometrically as described under "Non-aqueous titration", Method A (vol. 1, p. 131). Each ml of perchloric acid (0.1 mol/l) VS is equivalent to 41.35 mg of $C_{15}H_{21}N_3O_2,C_7H_6O_3$.

PILOCARPINI HYDROCHLORIDUM

Pilocarpine hydrochloride

Molecular formula. $C_{11}H_{16}N_2O_2$,HCl

Relative molecular mass. 244.7

Graphic formula.

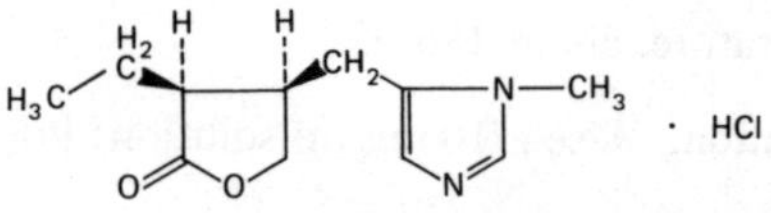

Chemical name. Pilocarpine monohydrochloride; (3S-cis)-3-ethyldihydro-4-[(1-methyl-1H-imidazol-5-yl)methyl]-2(3H)-furanone monohydrochloride; CAS Reg. No. 54-71-7.

Description. Colourless crystals or a white, crystalline powder; odourless or almost odourless.

Solubility. Very soluble in water; freely soluble in ethanol (~750 g/l) TS; slightly soluble in chloroform R; insoluble in ether R.

Category. Parasympathomimetic; miotic.

Storage. Pilocarpine hydrochloride should be kept in a tightly closed container, protected from light.

Additional information. Pilocarpine hydrochloride is very poisonous; it is hygroscopic and is affected by light. Even in the absence of light, Pilocarpine hydrochloride is gradually degraded on exposure to a humid atmosphere, the decomposition being faster at higher temperatures.

REQUIREMENTS

General requirement. Pilocarpine hydrochloride contains not less than 98.5% and not more than 101.0% of $C_{11}H_{16}N_2O_2$,HCl, calculated with reference to the dried substance.

Identity tests

A.   Dissolve 10 mg in 5 ml of water, add 2 drops of sulfuric acid (~100 g/l) TS, 1 ml of hydrogen peroxide (~60 g/l) TS, 1 ml of toluene R, and 1 drop of potassium dichromate (100 g/l) TS, and shake well; the toluene layer acquires a violet colour, whereas the aqueous layer remains yellow.

B.   A 0.05 g/ml solution yields reaction B described under "General identification tests" as characteristic of chlorides (vol. 1, p. 113).

C.   Melting temperature, about 203 °C.

Specific optical rotation.   Use a 50 mg/ml solution; $[\alpha]_D^{20\,°C} = +89$ to $+93\,°$.

Nitrates.   Dissolve 0.05 g in 5 ml of water and carefully add the solution to 5 ml of a 1 mg/ml solution of diphenylamine R in sulfuric acid (~1760 g/l) TS, ensuring that the liquids do not mix; no blue colour is produced at the interface of the two liquids.

Clarity and colour of solution.   A solution of 1.0 g in 10 ml of water is clear and colourless.

Sulfated ash.   Not more than 3.0 mg/g.

Loss on drying.   Dry to constant weight at 105 °C; it loses not more than 20 mg/g.

pH value.   pH of a 5.0 mg/ml solution, 3.8–5.2.

Related alkaloids.   Carry out the tests as described under "Thin-layer chromatography" (vol. 1, p. 83), using silica gel R1 as the coating substance and a mixture of 25 volumes of chloroform R, 20 volumes of acetone R, and 0.4 volumes of ammonia (~260 g/l) TS as the mobile phase. Apply separately to the plate 5 µl of each of 2 solutions containing (A) 50 mg of the test substance per ml and (B) 1.0 mg of the test substance per ml. After removing the plate from the chromatographic chamber, allow it to dry in air, spray with potassium iodobismuthate TS2, and examine the chromatogram in daylight. Any spot obtained with solution A, other than the principal spot, is not more intense than that obtained with solution B.

Assay.   Dissolve about 0.5 g, accurately weighed, in 30 ml of glacial acetic acid R1, add 10 ml of mercuric acetate/acetic acid TS, and titrate with perchloric acid (0.1 mol/l) VS as described under "Non-aqueous titration", Method A (vol. 1, p. 131). Each ml of perchloric acid (0.1 mol/l) VS is equivalent to 24.47 mg of $C_{11}H_{16}N_2O_2$,HCl.

PILOCARPINI NITRAS

Pilocarpine nitrate

Molecular formula. $C_{11}H_{16}N_2O_2,HNO_3$

Relative molecular mass. 271.3

Graphic formula.

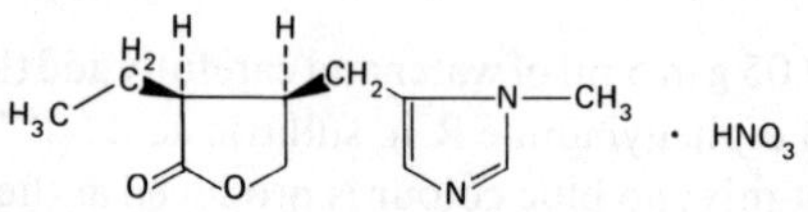

Chemical name. Pilocarpine mononitrate; (3S-cis)-3-ethyldihydro-4-[(1-methyl-1H-imidazol-5-yl)methyl]-2(3H)-furanone mononitrate; CAS Reg. No. 148-72-1.

Description. Colourless crystals or a white, crystalline powder; odourless.

Solubility. Freely soluble in water; sparingly soluble in ethanol (~750 g/l) TS; practically insoluble in chloroform R and ether R.

Category. Parasympathomimetic; miotic.

Storage. Pilocarpine nitrate should be kept in a tightly closed container, protected from light.

Additional information. Pilocarpine nitrate is very poisonous; it is affected by light. Even in the absence of light, Pilocarpine nitrate is gradually degraded on exposure to a humid atmosphere, the decomposition being faster at higher temperatures.

REQUIREMENTS

General requirement. Pilocarpine nitrate contains not less than 98.5% and not more than 101.0% of $C_{11}H_{16}N_2O_2,HNO_3$, calculated with reference to the dried substance.

Identity tests

A.   Dissolve 10 mg in 5 ml of water, add 2 drops of sulfuric acid ($\sim$100 g/l) TS, 1 ml of hydrogen peroxide ($\sim$60 g/l) TS, 1 ml of toluene R, and 1 drop of potassium dichromate (100 g/l) TS, and shake well; the toluene layer acquires a violet colour, whereas the aqueous layer remains yellow.

B.   To 2 ml of a 0.05 g/ml solution add 2 ml of ferrous sulfate (15 g/l) TS; it yields reaction A described under "General identification tests" as characteristic of nitrates (vol. 1, p. 114).

C.   Melting temperature, about 176 °C with decomposition.

Specific optical rotation.   Use a 50 mg/ml solution; $[\alpha]_D^{20\,°C} = +80$ to $+83$ °.

Chlorides.   Dissolve 0.7 g in a mixture of 2 ml of nitric acid ($\sim$130 g/l) TS and 30 ml of water, and proceed as described under "Limit test for chlorides" (vol. 1, p. 116); the chloride content is not more than 0.35 mg/g.

Clarity and colour of solution.   A solution of 1.0 g in 10 ml of water is clear and colourless.

Sulfated ash.   Not more than 2.0 mg/g.

Loss on drying.   Dry to constant weight at 105 °C; it loses not more than 20 mg/g.

pH value.   pH of a 5.0 mg/ml solution in water, 3.5–4.5.

Related alkaloids.   Carry out the test as described under "Thin-layer chromatography" (vol. 1, p. 83), using silica gel R1 as the coating substance and a mixture of 25 volumes of chloroform R, 20 volumes of acetone R, and 0.4 volume of ammonia ($\sim$260 g/l) TS as the mobile phase.   Apply separately to the plate 5 μl of each of 2 solutions containing (A) 50 mg of the test substance per ml and (B) 1.0 mg of the test substance per ml.   After removing the plate from the chromatographic chamber, allow it to dry in air, spray with potassium iodobismuthate TS2, and examine the chromatogram in daylight.   Any spot obtained with solution A, other than the principal spot, is not more intense than that obtained with solution B.

Assay.   Dissolve about 0.55 g, accurately weighed, in 30 ml of glacial acetic acid R1, and titrate with perchloric acid (0.1 mol/l) VS as described under "Non-aqueous titration", Method A (vol.1, p. 131).   Each ml of perchloric acid (0.1 mol/l) VS is equivalent to 27.13 mg of $C_{11}H_{16}N_2O_2$,HNO_3.

PIPERAZINI ADIPAS

Piperazine adipate

Molecular formula. $C_4H_{10}N_2,C_6H_{10}O_4$ or $C_{10}H_{20}N_2O_4$

Relative molecular mass.   232.3

Graphic formula.

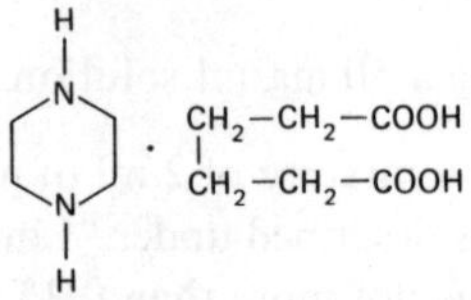

$$
\begin{array}{c}
\text{H} \\
| \\
\text{N} \\
\diagup \quad \diagdown \\
\diagdown \quad \diagup \\
\text{N} \\
| \\
\text{H}
\end{array}
\cdot
\begin{array}{l}
\text{CH}_2-\text{CH}_2-\text{COOH} \\
| \\
\text{CH}_2-\text{CH}_2-\text{COOH}
\end{array}
$$

Chemical name.   Piperazine hexanedioate (1:1); hexahydro-1,4-diazine adipate (1:1); CAS Reg. No. 142-88-1.

Description.   Colourless crystals or a white, crystalline powder; odourless.

Solubility.   Soluble in water; practically insoluble in ethanol ($\sim$750 g/l) TS, ether R, and chloroform R.

Category.   Anthelmintic.

Storage.   Piperazine adipate should be kept in a well-closed container.

REQUIREMENTS

General requirement.   Piperazine adipate contains not less than 98.0% and not more than 101.0% of $C_4H_{10}N_2,C_6H_{10}O_4$, calculated with reference to the dried substance.

Identity tests

A.   Dissolve 0.1 g in 5 ml of water, add 0.5 g of sodium hydrogen carbonate R, 0.5 ml of freshly prepared potassium ferricyanide (50 g/l) TS, and 0.1 ml of mercury R. Shake vigorously for 1 minute, and allow to stand for 20 minutes; a reddish colour slowly develops.

B.   Dissolve 0.5 g in 10 ml of water and add 5 ml of hydrochloric acid (~250 g/l) TS.   Extract 3 times with ether R, using 10 ml each time, and keep the aqueous layer for test C.   Evaporate the ether extracts to dryness and dry at 105 °C; melting temperature, about 152 °C (adipic acid).

C.   Cautiously heat the aqueous layer obtained from test B to eliminate any dissolved ether.   Cool and add 0.5 g of sodium nitrite R.   Heat to boiling and cool in ice for 15 minutes, stirring if necessary to induce crystallization.   Filter, wash with 10 ml of ice-water and dry the precipitate at 105 °C; melting temperature, about 158 °C (N,N'-dinitrosopiperazine).

Heavy metals.   Use 1.0 g for the preparation of the test solution as described under "Limit test for heavy metals", Procedure 1 (vol. 1, p. 118); determine the heavy metals content according to Method A (vol. 1, p. 119); not more than 20 μg/g.

Sulfated ash.   Not more than 1.0 mg/g.

Loss on drying.   Dry to constant weight at 105 °C; it loses not more than 5.0 mg/g.

pH value.   pH of a 0.05 g/ml solution, 5.0–6.0.

Primary amines.   For the preparation of the test solution dissolve 0.25 g in sufficient water to produce 50 ml.   Transfer 0.5 ml of this solution to a test-tube. Separately transfer to a second test-tube 0.5 ml of a solution containing 10 μg/ml of ethylenediamine R to serve as a reference solution.   To both tubes add 0.5 ml of ethanol (~750 g/l) TS, 1 ml of diethoxytetrahydrofuran/acetic acid TS, heat on a water-bath at 80 °C for 30 minutes, cool in ice, and add 3 ml of 4-dimethylami- nobenzaldehyde TS4.   Measure the absorbance at about 570 nm, 7–10 minutes after the addition of the last reagent, against a solvent cell containing the reagents prepared in a similar manner.   The absorbance of the test solution is not more intense than that of the reference solution.

Assay.   Dissolve about 0.20 g, accurately weighed, in 3.5 ml of sulfuric acid (0.5 mol/l) VS and 10 ml of water; add 100 ml of trinitrophenol (7 g/l) TS, heat on a water-bath for 15 minutes, and allow to stand for 1 hour.   Filter, wash the residue with successive quantities of trinitrophenol (7 g/l) TS, using 10 ml each time, until the washings are free from sulfates.   Finally, wash with dehydrated ethanol R, and dry the residue to constant weight at 105 °C.   Each g of residue is equivalent to 426.8 mg of $C_4H_{10}N_2,C_6H_{10}O_4$.

PIPERAZINI CITRAS
Piperazine citrate

Molecular formula. $(C_4H_{10}N_2)_3,2C_6H_8O_7$ or $C_{24}H_{46}N_6O_{14}$ (anhydrous)

Relative molecular mass. 642.7 (anhydrous)

Graphic formula.

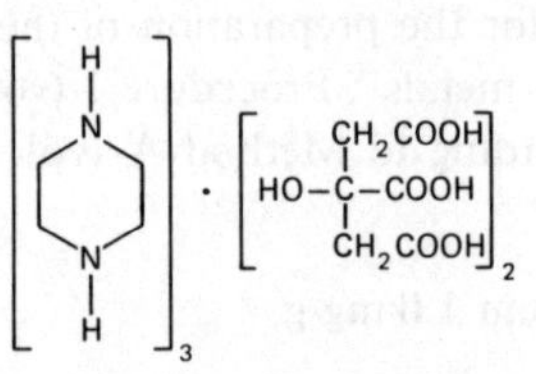

Chemical name. Piperazine 2-hydroxy-1,2,3-propanetricarboxylate (3:2); hexahydro-1,4-diazine citrate (3:2); CAS Reg. No. 144-29-6 (anhydrous).

Description. A fine, white, granular powder; almost odourless.

Solubility. Soluble in 1.5 parts of water; practically insoluble in ethanol (~750 g/l) TS and ether R.

Category. Anthelmintic.

Storage. Piperazine citrate should be kept in a well-closed container, protected from light.

Additional information. Piperazine citrate contains a variable amount of water of crystallization.

REQUIREMENTS

General requirement. Piperazine citrate contains not less than 98.0% and not more than 101.0% of $(C_4H_{10}N_2)_3,2C_6H_8O_7$, calculated with reference to the anhydrous substance.

Identity tests

A. Dissolve 0.1 g in 5 ml of water, add 0.5 g of sodium hydrogen carbonate R, 0.5 ml of freshly prepared potassium ferricyanide (50 g/l) TS, and 0.1 ml of mercury R. Shake vigorously for 1 minute, and allow to stand for 20 minutes; a reddish colour slowly develops.

B.   A 20 mg/ml solution yields reaction A described under "General identification tests" as characteristic of citrates (vol. 1, p. 113).

C.   Melting temperature, after drying at 105 °C, about 185 °C.

D.   Dissolve 0.2 g in 5 ml of hydrochloric acid (~70 g/l) TS, and add 0.5 g of sodium nitrite R.   Cool in ice for 15 minutes, stir if necessary to induce crystallization, filter, wash with 10 ml of ice-water, and dry the precipitate at 105 °C; melting temperature, about 158 °C (*N,N'*-dinitrosopiperazine).

Heavy metals.   Use 1.0 g for the preparation of the test solution as described under "Limit test for heavy metals", Procedure 1 (vol. 1, p. 118); determine the heavy metals content according to Method A (vol. 1, p. 119); not more than 20 μg/g.

Sulfated ash.   Not more than 1.0 mg/g.

Water.   Determine as described under "Determination of water by the Karl Fischer method", Method A (vol. 1, p. 135), using about 0.2 g of the substance; the water content is not less than 0.10 g/g and not more than 0.14 g/g.

pH value.   pH of a 0.05 g/ml solution, 5.0–6.0.

Primary amines.   For the preparation of the test solution dissolve 0.25 g in sufficient water to produce 50 ml.   Transfer 0.5 ml of this solution to a test-tube. Separately transfer to a second test-tube 0.5 ml of a solution containing 10 μg/ml of ethylenediamine R to serve as a reference solution.   To both tubes add 0.5 ml of ethanol (~750 g/l) TS, 1 ml of diethoxytetrahydrofuran/acetic acid TS, heat on a water-bath at 80 °C for 30 minutes, cool in ice, and add 3 ml of 4-dimethylaminobenzaldehyde TS4.   Measure the absorbance at about 570 nm, 7–10 minutes after the addition of the last reagent, against a solvent cell containing the reagents prepared in a similar manner.   The absorbance of the test solution is not more intense than that of the reference solution.

Assay.   Dissolve about 0.20 g, accurately weighed, in 3.5 ml of sulfuric acid (0.5 mol/l) VS and 10 ml of water, add 100 ml of trinitrophenol (7 g/l) TS, heat on a water-bath for 15 minutes, and allow to stand for 1 hour.   Filter, wash the residue with successive quantities of trinitrophenol (7 g/l) TS, using 10 ml each time, until the washings are free from sulfates.   Finally, wash with dehydrated ethanol R, and dry the residue to constant weight at 105 °C.   Each g of residue is equivalent to 393.5 mg of $(C_4H_{10}N_2)_3,2C_6H_8O_7$.

PREDNISOLONUM

Prednisolone

Molecular formula. $C_{21}H_{28}O_5$

Relative molecular mass. 360.5

Graphic formula.

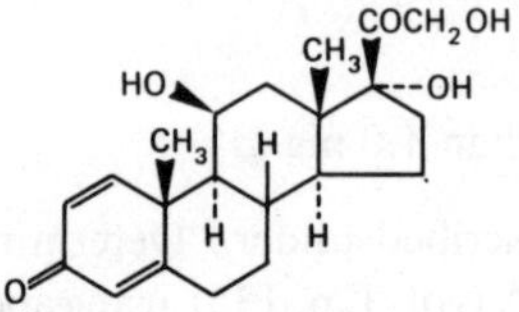

Chemical name. 11β,17,21-Trihydroxypregna-1,4-diene-3,20-dione; CAS Reg. No. 50-24-8.

Description. A white or almost white, crystalline powder; odourless.

Solubility. Soluble in 1300 parts of water and in 30 parts of dehydrated ethanol R; soluble in methanol R and dioxan R.

Category. Adrenocortical steroid.

Storage. Prednisolone should be kept in a tightly closed container, protected from light.

Additional information. Prednisolone is hygroscopic; it has a melting temperature of about 230 °C with decomposition.

REQUIREMENTS

General requirement. Prednisolone contains not less than 97.0% and not more than 102.0% of $C_{21}H_{28}O_5$, calculated with reference to the dried substance.

Identity tests

• Either test A or test B may be applied.

A. Carry out the examination as described under "Spectrophotometry in the infrared region" (vol. 1, p. 40). The infrared absorption spectrum is concordant with the spectrum obtained from prednisolone RS or with the *reference spectrum* of prednisolone.

B.   Carry out the test as described under "Thin-layer chromatography", (vol. 1, p. 83), using kieselguhr R1 as the coating substance and a mixture of 10 volumes of formamide R and 90 volumes of acetone R to impregnate the plate, dipping it about 5 mm beneath the surface of the liquid.   After the solvent has reached a height of at least 16 cm, remove the plate from the chromatographic chamber and allow it to stand at room temperature until the solvent has completely evaporated. Use the impregnated plate within 2 hours, carrying out the chromatography in the same direction as the impregnation.   Use chloroform R as the mobile phase. Apply separately to the plate 2 μl of each of 2 solutions in a mixture of 9 volumes of chloroform R and 1 volume of methanol R containing (A) 2.5 mg of the test substance per ml and (B) 2.5 mg of prednisolone RS per ml.   Develop the plate for a distance of 15 cm.   After removing the plate from the chromatographic chamber, allow it to dry in air until the solvents have evaporated, heat at 120 °C for 15 minutes, spray with sulfuric acid/ethanol TS, and then heat at 120 °C for 10 minutes.   Allow to cool, and examine the chromatogram in daylight and in ultraviolet light (365 nm).   The principal spot obtained with solution A corresponds in position, appearance, and intensity with that obtained with solution B.

Specific optical rotation.   Use a 10 mg/ml solution in dioxan R; $[\alpha]_D^{20\,°C} = +96$ to +103 °.

Loss on drying.   Dry to constant weight at 105 °C; it loses not more than 10 mg/g.

Related substances.   Carry out the test as described under "Thin-layer chromatography" (vol. 1, p. 83), using silica gel R2 as the coating substance and a mixture of 77 volumes of dichloromethane R, 15 volumes of ether R, 8 volumes of methanol R, and 1.2 volumes of water as the mobile phase.   Apply separately to the plate 1 μl of each of 2 solutions in a mixture of 9 volumes of chloroform R and 1 volume of methanol R containing (A) 15 mg of the test substance per ml and (B) 0.30 mg of the test substance per ml.   After removing the plate from the chromatographic chamber, allow it to dry in air until the solvents have evaporated and heat at 105 °C for 10 minutes; cool, and examine the chromatogram in ultraviolet light (254 nm).   Any spot obtained with solution A, other than the principal spot, is not more intense than that obtained with solution B.

Assay.   Dissolve about 20 mg, accurately weighed, in sufficient ethanol (~750 g/l) TS to produce 100 ml; dilute 5.0 ml of this solution to 100 ml with the same solvent.   Measure the absorbance of a 1-cm layer of the diluted solution at the maximum at about 242 nm.   Calculate the amount of $C_{21}H_{28}O_5$ in the substance being tested by comparison with prednisolone RS, similarly and concurrently examined.   In an adequately calibrated spectrophotometer the absorbance of the reference solution should be 0.44 ± 0.02 (preferably use 2-cm cells for the measurement and calculate the absorbance of a 1-cm layer).

PRIMAQUINI DIPHOSPHAS

Primaquine diphosphate

Molecular formula. $C_{15}H_{21}N_3O,2H_3PO_4$.

Relative molecular mass. 455.3

Graphic formula.

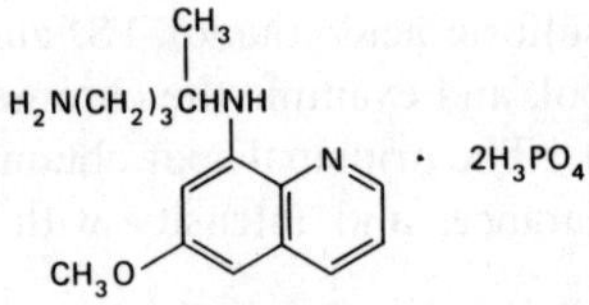

Chemical name. 8-[(4-Amino-1-methylbutyl)amino]-6-methoxyquinoline phosphate (1:2); N^4-(6-methoxy-8-quinolinyl)-1,4-pentanediamine phosphate (1:2); CAS Reg. No. 63-45-6.

Description. An orange-red, crystalline powder; odourless or almost odourless.

Solubility. Soluble in water; practically insoluble in ethanol (~750 g/l) TS, chloroform R, and ether R.

Category. Antimalarial.

Storage. Primaquine diphosphate should be kept in a well-closed container, protected from light.

REQUIREMENTS

General requirement. Primaquine diphosphate contains not less than 98.0% and not more than 102.0% of $C_{15}H_{21}N_3O,2H_3PO_4$, calculated with reference to the dried substance.

Identity tests

• Either tests A and C or tests B, C, and D may be applied.

A. Carry out the examination as described under "Spectrophotometry in the infrared region" (vol. 1, p. 40). The infrared absorption spectrum is concordant with the spectrum obtained from primaquine diphosphate RS or with the *reference spectrum* of primaquine diphospate.

B. Dissolve 10 mg in 5 ml of water and add 1 ml of ceric ammonium sulfate/nitric acid TS; a deep violet colour is immediately produced (distinction from chloroquine).

C. To 1 ml of a 20 mg/ml solution add 3 ml of nitric acid (~130 g/l) TS; it yields reaction A described under "General identification tests" as characteristic of orthophosphates (vol. 1, p. 114).

D. Melting temperature, about 202 °C.

Loss on drying. Dry to constant weight at 105 °C; it loses not more than 10 mg/g.

pH value. pH of a 10 mg/ml solution, 2.5–3.5.

Related substances. Carry out the test as described under "Thin-layer chromatography" (vol. 1, p. 83), using silica gel R1 as the coating substance and a mixture of 3 volumes of dimethylamine/ethanol TS, 4 volumes of acetone R and 5 volumes of chloroform R as the mobile phase. To 5 ml of a solution containing 20 mg of the test substance per ml add 5 ml of chloroform R and 0.5 ml of ammonia (~35 g/l) TS and shake. Separate the chloroform layer, filter and apply 5 μl of this solution to the plate. After removing the plate from the chromatographic chamber, allow it to dry in air, and examine the chromatogram in ultraviolet light (365 nm). Only a single fluorescent spot is obtained.

Assay. Carry out the assay as described under "Nitrite titration" (vol. 1, p. 133), using about 0.9 g, accurately weighed, and 50 ml of hydrochloric acid (~70 g/l) TS. Each ml of sodium nitrite (0.1 mol/l) VS is equivalent to 45.53 mg of $C_{15}H_{21}N_3O,2H_3PO_4$.

PROCAINAMIDI HYDROCHLORIDUM

Procainamide hydrochloride

Molecular formula. $C_{13}H_{21}N_3O,HCl$

Relative molecular mass. 271.8

Graphic formula.

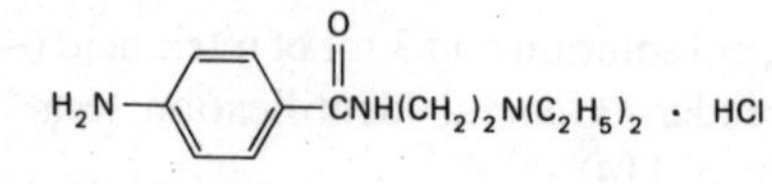

$$H_2N-\!\!\!\left\langle\ \right\rangle\!\!\!-CNH(CH_2)_2N(C_2H_5)_2 \cdot HCl$$

Chemical name. p-Amino-N-[2-(diethylamino)ethyl]benzamide monohydrochloride; 4-amino-N-[2-(diethylamino)ethyl]benzamide monohydrochloride; CAS Reg. No. 614-39-1.

Description. A white to yellowish white, crystalline powder; odourless.

Solubility. Very soluble in water; freely soluble in ethanol (~750 g/l) TS; slightly soluble in chloroform R; very slightly soluble in ether R.

Category. Antiarrhythmic.

Storage. Procainamide hydrochloride should be kept in a tightly closed container, protected from light.

Additional information. Procainamide hydrochloride is hygroscopic. Even in the absence of light, Procainamide hydrochloride is gradually degraded on exposure to a humid atmosphere, the decomposition being faster at higher temperatures.

REQUIREMENTS

General requirement. Procainamide hydrochloride contains not less than 98.0% and not more than 101.0% of $C_{13}H_{21}N_3O,HCl$, calculated with reference to the dried substance.

Identity tests

A. Dissolve 1 g in 10 ml of water, add 10 ml of sodium hydroxide (~200 g/l) TS, and extract with 10 ml of chloroform R. To the extract add 10 ml of toluene R, dry over anhydrous sodium sulfate R, and filter. Mix the filtrate with 5 ml of anhydrous pyridine R, add 1 ml of benzoyl chloride R drop by drop, heat on a water-bath for 30 minutes, and pour into a mixture of 50 ml of water and 50 ml of sodium hydroxide (~200 g/l) TS. Extract with 10 ml of ether R, wash the extract with 20 ml of water, dilute with 30 ml of ether R, and allow to crystallize. Recrystallize from ethanol (~375 g/l) TS; melting temperature, about 185 °C (benzoyl procainamide).

B.   Dissolve 0.1 g in 2 ml of water and add 2 ml of potassium ferrocyanide (45 g/l) TS. Add a few drops of hydrochloric acid (~70 g/l) TS to acidify slightly and heat; a light green precipitate is produced.

C.   A 0.05 g/ml solution yields reaction B described under "General identification tests" as characteristic of chlorides (vol. 1, p. 113).

Melting range.   165–169 °C.

Heavy metals.   Use 1.0 g for the preparation of the test solution as described under "Limit test for heavy metals", Procedure 3 (vol.1, p. 118); determine the heavy metals content according to Method A (vol. 1, p. 119); not more than 20 μg/g.

Sulfated ash.   Not more than 1.0 mg/g.

Loss on drying.   Dry to constant weight at 105 °C; it loses not more than 3.0 mg/g.

pH value.   pH of a 0.10 g/ml solution in carbon-dioxide-free water R, 5.0–6.5.

Related substances.   Carry out the test as described under "Thin-layer chromatography" (vol. 1, p. 83), using silica gel R2 as the coating substance and a mixture of 4 volumes of 1-butanol R, 1 volume of glacial acetic acid R, and 2 volumes of water as the mobile phase. Apply separately to the plate 2 μl of each of 2 solutions in ethanol (~750 g/l) TS containing (A) 50 mg of the test substance per ml and (B) 0.25 mg of the test substance per ml. After removing the plate from the chromatographic chamber, allow it dry in air, and examine the chromatogram in ultraviolet light (254 nm). Any spot obtained with solution A, other than the principal spot, is not more intense than that obtained with solution B.

Assay.   Dissolve about 0.25 g, accurately weighed, in 5 ml of acetic anhydride R and 15 ml of glacial acetic acid R1. Heat the solution until boiling. Add 20 ml of dioxan R and 20 ml of mercuric acetate/acetic acid TS and titrate with perchloric acid (0.1 mol/l) VS as described under "Non-aqueous titration", Method A (vol. 1, p. 131). Each ml of perchloric acid (0.1 mol/l) VS is equivalent to 27.18 mg of $C_{13}H_{21}N_3O,HCl$.

PROCAINI HYDROCHLORIDUM
Procaine hydrochloride

Molecular formula. $C_{13}H_{20}N_2O_2,HCl$

Relative molecular mass. 272.8

Graphic formula.

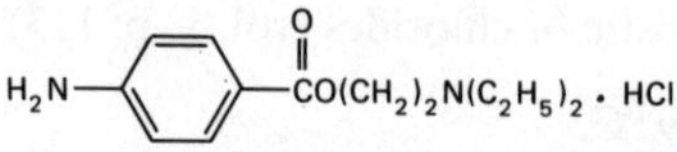

$$H_2N-\underset{}{\bigcirc}-CO(CH_2)_2N(C_2H_5)_2 \cdot HCl$$

Chemical name. 2-(Diethylamino)ethyl p-aminobenzoate monohydrochloride; 2-(diethylamino)ethyl 4-aminobenzoate monohydrochloride; CAS Reg. No. 51-05-8.

Description. Colourless crystals or a white, crystalline powder; odourless.

Solubility. Soluble in 1 part of water and in 25 parts of ethanol (~750 g/l) TS; slightly soluble in chloroform R; practically insoluble in ether R.

Category. Local anaesthetic.

Storage. Procaine hydrochloride should be kept in a tightly closed container, protected from light.

Additional information. Procaine hydrochloride causes local numbness after being placed on the tongue. Even in the absence of light, Procaine hydrochloride is gradually degraded on exposure to a humid atmosphere, the decomposition being faster at higher temperatures.

REQUIREMENTS

General requirement. Procaine hydrochloride contains not less than 99.0% and not more than 101.0% of $C_{13}H_{20}N_2O_2,HCl$, calculated with reference to the dried substance.

Identity tests

• Either tests A and D or tests B, C, and D may be applied.

A. Carry out the examination as described under "Spectrophotometry in the infrared region" (vol. 1, p. 40). The infrared absorption spectrum is concordant with the spectrum obtained from procaine hydrochloride RS or with the *reference spectrum* of procaine hydrochloride.

B.   About 0.05 g yields the reaction described for the identification of primary aromatic amines under "General identification tests" (vol. 1, p. 111), producing a vivid red precipitate.

C.   Dissolve 0.05 g in 5 ml of water, add 5 drops of sulfuric acid (~100 g/l) TS and 2 drops of potassium permanganate (0.02 mol/l) VS; the violet colour produced disappears quickly.
D.   A 0.05 g/ml solution yields reaction B described under "General identification tests" as characteristic of chlorides (vol. 1, p. 113).

Melting range.   154–158 °C.

Heavy metals.   Use 1.0 g for the preparation of the test solution as described under "Limit test for heavy metals", Procedure 1 (vol. 1, p.118); determine the heavy metals content according to Method A (vol. 1, p. 119); not more than 20 μg/g.

Clarity and colour of solution.   A solution of 1.0 g in 10 ml of carbon-dioxide-free water R is clear and colourless.

Sulfated ash.   Not more than 1.5 mg/g.

Loss on drying.   Dry to constant weight at 105 °C; it loses not more than 10 mg/g.

pH value.   pH of a 10 mg/ml solution in carbon-dioxide-free water R, 5.0–6.5.

Related substances.   Carry out the test as described under "Thin-layer chromatography" (vol. 1, p. 83), using silica gel R2 as the coating substance and a mixture of 80 volumes of dibutyl ether R, 16 volumes of hexane R, and 4 volumes of glacial acetic acid R as the mobile phase.   Apply separately to the plate 5 μl of each of 2 solutions containing (A) 0.10 g of the test substance per ml and (B) 0.050 mg of 4-aminobenzoic acid R per ml.   After removing the plate from the chromatographic chamber, allow it to dry at 105 °C for 10 minutes, and examine the chromatogram in ultraviolet light (254 nm).   Any spot obtained with solution A, other than the principal spot, is not more intense than that obtained with solution B.   The principal spot remains at the point of application.

Assay.   Carry out the assay as described under "Nitrite titration" (vol. 1, p. 133); dissolve about 0.5 g, accurately weighed, in 50 ml of hydrochloric acid (~70 g/l) TS, add 0.1 g of potassium bromide R, and titrate with sodium nitrite (0.1 mol/l) VS.   Each ml of sodium nitrite (0.1 mol/l) VS is equivalent to 27.28 mg of $C_{13}H_{20}N_2O_2$,HCl.

PROGESTERONUM
Progesterone

Molecular formula. $C_{21}H_{30}O_2$

Relative molecular mass. 314.5

Graphic formula.

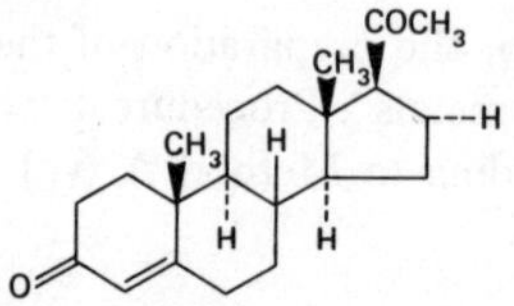

Chemical name. Pregn-4-ene-3,20-dione; CAS Reg. No. 57-83-0.

Description. Colourless crystals or a white to slightly yellowish white, crystalline powder; odourless.

Solubility. Practically insoluble in water; soluble in 8 parts of ethanol (~750 g/l) TS.

Category. Progestational steroid.

Storage. Progesterone should be kept in a well-closed container, protected from light.

Additional information. Progesterone may exist in 2 polymorphic forms, one of which melts at about 130 °C, the other at about 121 °C.

REQUIREMENTS

General requirement. Progesterone contains not less than 97.0% and not more than 102.0% of $C_{21}H_{30}O_2$, calculated with reference to the dried substance.

Identity tests

• Either test A or test B may be applied.
A. Carry out the examination as described under "Spectrophotometry in the infrared region" (vol. 1, p. 40). The infrared absorption spectrum is concordant with the spectrum obtained from progesterone RS or with the *reference spectrum* of progesterone. If the spectrum obtained from the solid state of the test substance is not concordant with the spectrum obtained from the reference substance, compare

the spectra using solutions in chloroform R containing 30 mg/ml and a path length of 0.2 mm.

B.   Carry out the test as described under "Thin-layer chromatography" (vol. 1, p. 83), using kieselguhr R1 as the coating substance and a mixture of 10 volumes of propylene glycol R and 90 volumes of acetone R to impregnate the plate, dipping it about 5 mm beneath the surface of the liquid. After the solvent has reached the height of at least 16 cm, remove the plate from the chromatographic chamber and allow it to stand at room temperature until the solvent has completely evaporated. Use the impregnated plate within 2 hours, carrying out the chromatography in the same direction as the impregnation. As the mobile phase, use a mixture of 50 volumes of cyclohexane R and 50 volumes of light petroleum R. Apply separately to the plate 5 μl of each of 2 solutions in a mixture of 9 volumes of chloroform R and 1 volume of methanol R containing (A) 1.0 mg of the test substance per ml and (B) 1.0 mg of progesterone RS per ml. Develop the plate for a distance of 15 cm. After removing the plate from the chromatographic chamber allow it to dry in air until the solvents have evaporated, heat at 120 °C for 15 minutes, spray with 4-toluenesulfonic acid/ethanol TS, and then heat at 120 °C for 10 minutes. Allow to cool and examine the chromatogram in daylight and in ultraviolet light (365 nm). The principal spot obtained with solution A corresponds in position, appearance, and intensity with that obtained with solution B.

Specific optical rotation. Use a 10 mg/ml solution in dehydrated ethanol R; $[\alpha]_D^{20\,°C} = +186$ to $+196$ °.

Loss on drying. Dry to constant weight at 105 °C; it loses not more than 5.0 mg/g.

Related substances. Carry out the test as described under "Thin-layer chromatography" (vol. 1, p. 83), using silica gel R2 as the coating substance and a mixture of 2 parts of chloroform R and 1 part of ethyl acetate R as the mobile phase. Apply separately to the plate 10 μl of each of 2 solutions in a mixture of 1 volume of ethanol (~750 g/l) TS and 1 volume of chloroform R containing (A) 10 mg of the test substance per ml and (B) 0.10 mg of the test substance per ml. After removing the plate from the chromatographic chamber, allow it to dry in air until the solvents have evaporated, and examine the chromatogram in ultraviolet light (254 nm). Any spot obtained with solution A, other than the principal spot, is not more intense than that obtained with solution B.

Assay. Dissolve about 20 mg, accurately weighed, in sufficient methanol R to produce 100 ml; dilute 5.0 ml of this solution to 100 ml with the same solvent. Measure the absorbance of a 1-cm layer of the diluted solution at the maximum at about 240 nm. Calculate the amount of $C_{21}H_{30}O_2$ in the substance being tested by comparison with progesterone RS, similarly and concurrently examined. In an adequately calibrated spectrophotometer the absorbance of the reference solution should be 0.54 ± 0.03.

PROPRANOLOLI HYDROCHLORIDUM

Propranolol hydrochloride

Molecular formula. $C_{16}H_{21}NO_2,HCl$

Relative molecular mass. 295.8

Graphic formula.

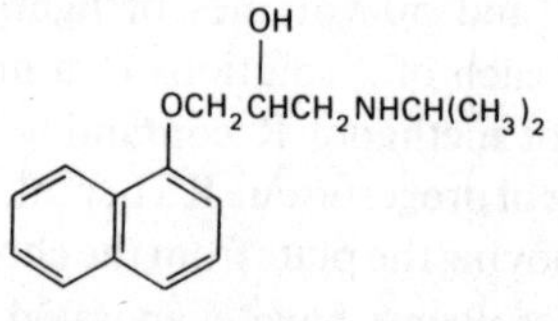

$$\underset{\text{OCH}_2\text{CHCH}_2\text{NHCH(CH}_3)_2}{\overset{\text{OH}}{|}}$$

· HCl

Chemical name. (±)-1-(Isopropylamino)-3-(1-naphthyloxy)-2-propanol hydrochloride; (±)-1-[(1-methylethyl)amino]-3-(1-naphthalenyloxy)-2-propanol hydrochloride; CAS Reg. No. 3506-09-0.

Description. A white or almost white, crystalline powder; odourless.

Solubility. Soluble in water and in ethanol (~750 g/l) TS; slightly soluble in chloroform R; practically insoluble in ether R.

Category. Antiadrenergic.

Storage. Propranolol hydrochloride should be kept in a well-closed container, protected from light.

REQUIREMENTS

General requirement. Propranolol hydrochloride contains not less than 98.0% and not more than 101.0% of $C_{16}H_{21}NO_2,HCl$, calculated with reference to the dried substance.

Identity tests

A. Carry out the examination as described under "Spectrophotometry in the infrared region" (vol. 1, p. 40). The infrared absorption spectrum is concordant with the spectrum obtained from propranolol hydrochloride RS or with the *reference spectrum* of propranolol hydrochloride.

B. The absorption spectrum of a 20 µg/ml solution in methanol R, when observed between 230 nm and 350 nm, is qualitatively similar to that of a 20 µg/ml solution in methanol R of propranolol hydrochloride RS (maxima occur at about 290 nm, 306 nm, and 319 nm). The absorbances of the solutions at their respective maxima do not differ from each other by more than 3%. The absorbances of a 1-cm layer at those wavelengths are about 0.42, 0.25 and 0.15 (preferably use 2-cm cells for the measurement and calculate the absorbances of 1-cm layers).

C. A 20 mg/ml solution yields reaction B described under "General identification tests" as characteristic of chlorides (vol. 1, p. 113).

Melting range. 161–165 °C.

Specific optical rotation. Use a 0.10 g/ml solution; the substance is optically inactive.

Clarity and colour of solution. A solution of 0.20 g in 10 ml of water is clear and not more intensely coloured than standard colour solution Yw2 when compared as described under "Colour of liquids" (vol. 1, p. 50).

Sulfated ash. Not more than 1.0 mg/g.

Loss on drying. Dry to constant weight at 105 °C; it loses not more than 5.0 mg/g.

pH value. pH of a 10 mg/ml solution, 5.0–6.0.

Related substances. Carry out the test as described under "Thin-layer chromatography" (vol. 1, p. 83), using silica gel R2 as the coating substance and a mixture of 140 volumes of dichloroethane R, 60 volumes of methanol R, 2.5 volumes of water, and 2.5 volumes of anhydrous formic acid R as the mobile phase. Apply separately to the plate 10 μl of each of 2 solutions in chloroform R containing (A) 10 mg of the test substance per ml and (B) 0.050 mg of the test substance per ml. Develop the plate for a distance of 10 cm. After removing the plate from the chromatographic chamber, allow it to dry in air, and examine the chromatogram in ultraviolet light (254 nm). Any spot obtained with solution A, other than the principal spot, is not more intense than that obtained with solution B.

Assay. Dissolve about 0.6 g, accurately weighed, in 50 ml of glacial acetic acid R1, and add 10 ml of mercuric acetate/acetic acid TS, warming slightly if necessary to effect solution. Cool and titrate with perchloric acid (0.1 mol/l) VS as described under "Non-aqueous titration", Method A (vol. 1, p. 131). Each ml of perchloric acid (0.1 mol/l) VS is equivalent to 29.58 mg of $C_{16}H_{21}NO_2$,HCl.

PROPYLTHIOURACILUM

Propylthiouracil

Molecular formula. $C_7H_{10}N_2OS$

Relative molecular mass. 170.2

Graphic formula.

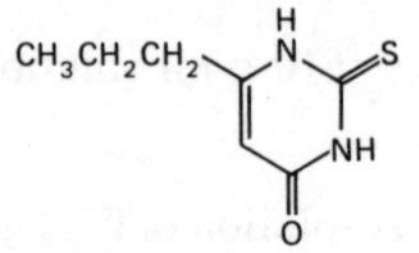

Chemical name. 6-Propyl-2-thiouracil; 2,3-dihydro-6-propyl-2-thioxo-4(1*H*)-pyrimidinone; 6-propyl-2-thio-2,4(1*H*,3*H*)-pyrimidinedione; CAS Reg. No. 51-52-5.

Description. Colourless or pale cream-coloured crystals or a white or cream-coloured, crystalline powder; odourless.

Solubility. Very slightly soluble in water; sparingly soluble in ethanol (~750 g/l) TS; slightly soluble in chloroform R and ether R.

Category. Antithyroid substance.

Storage. Propylthiouracil should be kept in a well-closed container, protected from light.

Additional information. Propylthiouracil has a bitter taste.

REQUIREMENTS

General requirement. Propylthiouracil contains not less than 98.0% and not more than 100.5% of $C_7H_{10}N_2OS$, calculated with reference to the dried substance.

Identity tests

• Either test A alone or tests B, C, and D may be applied.

A. Carry out the examination as described under "Spectrophotometry in the infrared region" (vol. 1, p. 40). The infrared absorption spectrum is concordant with the *reference spectrum* of propylthiouracil.

B.   Dissolve 0.05 g in 5 ml of boiling water and to the hot solution add a freshly prepared solution of 20 mg of hydroxylamine hydrochloride R and 0.04 g of anhydrous sodium carbonate R in 5 ml of water, to which 0.4 ml of sodium nitroprusside (45 g/l) TS has been added; a greenish blue colour is produced.

C.   To 25 mg add bromine TS1, drop by drop, until the substance is completely dissolved.   Warm until the colour is discharged, cool, and add 10 ml of barium hydroxide (15 g/l) TS; a white precipitate is produced (distinction from thiouracil, which yields a white precipitate that turns purple within 1 minute).

D.   Melting temperature, about 220 °C.

Heavy metals.   Use 1.0 g for the preparation of the test solution as described under "Limit test for heavy metals", Procedure 3 (vol. 1, p. 118); determine the heavy metals content according to Method A (vol. 1, p. 119); not more than 20 μg/g.

Sulfated ash.   Not more than 1.0 mg/g.

Loss on drying.   Dry to constant weight at 105 °C; it loses not more than 5.0 mg/g.

Thiourea.   Boil 0.50 g with 50 ml of water under a reflux condenser until dissolved and dilute 5 ml of the hot solution to 50 ml with water.   Place 10 ml of this solution in a test-tube and add to it 1 ml of thiourea (0.1 g/l) TS.   Cool the remainder of the hot solution, filter, and place 10 ml of the filtrate in a second test-tube, to serve as a reference.   To each tube add 0.5 g of sodium acetate R and 5 ml of silver nitrate (0.1 mol/l) VS and heat in a water-bath for 5 minutes.   The colour produced in the test solution, when viewed transversely against a white background, is not more intense than that of the reference solution when compared as described under "Colour of liquids" (vol. 1, p. 50).

Assay.   Transfer about 0.3 g, accurately weighed, to a 500-ml flask and add 30 ml of water.   Add from a burette about 30 ml of sodium hydroxide (0.1 mol/l) VS, heat to boiling, and shake the flask until solution is complete.   Wash down any particles on the wall of the flask with a small volume of water, then add about 50 ml of silver nitrate (0.1 mol/l) VS while mixing, and boil gently for 5 minutes.   Add 1–2 ml of bromothymol blue/ethanol TS, and continue to titrate with sodium hydroxide (0.1 mol/l) VS until a permanent blue-green colour is produced.   Each ml of sodium hydroxide (0.1 mol/l) VS is equivalent to 8.51 mg of $C_7H_{10}N_2OS$.

PYRIDOSTIGMINI BROMIDUM
Pyridostigmine bromide

Molecular formula. $C_9H_{13}BrN_2O_2$

Relative molecular mass. 261.1

Graphic formula.

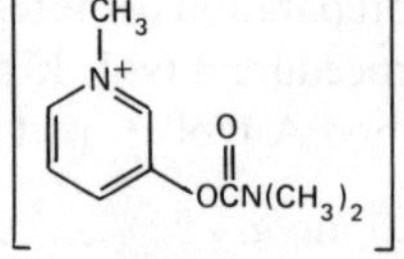

Chemical name. 3-Hydroxy-1-methylpyridinium bromide dimethylcarbamate; 3-[[(dimethylamino)carbonyl]oxy]-1-methylpyridinium bromide; CAS Reg. No. 101-26-8.

Description. A white or almost white, crystalline powder; odour, agreeable, characteristic.

Solubility. Soluble in less than 1 part of water and ethanol (~750 g/l) TS; freely soluble in chloroform R; practically insoluble in ether R.

Category. Cholinergic.

Storage. Pyridostigmine bromide should be kept in a well-closed container, protected from light.

Additional information. Pyridostigmine bromide is deliquescent.

REQUIREMENTS

General requirement. Pyridostigmine bromide contains not less than 98.5% and not more than 101.0% of $C_9H_{13}BrN_2O_2$, calculated with reference to the dried substance.

Identity tests

A. The absorption spectrum of a 25 μg/ml solution, when observed between 230 nm and 350 nm, exhibits a maximum at about 270 nm; the absorbance of a 1-cm layer at this wavelength is about 0.46 (preferably use 2-cm cells for the measurement and calculate the absorbance of a 1-cm layer).

B. See the test described below under "Related substances". The principal spot obtained with solution B corresponds in position, appearance, and intensity with that obtained with solution C.

C. To 0.1 g add 0.6 ml of sodium hydroxide (~80 g/l) TS; an orange colour is produced. Warm the solution; the colour changes to yellow and the vapours evolved turn moistened red litmus paper blue.

D. A 20 mg/ml solution yields reaction A described under "General identification tests" as characteristic of bromides (vol. 1, p. 112).

Melting range. 153–156 °C.

Sulfated ash. Not more than 1.0 mg/g.

Loss on drying. Dry to constant weight at 105 °C under reduced pressure (not exceeding 0.6 kPa or about 5 mm of mercury); it loses not more than 20 mg/g.

Related substances. Carry out the test as described under "Thin-layer chromatography" (vol. 1, p. 83), using silica gel R1 as the coating substance and a mixture of 67 volumes of water, 30 volumes of methanol R, and 3 volumes of diethylamine R as the mobile phase. Apply separately to the plate 10 μl of each of 3 solutions containing (A) 20 mg of the test substance per ml, (B) 0.10 mg of the test substance per ml, and (C) 0.10 mg of pyridostigmine bromide RS per ml. After removing the plate from the chromatographic chamber, allow it to dry in a current of warm air, spray it with nitroaniline TS2 and then with sodium hydroxide (0.1 mol/l) VS. Dry the plate again in a current of warm air, spray it with potassium iodobismuthate TS2, and examine the chromatogram in daylight. Any spot obtained with solution A, other than the principal spot, is not more intense than that obtained with solution B.

Assay. Dissolve about 0.5 g, accurately weighed, in 30 ml of glacial acetic acid R1, add 10 ml of mercuric acetate/acetic acid TS and 2 drops of quinaldine red/ethanol TS as indicator, and titrate with perchloric acid (0.1 mol/l) VS as described under "Non-aqueous titration", Method A (vol. 1, p. 131). Each ml of perchloric acid (0.1 mol/l) VS is equivalent to 26.11 mg of $C_9H_{13}BrN_2O_2$.

PYRIDOXINI HYDROCHLORIDUM

Pyridoxine hydrochloride

Molecular formula. $C_8H_{11}NO_3,HCl$

Relative molecular mass. 205.6

Graphic formula.

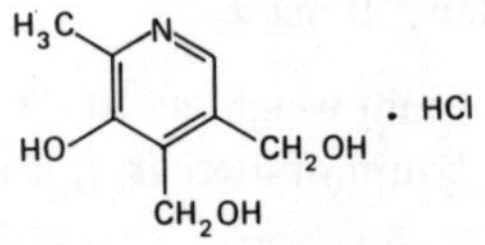

Chemical name. 5-Hydroxy-6-methyl-3,4-pyridinedimethanol hydrochloride; 3-hydroxy-4,5-bis(hydroxymethyl)-2-methylpyridine hydrochloride; CAS Reg. No. 58-56-0.

Description. Colourless crystals or a white, crystalline powder.

Solubility. Freely soluble in water; slightly soluble in ethanol (~750 g/l) TS; practically insoluble in chloroform R and ether R.

Category. Vitamin.

Storage. Pyridoxine hydrochloride should be kept in a tightly closed container, protected from light.

Additional information. Even in the absence of light, Pyridoxine hydrochloride is gradually degraded on exposure to a humid atmosphere, the decomposition being faster at higher temperatures.

REQUIREMENTS

General requirement. Pyridoxine hydrochloride contains not less than 98.5% and not more than 101.0% of $C_8H_{11}NO_3,HCl$, calculated with reference to the dried substance.

Identity tests

A.   The absorption spectrum of a 10 μg/ml solution in hydrochloric acid
(0.1 mol/l) VS, when observed between 230 nm and 350 nm, exhibits a maximum
at about 290 nm; the absorbance of a 1-cm layer at this wavelength is about 0.43
(preferably use 2-cm cells for the measurement and calculate the absorbance of a
1-cm layer).

B.   The absorption spectrum of a 0.5 mg/ml solution in phosphate buffer pH 6.9,
TS, when observed between 230 nm and 350 nm, exhibits maxima at about 254 nm
and 324 nm; the absorbances of a 1-cm layer at the maximum wavelengths are
about 0.18 and 0.35, respectively (preferably use 2-cm cells for the measurement
and calculate the absorbances of 1-cm layers).

C.   In each of two test-tubes A and B, place 1 ml of a 0.1 mg/ml solution and 2 ml
of sodium acetate (150 g/l) TS. To tube A add 1 ml of water and to tube B 1 ml of
boric acid (50 g/l) TS and mix. Cool both tubes to about 20 °C and rapidly add to
each tube 1 ml of 2,6-dichloroquinone chlorimide/ethanol TS; a blue colour is
produced in tube A, whereas in tube B no blue colour is observed.

D.   A 0.05 g/ml solution yields reaction B described under "General identification tests" as characteristic of chlorides (vol. 1, p. 113).

Heavy metals.   Use 0.5 g for the preparation of the test solution as described under
"Limit test for heavy metals", Procedure 3 (vol. 1, p. 118); determine the heavy
metals content according to Method A (vol. 1, p. 119); not more than 40 μg/g.

Clarity and colour of solution.   A solution of 0.50 g in 10 ml of water is clear and
colourless.

Sulfated ash.   Not more than 1.0 mg/g.

Loss on drying.   Dry to constant weight at ambient temperature under reduced
pressure (not exceeding 0.6 kPa or about 5 mm of mercury) over silica gel,
desiccant, R; it loses not more than 5.0 mg/g.

pH value.   pH of a 10 mg/ml solution, 2.3–3.5.

Assay.   Dissolve about 0.4 g, accurately weighed, in 30 ml of glacial acetic acid
R1, add 10 ml of mercuric acetate/acetic acid TS, and titrate with perchloric acid
(0.1 mol/l) VS as described under "Non-aqueous titration", Method A (vol. 1, p.
131). Each ml of perchloric acid (0.1 mol/l) VS is equivalent to 20.56 mg of
$C_8H_{11}NO_3$,HCl.

QUININI HYDROCHLORIDUM

Quinine hydrochloride

Molecular formula. $C_{20}H_{24}N_2O_2,HCl,2H_2O$

Relative molecular mass. 396.9

Graphic formula.

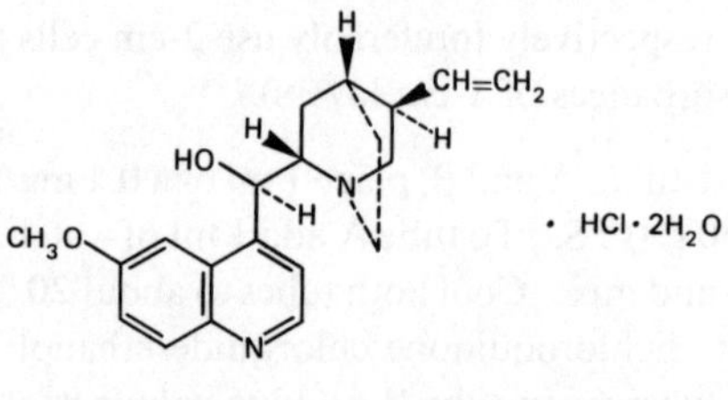

$\cdot \ HCl \cdot 2H_2O$

Chemical name. $(8\alpha,9R)$-6'-Methoxycinchonan-9-ol monohydrochloride (salt) dihydrate; $(8\alpha,9R)$-9-hydroxy-6'-methoxycinchonan hydrochloride (1:1) (salt) dihydrate; CAS Reg. No. 6119-47-7.

Description. Silky, colourless crystals, often grouped in clusters; odourless.

Solubility. Soluble in water; freely soluble in ethanol ($\sim$750 g/l) TS; very slightly soluble in ether R.

Category. Antimalarial.

Storage. Quinine hydrochloride should be kept in a well-closed container, protected from light.

Additional information. Quinine hydrochloride has a very bitter taste; it is freely soluble in chloroform R giving a turbid solution.

REQUIREMENTS

General requirement. Quinine hydrochloride contains not less than 98.5% and not more than 101.0% of $C_{20}H_{24}N_2O_2,HCl$, calculated as total alkaloids and with reference to the dried substance.

Identity tests

A. Dissolve 0.1 g in 2.5 ml of water; the solution is not fluorescent. Dilute 0.5 ml of this solution to 100 ml with water and add 2 drops of sulfuric acid ($\sim$100 g/l) TS; a strong blue fluorescence is produced.

B. To 5 ml of a 1 mg/ml solution add 2–3 drops of bromine TS1 and 5 drops of ammonia (~100 g/l) TS; an emerald-green colour is produced.

C. A 10 mg/ml solution yields reaction B described under "General identification tests" as characteristic of chlorides (vol. 1, p. 113).

Specific optical rotation. Use a 20 mg/ml solution in hydrochloric acid (0.1 mol/l) VS and calculate with reference to the dried substance; $[\alpha]_D^{20\,°C} = -240$ to $-258°$.

Barium. To 15 ml of a 0.3 g/ml solution add 1 ml of sulfuric acid (~100 g/l) TS; the solution remains clear for not less than 15 minutes.

Sulfates. Dissolve 0.5 g in 20 ml of water and proceed as described under "Limit test for sulfates" (vol. 1, p. 116); the sulfate content is not more than 1 mg/g.

Clarity and colour of solution. A solution of 0.10 g in 10 ml of water is clear and colourless.

Sulfated ash. Not more than 1.0 mg/g.

Loss on drying. Dry to constant weight at 105 °C; it loses not less than 60 mg/g and not more than 100 mg/g.

pH value. pH of a 10 mg/ml solution in carbon-dioxide-free water R, 6.0–7.0.

Related cinchona alkaloids. Carry out the test as described under "Thin-layer chromatography" (vol. 1, p. 83), using silica gel R1 as the coating substance and a mixture of 20 volumes of toluene R, 12 volumes of ether R, and 5 volumes of diethylamine R as the mobile phase. Apply separately to the plate 4 µl of each of 2 solutions in methanol R containing (A) 10 mg of the test substance per ml and (B) 0.25 mg of cinchonidine R per ml. After removing the plate from the chromatographic chamber, heat it at 105 °C for 30 minutes, allow it to cool, spray with potassium iodoplatinate TS, and examine the plate in daylight. Any spot obtained with solution A, other than the principal spot, is not more intense than that obtained with solution B.

Limit of dihydroquinine. Dissolve about 0.2 g, accurately weighed, in 20 ml of water. Add 0.5 g of potassium iodide R, 10 ml of hydrochloric acid (~70 g/l) TS and 2 drops of methyl red/ethanol TS. Titrate with potassium bromate (0.0167 mol/l) VS until the colour is discharged. Add 0.5 g of potassium iodide R, stopper the flask, and allow to stand for 5 minutes. Titrate the liberated iodine with sodium thiosulfate (0.1 mol/l) VS, adding 2 ml of starch TS when the solution has reached a light yellow coloration. Each ml of potassium bromate (0.0167 mol/l) VS is equivalent to 18.04 mg of $C_{20}H_{24}N_2O_2,HCl$. Express the results of both the above determination and the assay in percentages. The difference between the two is not more than 10%.

Assay. Dissolve about 0.35 g, accurately weighed, in 50 ml of glacial acetic acid R1, add 20 ml of acetic anhydride R and 10 ml of mercuric acetate/acetic acid TS, and titrate with perchloric acid (0.1 mol/l) VS as described under "Non-aqueous titration", Method A (vol. 1, p. 131). Each ml of perchloric acid (0.1 mol/l) VS is equivalent to 18.04 mg of $C_{20}H_{24}N_2O_2,HCl$.

QUININI SULFAS

Quinine sulfate

Molecular formula. $(C_{20}H_{24}N_2O_2)_2,H_2SO_4,2H_2O$

Relative molecular mass.   783.0

Graphic formula.

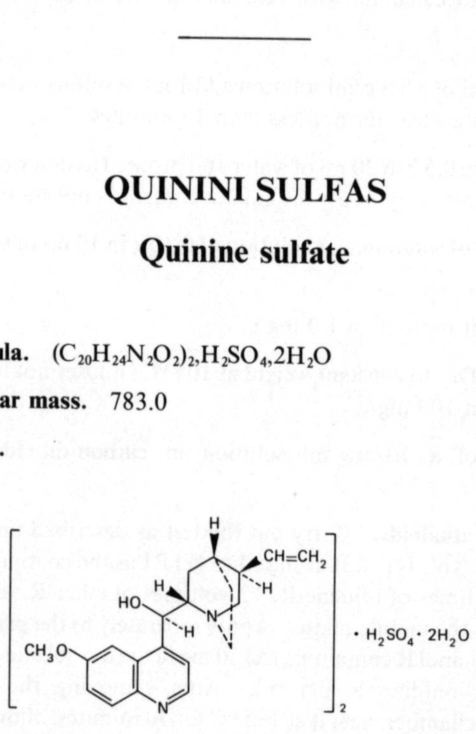

Chemical name. $(8\alpha,9R)$-6'-Methoxycinchonan-9-ol sulfate (2:1) (salt) dihydrate; $(8\alpha,9R)$-9-hydroxy-6'-methoxycinchonan sulfate (2:1) (salt) dihydrate; CAS Reg. No. 6591-63-5.

Description.   Colourless, needle-like crystals; odourless.

Solubility.   Slightly soluble in water, ethanol ($\sim$750 g/l) TS, ether R, and chloroform R.

Category.   Antimalarial.

Storage.   Quinine sulfate should be kept in a well-closed container, protected from light.

Additional information.   Quinine sulfate has a very bitter taste.

REQUIREMENTS

General requirement. Quinine sulfate contains not less than 99.0% and not more than 101.0% of $(C_{20}H_{24}N_2O_2)_2,H_2SO_4$, calculated as total alkaloids and with reference to the dried substance.

Identity tests

A. Dissolve 5 mg in 10 ml of water and add 1 drop of sulfuric acid (~100 g/l) TS; a strong blue fluorescence is produced.

B. To 5 ml of a 1 mg/ml solution add 2–3 drops of bromine TS1 and 5 drops of ammonia (~100 g/l) TS; an emerald-green colour is produced.

C. A 20 mg/ml solution yields reaction A described under "General identification tests" as characteristic of sulfates (vol. 1, p. 115).

Specific optical rotation. Use a 30 mg/ml solution in sulfuric acid (~100 g/l) TS and calculate with reference to the dried substance; $[\alpha]_D^{20\,°C} = -240$ to $-250\,°$.

Clarity and colour of solution. Dissolve 20 mg in 5 ml of hydrochloric acid (0.1 mol/l) VS and add sufficient water to produce 10 ml. This solution is clear and not more intensely coloured than standard colour solution Yw2 when compared as described under "Colour of liquids" (vol. 1, p. 50).

Sulfated ash. Not more than 1.0 mg/g.

Loss on drying. Dry to constant weight at 105 °C; it loses not less than 30 mg/g and not more than 50 mg/g.

pH value. pH of a 10 mg/ml suspension in carbon-dioxide-free water R, 5.7–6.6.

Related cinchona alkaloids. Carry out the test as described under "Thin-layer chromatography" (vol. 1, p. 83), using silica gel R1 as the coating substance and a mixture of 20 volumes of toluene R, 12 volumes of ether R, and 5 volumes of diethylamine R as the mobile phase. Apply separately to the plate 4 μl of each of 2 solutions in methanol R containing (A) 10 mg of the test substance per ml and (B) 0.25 mg of cinchonidine R per ml. After removing the plate from the chromatographic chamber, heat it at 105 °C for 30 minutes, allow it to cool, spray with potassium iodoplatinate TS and examine the chromatogram in daylight. Any spot obtained with solution A, other than the principal spot, is not more intense than that obtained with solution B.

Limit of dihydroquinine. Dissolve about 0.2 g, accurately weighed, in 20 ml of water. Add 0.5 g of potassium iodide R, 10 ml of hydrochloric acid (~70 g/l) TS and 2 drops of methyl red/ethanol TS. Titrate with potassium bromate (0.0167 mol/l) VS until the colour is discharged. Add 0.5 g of potassium iodide R, stopper the flask and allow to stand for 5 minutes. Titrate the liberated iodine with sodium thiosulfate (0.1 mol/l) VS, adding 2 ml of starch TS when the solution has reached a light yellow coloration. Each ml of potassium bromate (0.0167 mol/l) VS is equivalent to 24.90 mg of $(C_{20}H_{24}N_2O_2)_2,H_2SO_4$. Express the results of both the above determination and the assay in percentages. The difference between the two is not more than 10%.

Assay. Dissolve about 0.20 g, accurately weighed, in 30 ml of glacial acetic acid R1, add 20 ml of acetic anhydride R, and titrate with perchloric acid (0.1 mol/l) VS as described under "Non-aqueous titration", Method A (vol. 1, p. 131). Each ml of perchloric acid (0.1 mol/l) VS is equivalent to 24.90 mg of $(C_{20}H_{24}N_2O_2)_2,H_2SO_4$.

RESERPINUM

Reserpine

Molecular formula. $C_{33}H_{40}N_2O_9$

Relative molecular mass. 608.7

Graphic formula.

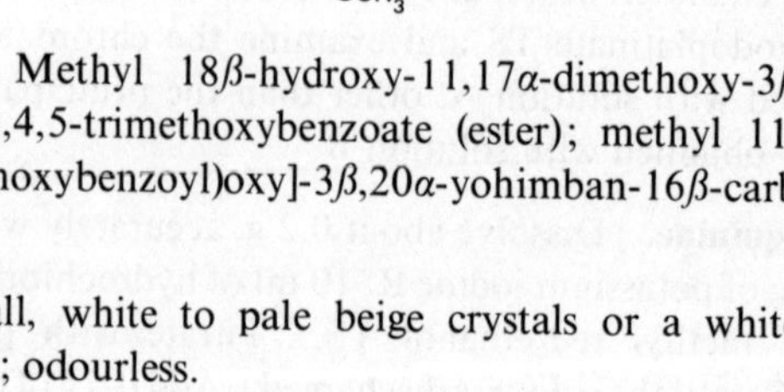

Chemical name. Methyl 18β-hydroxy-11,17α-dimethoxy-3β,20α-yohimban-16β-carboxylate 3,4,5-trimethoxybenzoate (ester); methyl 11,17α-dimethoxy-18β-[(3,4,5-trimethoxybenzoyl)oxy]-3β,20α-yohimban-16β-carboxylate; CAS Reg. No. 50-55-5.

Description. Small, white to pale beige crystals or a white to pale beige, crystalline powder; odourless.

Solubility. Practically insoluble in water; soluble in 90 parts of acetone R and in 6 parts of chloroform R; very slightly soluble in methanol R, ethanol ($\sim$750 g/l) TS, and ether R.

Category. Neuroleptic; hypotensive.

Storage. Reserpine should be kept in a well-closed container, protected from light.

Additional information. Reserpine darkens slowly on exposure to light, but more rapidly in solution.

REQUIREMENTS

General requirement. Reserpine contains not less than 98.0% and not more than 102.0% of $C_{33}H_{40}N_2O_9$, calculated with reference to the dried substance.

Identity tests

- Either test A alone or tests B and C may be applied.

A. Carry out the examination as described under "Spectrophotometry in the infrared region" (vol. 1, p. 40). The infrared absorption spectrum is concordant with the spectrum obtained from reserpine RS or with the *reference spectrum* of reserpine.

B. To 1 mg add 0.2 ml of a freshly prepared 10 g/l solution of vanillin R in hydrochloric acid ($\sim$250 g/l) TS; a pink colour is produced in about 2 minutes.

C. Mix 0.5 mg with 5 mg of 4-dimethylaminobenzaldehyde R and 0.2 ml of glacial acetic acid R and add 0.2 ml of sulfuric acid ($\sim$1760 g/l) TS; a green colour is produced. Add 1 ml of glacial acetic acid R; the colour changes to red.

Specific optical rotation. Use a 10 mg/ml solution in chloroform R; $[\alpha]_D^{20\,°C} = $ −113 to −127 °.

Sulfated ash. Not more than 1.0 mg/g.

Loss on drying. Dry to constant weight at 60 °C under reduced pressure (not exceeding 0.6 kPa or about 5 mm of mercury); it loses not more than 10 mg/g.

Oxidation products. Measure the absorbance of a 1-cm layer of a 0.2 mg/ml solution in glacial acetic acid R at the maximum at about 388 nm; not greater than 0.10 (preferably use 2-cm cells for the measurement and calculate the absorbance of a 1-cm layer).

Assay

• The solutions must be protected from air and light throughout the assay.

Moisten about 25 mg, accurately weighed, with 2 ml of ethanol (~750 g/l) TS, add 2 ml of sulfuric acid (0.25 mol/l) VS and 10 ml of ethanol (~750 g/l) TS, and warm gently to effect solution. Cool, dilute to 100.0 ml with ethanol (~750 g/l) TS, and dilute 5.0 ml of this solution to 50.0 ml with the same solvent. Transfer 10.0 ml of the solution to a boiling tube, add 2.0 ml of sulfuric acid (0.25 mol/l) VS and 2.0 ml of freshly prepared sodium nitrite (3 g/l) TS, mix, and heat in a water-bath at 55 °C for 30 minutes. Cool, add 1.0 ml of freshly prepared sulfamic acid (50 g/l) TS, and dilute to 25.0 ml with ethanol (~750 g/l) TS. Measure the absorbance of a 1-cm layer at the maximum at about 390 nm, against a solvent cell containing a solution prepared by treating a further 10.0 ml of the solution in the same manner but omitting the sodium nitrite. Calculate the amount of $C_{33}H_{40}N_2O_9$ in the substance being tested by comparison with reserpine RS, similarly and concurrently examined. In an adequately calibrated spectrophotometer the absorbance of the reference solution should be 0.24 ± 0.01 (preferably use 2-cm cells for the measurement and calculate the absorbance of a 1-cm layer).

RIBOFLAVINUM

Riboflavin

Molecular formula. $C_{17}H_{20}N_4O_6$

Relative molecular mass. 376.4

Graphic formula.

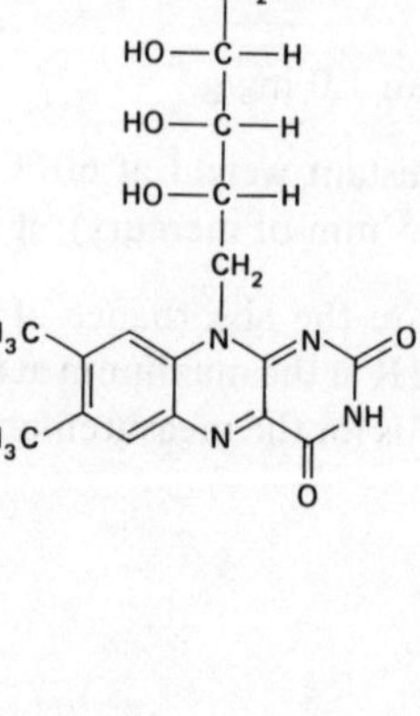

Chemical name. 7.8-Dimethyl-10-(D-*ribo*-2,3,4,5-tetrahydroxypentyl)iso-alloxazine; CAS Reg. No. 83-88-5.

Description. A yellow to orange-yellow, crystalline powder; odourless or almost odourless.

Solubility. Very slightly soluble in water; practically insoluble in ethanol (~750 g/l) TS, chloroform R, ether R, and acetone R.

Category. Vitamin.

Storage. Riboflavin should be kept in a tightly closed container, protected from light.

Additional information. Riboflavin has a bitter taste. Solutions of Riboflavin, especially in dilute solutions of alkalis, deteriorate rapidly when exposed to light.

REQUIREMENTS

General requirement. Riboflavin contains not less than 98.0% and not more than 102.0% of $C_{17}H_{20}N_4O_6$, calculated with reference to the dried substance.

Identity tests

A. Carry out the examination as described under "Spectrophotometry in the infrared region" (vol. 1, p. 40). The infrared absorption spectrum is concordant with the spectrum obtained from riboflavin RS or with the *reference spectrum* of riboflavin.

B. Dissolve 1 mg in 100 ml of water. The solution has a pale greenish yellow colour by transmitted light and an intense yellowish green fluorescence by reflected light. The addition of mineral acids or alkalis destroys the fluorescence.

Sulfated ash. Not more than 3.0 mg/g.

Loss on drying. Dry to constant weight at 105 °C; it loses not more than 15 mg/g.

Lumiflavin. Shake 25 mg with 10 ml of ethanol-free chloroform R for 5 minutes and filter. Measure the absorbance of the filtrate in a 1-cm layer at the maximum at about 440 nm against a solvent cell containing ethanol-free chloroform R; the absorbance does not exceed 0.025 (preferably use 2-cm cells for the measurement and calculate the absorbance of a 1-cm layer).

Assay
• The operations must be carried out in subdued light.
To about 0.075 g, accurately weighed, add 150 ml of water and 2 ml of glacial acetic acid R and heat on a water-bath, shaking the flask frequently until the

riboflavin is dissolved. Cool, dilute with sufficient water to produce 1000 ml; to 10.0 ml of this solution, add 1 ml of sodium acetate (50 g/l) TS and sufficient water to produce 50.0 ml. Measure the absorbance of a 1-cm layer of the diluted solution at the maximum at about 444 nm. Calculate the amount of $C_{17}H_{20}N_4O_6$ in the substance being tested by comparison with riboflavin RS, similarly and concurrently examined. In an adequately calibrated spectrophotometer the absorbance of the reference solution should be 0.48 ± 0.02 (preferably use 2-cm cells for the measurement and calculate the absorbance of a 1-cm layer).

STREPTOMYCINI SULFAS

Streptomycin sulfate

Streptomycin sulfate (non-injectable)
Streptomycin sulfate, sterile

Molecular formula. $(C_{21}H_{39}N_7O_{12})_2, 3H_2SO_4$

Relative molecular mass.   1457

Graphic formula.

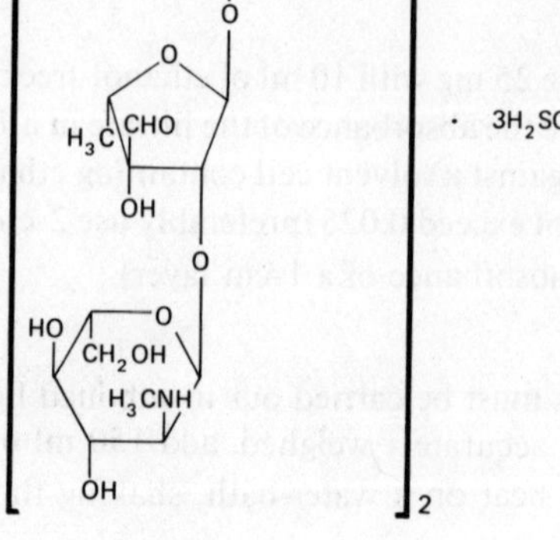

Chemical name. *O*-2-Deoxy-2-(methylamino)-α-L-glucopyranosyl-(1→2)-*O*-5-deoxy-3-*C*-formyl-α-L-lyxofuranosyl-(1→4)-*N*,*N'*-bis(aminoiminomethyl)-D-streptamine sulfate (2:3) (salt); CAS Reg. No. 3810-74-0.

Description. A white or almost white powder; odourless or with a slight odour.

Solubility. Very soluble in water; practically insoluble in ethanol (~750 g/l) TS, chloroform R, and ether R.

Category. Antibiotic.

Storage. Streptomycin sulfate should be kept in a well-closed container, protected from moisture, and stored at a temperature not exceeding 30 °C.

Labelling. The designation sterile Streptomycin sulfate indicates that the substance complies with the additional requirements for sterile Streptomycin sulfate and may be used for parenteral administration or for other sterile applications.

Additional information. Streptomycin sulfate is hygroscopic, but it is stable in air and on exposure to light.

REQUIREMENTS

General requirement. Streptomycin sulfate contains not less than 90.0% of $(C_{21}H_{39}N_7O_{12})_2,3H_2SO_4$ and not less than 720 International Units per mg, both calculated with reference to the dried substance.

Identity tests

A. Dissolve 20 mg in 5 ml of water and boil for a few minutes with 10 drops of sodium hydroxide (1 mol/l) VS; add 3 drops of hydrochloric acid (~250 g/l) TS and 1 ml of ferric chloride (25 g/l) TS; an intense violet colour is produced.

B. Dissolve 0.1 g in 2 ml of water, add 1 ml of 1-naphthol TS1 and 2 ml of a mixture of equal volumes of sodium hypochlorite (~40 g/l) TS and water; a red colour is produced.

C. A 20 mg/ml solution yields reaction A described under "General identification tests" as characteristic of sulfates (vol. 1, p. 115).

Clarity and colour of solution. A solution of 1.0 g in 10 ml of water is clear and not more intensely coloured than standard colour solution Yw4 when compared as described in "Colour of liquids" (vol. 1, p. 50).

Loss on drying. Dry at 60 °C under reduced pressure (not exceeding 0.6 kPa or about 5 mm of mercury) for 3 hours; it loses not more than 70 mg/g.

pH value. pH of a 0.25 g/ml solution in carbon-dioxide-free water R, 4.5–7.0.

Methanol. Transfer 0.2 g, accurately weighed, to a flask, dissolve in 5 ml of water and add 0.05 ml of sulfuric acid (0.05 mol/l) VS; connect the flask to a distillation apparatus, distil and collect about 2.5 ml of distillate in a 10-ml test-tube. Transfer the distillate to a conical flask, rinsing the test-tube twice with water, using 1 ml each time, and add 25 ml of potassium dichromate (0.0167 mol/l) VS. Cautiously add 10 ml of sulfuric acid (~1760 g/l) TS and heat the resulting solution for 30 minutes on a water-bath; cool and dilute to about 500 ml with water. Add 12.5 ml of potassium iodide (80 g/l) TS, allow to stand for 5 minutes, and then titrate with sodium thiosulfate (0.1 mol/l) VS, using starch TS as indicator, added towards the end of the titration, the endpoint being reached when the dark blue colour turns pale green. Repeat the operation without the substance being tested; the difference between the volumes used for the two titrations represents the amount of sodium thiosulfate (0.1 mol/l) VS, equivalent to the methanol present. Each ml of sodium thiosulfate (0.1 mol/l) VS is equivalent to 0.534 mg of CH_4O; the methanol content is not more than 40 mg/g, calculated as CH_4O.

Assay

For streptomycin sulfate. Dissolve about 0.10 g, accurately weighed, in sufficient water to produce 100 ml. To 5 ml add 5 ml of sodium hydroxide (0.2 mol/l) VS and heat in a water-bath for exactly 10 minutes. Cool in ice for exactly 5 minutes, add 3 ml of ferric ammonium sulfate TS2 and sufficient water to produce 25 ml, and mix. Exactly 20 minutes after the addition of the ferric ammonium sulfate TS2 measure the absorbance of a 1-cm layer at the maximum at about 525 nm, against a solvent cell containing a solution prepared in the same manner but omitting the substance being examined. Calculate the content of $(C_{21}H_{39}N_7O_{12})_2,3H_2SO_4$ in the substance, using the absorptivity value of 1.18 $(E^{1\%}_{1\,cm} = 11.8)$.

For potency. Carry out the assay as described under "Microbiological assay of antibiotics" (vol. 1, p. 145), using either (a) Bacillus subtilis (NCTC 8236, or ATCC 11774) as the test organism, culture medium Cm1 with a final pH of 7.9–8.0, sterile phosphate buffer pH 8.0, TS1 or TS2, an appropriate concentration of streptomycin (usually between 5 and 20 IU), and an incubation temperature of 36–39 °C, or (b) Bacillus subtilis (ATCC 6633) as the test organism, culture medium Cm1 with a final pH of 8.0–8.1, sterile phosphate buffer pH 8.0, TS1 or TS2, an appropriate concentration of streptomycin (usually between 3 and 15 IU), and an incubation temperature of 35–37 °C. The precision of the assay is such that the fiducial limits of error of the estimated potency ($P = 0.95$) are not less than 95% and not more than 105% of the estimated potency. The upper fiducial limit of error of the estimated potency ($P = 0.95$) is not less than 720 IU per mg, calculated with reference to the dried substance.

Additional Requirements for Sterile Streptomycin Sulfate

Histamine-like substances. Carry out the test as described under "Test for histamine-like substances" (vol. 1, p. 157) using, per kg of body weight, a solution containing 3 mg of streptomycin base in 1 ml of saline TS.

Undue toxicity. Carry out the test as described under "Test for undue toxicity" (vol. 1, p. 154), using 0.5 ml of a solution in sterile water R containing a quantity equivalent to 3 mg of streptomycin base per ml.

Pyrogens. Carry out the test as described under "Test for pyrogens" (vol. 1, p. 155) injecting, per kg of the rabbit's weight, a solution containing 10 mg of streptomycin base in 5 ml of sterile water R.

Sterility. Complies with the "Sterility testing of antibiotics" (vol. 1, p. 152), applying the membrane filtration test procedure.

SULFAMETHOXAZOLUM

Sulfamethoxazole

Molecular formula. $C_{10}H_{11}N_3O_3S$

Relative molecular mass. 253.3

Graphic formula.

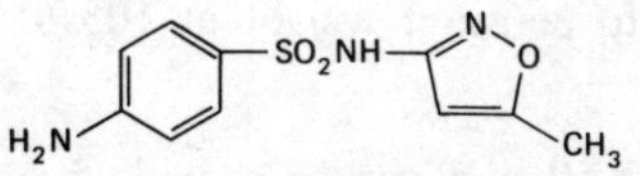

Chemical name. N^1-(5-Methyl-3-isoxazolyl)sulfanilamide: 4-amino-N-(5-methyl-3-isoxazolyl)benzenesulfonamide; CAS Reg. No. 723-46-6.

Description. A white or yellowish white, crystalline powder; odourless.

Solubility. Very slightly soluble in water; soluble in 50 parts of ethanol (~750 g/l) TS and in 3 parts of acetone R.

Category. Antibacterial.

Storage. Sulfamethoxazole should be kept in a well-closed container, protected from light.

REQUIREMENTS

General requirement.   Sulfamethoxazole contains not less than 99.0% and not more than 101.0% of $C_{10}H_{11}N_3O_3S$, calculated with reference to the dried substance.

Identity tests

• Either tests A and C or tests B and C may be applied.

A.   Carry out the examination as described under "Spectrophotometry in the infrared region" (vol. 1, p. 40). The infrared absorption spectrum is concordant with the spectrum obtained from sulfamethoxazole RS or with the *reference spectrum* of sulfamethoxazole.

B.   Dissolve 5 mg in 0.5 ml of sodium hydroxide (~80 g/l) TS and add 5 ml of water. Add 0.1 g of phenol R, heat to boiling, cool, and add 1 ml of sodium hypochlorite (~40 g/l) TS; a golden yellow colour is immediately produced and is persistent.

C.   About 0.1 g yields the reaction described for the identification of primary aromatic amines under "General identification tests" (vol. 1, p. 111), producing a red-orange precipitate.

Melting range.   168–172 °C.

Heavy metals.   Use 1.0 g for the preparation of the test solution as described under "Limit test for heavy metals", Procedure 3 (vol. 1, p. 118); determine the heavy metals content according to Method A (vol. 1, p. 119); not more than 20 μg/g.

Solution in alkali.   Dissolve 0.40 g in a mixture of 8.0 ml of water and 2.0 ml of sodium hydroxide (1 mol/l) VS; the solution is clear.

Sulfated ash.   Not more than 1.0 mg/g.

Loss on drying.   Dry to constant weight at 105 °C; it loses not more than 5.0 mg/g.

Acidity.   Heat 1.0 g with 50 ml of carbon-dioxide-free water R at about 70°C for 5 minutes, cool quickly to 20 °C, and filter; titrate 25 ml of the filtrate, phenolphthalein/ethanol TS being used as indicator; not more than 0.35 ml of sodium hydroxide (0.1 mol/l) VS is required to obtain the midpoint of the indicator.

Related substances.   Carry out the test as described under "Thin-layer chromatography" (vol. 1, p. 83), using silica gel R3 as the coating substance and a mixture of 20 volumes of chloroform R, 2 volumes of methanol R, and 1 volume of dimethylformamide R as the mobile phase. Apply separately to the plate 10 μl of each of 2 solutions in a mixture of 9 volumes of ethanol (~750 g/l) TS and 1 volume of ammonia (~260 g/l) TS containing (A) 2.5 mg of the test substance per ml and

(B) 12.5 μg of sulfanilamide RS per ml. After removing the plate from the chromatographic chamber, allow it to dry in air until the solvents have evaporated. Spray the dried plate with sulfuric acid/ethanol TS, heat at 105 °C for 30 minutes, and immediately expose to nitrous fumes in a closed chamber for 15 minutes (the nitrous fumes may be generated by adding sulfuric acid (~700 g/l) TS drop by drop to a solution containing 10 g of sodium nitrite R and 3 g of potassium iodide R in 100 ml). Place the plate in a current of warm air for 15 minutes and spray with N-(1-naphthyl)ethylenediamine hydrochloride/ethanol TS. If necessary, allow to dry before repeating the spraying and examine the chromatogram in daylight. Any spot obtained with solution A, other than the principal spot, is not more intense than that obtained with solution B.

Assay. Carry out the assay as described under "Nitrite titration" (vol. 1, p. 133), using about 0.5 g, accurately weighed, dissolved in a mixture of 40 ml of water and 20 ml of glacial acetic acid R; add 15 ml of hydrochloric acid (~70 g/l) TS and titrate with sodium nitrite (0.1 mol/l) VS. Each ml of sodium nitrite (0.1 mol/l) VS is equivalent to 25.33 mg of $C_{10}H_{11}N_3O_3S$.

SULFAMETHOXYPYRIDAZINUM

Sulfamethoxypyridazine

Molecular formula. $C_{11}H_{12}N_4O_3S$

Relative molecular mass. 280.3

Graphic formula.

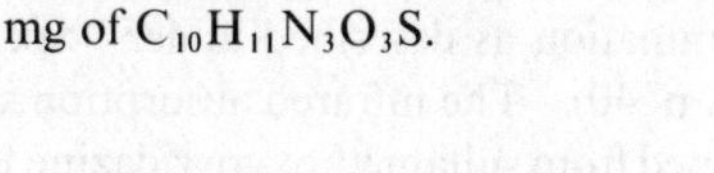

Chemical name. N^1-(6-Methoxy-3-pyridazinyl)sulfanilamide; 4-amino-N-(6-methoxy-3-pyridazinyl)benzenesulfonamide; CAS Reg. No. 80-35-3.

Description. A white or yellowish white, crystalline powder; odourless or almost odourless.

Solubility. Very slightly soluble in water; sparingly soluble in ethanol (~750 g/l) TS; soluble in acetone R.

Category. Antibacterial.

Storage. Sulfamethoxypyridazine should be kept in a well-closed container, protected from light.

Additional information. Sulfamethoxypyridazine becomes gradually coloured on exposure to light.

REQUIREMENTS

General requirement. Sulfamethoxypyridazine contains not less than 99.0% and not more than 101.0% of $C_{11}H_{12}N_4O_3S$, calculated with reference to the dried substance.

Identity tests

• Either test A alone or tests B and C may be applied.

A. Carry out the examination as described under "Spectrophotometry in the infrared region" (vol. 1, p. 40). The infrared absorption spectrum is concordant with the spectrum obtained from sulfamethoxypyridazine RS or with the *reference spectrum* of sulfamethoxypyridazine.

B. About 0.05 g yields the reaction described for the identification of primary aromatic amines under "General identification tests" (vol. 1, p. 111), producing a bright orange-red precipitate.

C. To 20 mg add 10 ml of sulfuric acid (~100 g/l) TS, mix to dissolve and carefully add 0.1 ml of potassium bromate (50 g/l) TS; a yellow colour that changes to amber is produced and a brown precipitate is gradually formed.

Melting range. 180–183 °C.

Heavy metals. Use 1.0 g for the preparation of the test solution as described under "Limit test for heavy metals", Procedure 3 (vol. 1, p. 118); determine the heavy metals content according to Method A (vol. 1, p. 119); not more than 20 μg/g.

Sulfated ash. Not more than 1.0 mg/g.

Loss on drying. Dry to constant weight at 105 °C; it loses not more than 5.0 mg/g.

Acidity. Heat 1.0 g with 50 ml of carbon-dioxide-free water R at about 70 °C for 5 minutes, cool quickly to 20 °C, and filter; 25 ml of the filtrate requires for titration to pH 7.0 not more than 0.35 ml of sodium hydroxide (0.1 mol/l) VS.

Related substances. Carry out the test as described under "Thin-layer chromatography" (vol. 1, p. 83), using silica gel R3 as the coating substance and a mixture of 20 volumes of chloroform R, 2 volumes of methanol R, and 1 volume of dimethylformamide R as the mobile phase. Apply separately to the plate 10 μl of each of 2 solutions in a mixture of 9 volumes of ethanol (~750 g/l) TS and 1 volume of ammonia (~260 g/l) TS containing (A) 2.5 mg of the test substance per ml and (B) 12.5 μg of sulfanilamide RS per ml. After removing the plate from the chromatographic chamber, allow it to dry in air until the solvents have evaporated. Spray the dried plate with sulfuric acid/ethanol TS, heat at 105 °C for 30 minutes, and immediately expose to nitrous fumes in a closed chamber for 15 minutes (the nitrous fumes may be generated by adding sulfuric acid (~700 g/l) TS drop by drop to a solution containing 10 g of sodium nitrite R and 3 g of potassium iodide R in 100 ml). Place the plate in a current of warm air for 15 minutes and spray with N-(1-naphthyl)ethylenediamine hydrochloride/ethanol TS. If necessary, allow to dry before repeating the spraying and examine the chromatogram in daylight. Any spot obtained with solution A, other than the principal spot, is not more intense than that obtained with solution B.

Assay. Carry out the assay as described under "Nitrite titration" (vol. 1, p. 133), using about 0.5 g, accurately weighed, dissolved in 50 ml of hydrochloric acid (~70 g/l) TS, and titrate with sodium nitrite (0.1 mol/l) VS. Each ml of sodium nitrite (0.1 mol/l) VS is equivalent to 28.03 mg of $C_{11}H_{12}N_4O_3S$.

TESTOSTERONI PROPIONAS

Testosterone propionate

Molecular formula. $C_{22}H_{32}O_3$

Relative molecular mass. 344.5

Graphic formula.

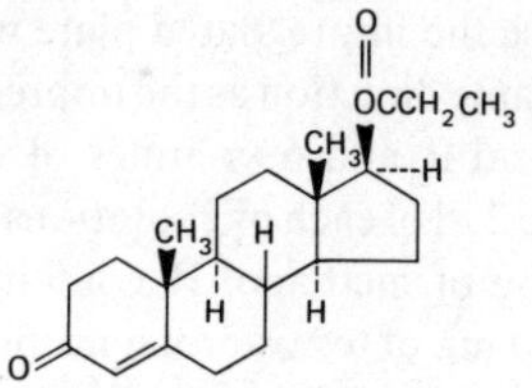

Chemical name. 17β-(1-Oxopropoxy)androst-4-en-3-one; 17β-hydroxyandrost-4-en-3-one propionate; CAS Reg. No. 57-85-2.

Description. Colourless or slightly yellowish crystals or a white or slightly yellowish powder; odourless.

Solubility. Practically insoluble in water; freely soluble in ethanol (~750 g/l) TS and ether R; very soluble in chloroform R; soluble in vegetable oils.

Category. Androgen.

Storage. Testosterone propionate should be kept in a well-closed container, protected from light.

REQUIREMENTS

General requirement. Testosterone propionate contains not less than 97.0% and not more than 102.0% of $C_{22}H_{32}O_3$, calculated with reference to the dried substance.

Identity tests

• Either test A or tests B and C may be applied.

A. Carry out the examination as described under "Spectrophotometry in the infrared region" (vol. 1, p. 40). The infrared absorption spectrum is concordant with the spectrum obtained from testosterone propionate RS or with the *reference spectrum* of testosterone propionate.

B. Carry out the test as described under "Thin-layer chromatography" (vol. 1, p. 83), using kieselguhr R1 as the coating subtance and a mixture of 10 volumes of liquid paraffin R and 90 volumes of light petroleum R to impregnate the plate, dipping it about 5 mm beneath the surface of the liquid. After the solvent has reached a height of at least 16 cm, remove the plate from the chromatographic chamber and allow it to stand at room temperature until the solvent has completely evaporated. Use the impregnated plate within 2 hours, carrying out the chromatography in the same direction as the impregnation. Use a mixture of 4 volumes of glacial acetic acid R and 6 volumes of water as the mobile phase. Apply separately to the plate 2 μl of each of 2 solutions in a mixture of 9 volumes of chloroform R and 1 volume of methanol R containing (A) 1.0 mg of the test substance per ml and (B) 1.0 mg of testosterone propionate RS per ml. Develop the plate for a distance of 12 cm. After removing the plate from the chromatographic chamber, allow it to dry in air until the solvents have evaporated, heat at 120 °C for 5–10 minutes, spray with 4-toluenesulfonic acid/ethanol TS, and then heat at 120 °C for 10 minutes. Allow to cool, and examine the chromatogram in daylight and in ultraviolet light (365 nm). The principal spot obtained with solution A corresponds in position, appearance, and intensity with that obtained with solution B.

C. Melting temperature, about 121 °C.

Specific optical rotation. Use a 10 mg/ml solution in dioxan R; $[\alpha]_D^{20\,°C}$ = +81 to +91°.

Solution in ethanol. A solution of 0.50 g in 10 ml of ethanol (~750 g/l) TS is clear and not more intensely coloured than standard colour solution Yw2 when compared as described under "Colour of liquids" (vol. 1, p. 50).

Loss on drying. Dry to constant weight at 105 °C; it loses not more than 5.0 mg/g.

Related substances. Carry out the test as described under "Thin-layer chromatography" (vol. 1, p. 83), using silica gel R1 as the coating substance and a mixture of 92 volumes of dichloroethane R, 8 volumes of methanol R, and 0.5 volumes of water as the mobile phase. Apply separately to the plate 5 μl of each of 2 solutions in a mixture of 9 volumes of chloroform R and 1 volume of methanol R containing (A) 20 mg of the test substance per ml and (B) 0.20 mg of the test substance per ml. After removing the plate from the chromatographic chamber, allow it to dry in air and heat at 110 °C for 10 minutes. Spray the hot plate with sulfuric acid/ethanol TS, again heat it at 110 °C for 10 minutes, and examine the chromatogram in ultraviolet light (365 nm). Any spot obtained with solution A, other than the principal spot, is not more intense than that obtained with solution B.

Assay. Dissolve about 20 mg, accurately weighed, in sufficient ethanol (~750 g/l) TS to produce 100 ml; dilute 5.0 ml of this solution to 100 ml with the same solvent. Measure the absorbance of a 1-cm layer of the diluted solution at the maximum at about 241 nm. Calculate the amount of $C_{22}H_{32}O_3$ in the substance being tested by comparison with testosterone propionate RS, similarly and concurrently examined. In an adequately calibrated spectrophotometer the absorbance of the reference solution should be 0.50 ± 0.03.

TETRACYCLINI HYDROCHLORIDUM

Tetracycline hydrochloride

Tetracycline hydrochloride (non-injectable)
Tetracycline hydrochloride, sterile

Molecular formula. $C_{22}H_{24}N_2O_8, HCl$

Relative molecular mass. 480.9

Graphic formula.

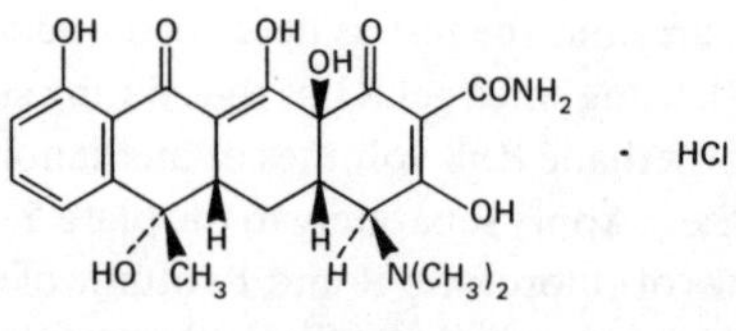

Chemical name. (4S,4aS,5aS,6S,12aS)-4-Dimethylamino-1,4,4a,5,5a,6,11,12a-octahydro-3,6,10,12,12a-pentahydroxy-6-methyl-1,11-dioxo-2-naphthacene-carboxamide monohydrochloride; [4S-(4α,4aα,5aα,6β,12aα)]-4-(dimethylami-no)-1,4,4a,5,5a,6,11,12a-octahydro-3,6,10,12,12a-pentahydroxy-6-methyl-1,11-dioxo-2-naphthacenecarboxamide monohydrochloride; CAS Reg. No. 64-75-5.

Description. A yellow, crystalline powder; odourless.

Solubility. Soluble in 10 parts of water and in 100 parts of ethanol (~750 g/l) TS; practically insoluble in acetone R, chloroform R, and ether R.

Category. Antibiotic.

Storage. Tetracycline hydrochloride should be kept in a tightly closed container, protected from light.

Labelling. The designation sterile Tetracycline hydrochloride indicates that the substance complies with the additional requirements for sterile Tetracycline hydrochloride and may be used for parenteral administration or for other sterile preparations.

Additional information. Tetracycline hydrochloride decomposes rapidly in solutions below pH 2, and less rapidly in solutions above pH 7. Even in the absence of light, Tetracycline hydrochloride is gradually degraded on exposure to a humid atmosphere, the decomposition being faster at higher temperatures.

REQUIREMENTS

General requirement. Tetracycline hydrochloride contains when tested according to assay A not less than 96.0% and not more than 102.0% of $C_{22}H_{24}N_2O_8,HCl$, and when tested according to assay B not less than 950 International Units per mg, both calculated with reference to the dried substance.

Identity tests

A. Carry out the test as described under "Thin-layer chromatography" (vol. 1, p. 83), but using an unlined chamber and a cellulose coating prepared as follows: To 0.275 g of carbomer R add 120 ml of water, let the mixture stand for 1 hour while shaking it from time to time; then add gradually while stirring a sufficient volume of sodium hydroxide (~80 g/l) TS to adjust to pH 7.0. To this mixture add 30 g of cellulose R1 and a sufficient quantity of water (usually 60–80 ml) to obtain a coating substance of suitable consistency. Coat the plates with a layer 0.4 mm thick, and allow them to dry at room temperature. The plates thus coated are used after a suitable treatment both for the identity test and the test of "related substances". For the identity test spray the plate with phosphate/citrate buffer pH 4.5, TS, until traces of moisture appear. Dry the plate at 50 °C for 30 minutes.

Prepare the following solutions immediately before use while protected from bright light: Dissolve 5.0 mg of the test substance, 5.0 mg of chlortetracycline hydrochoride RS, 5.0 mg of oxytetracycline hydrochloride RS, and 5.0 mg of tetracycline hydrochloride RS in sufficient methanol R to produce 10 ml; this constitutes solution A. Dissolve 5.0 mg of chlortetracycline hydrochloride RS and 5.0 mg of oxytetracycline hydrochloride RS in sufficient methanol R to produce 10 ml; this constitutes solution B. Dissolve 5.0 mg of chlortetracycline hydrochloride RS, 5.0 mg of oxytetracycline hydrochloride RS, and 5.0 mg of tetracycline hydrochloride RS in sufficient methanol R to produce 10 ml; this constitutes solution C.

Apply separately to the plate 1 μl of each of solutions A, B and C, and spray it very finely and uniformly with trimethylpyridine (50 g/l) TS until traces of humidity appear (about 8 ml).

Pour the mobile phase consisting of a mixture of 60 volumes of ethyl acetate R, 30 volumes of acetone R, and 6 volumes of water in the unlined chromatographic chamber. Place the plate in the chamber in such a manner that it is not in contact with the mobile phase. Allow the plate to become impregnated with the vapours for 1 hour. Then dip the plate into the mobile phase and allow the chromatogram to develop to a distance of 15 cm. After removing the plate from the chromatographic chamber, allow it to dry in air, expose it to the vapour of ammonia (~260 g/l) TS, and examine the chromatogram immediately in ultraviolet light (365 nm). Three principal clearly separated spots are obtained with solution A corresponding in position, appearance, and intensity with those obtained with solution C, two of which correspond with the spots obtained with solution B.

B.   To about 1 mg add 2 ml of sulfuric acid (~1760 g/l) TS; a red-violet colour is produced which on the addition of 0.1 ml of water changes to yellow.

C.   A 0.05 g/ml solution yields reaction B described under "General identification tests" as characteristic of chlorides (vol. 1, p. 113).

Specific optical rotation.   Use a 10 mg/ml solution in hydrochloric acid (0.01 mol/l) VS and calculate with reference to the dried substance; $[\alpha]_D^{20\,^\circ C} = -239$ to $-258°$.

Loss on drying.   Dry at 60°C under reduced pressure (not exceeding 0.6 kPa or about 5 mm of mercury) for 3 hours; it loses not more than 20 mg/g.

pH value.   pH of a 10 mg/ml solution, 1.8-2.8.

Related substances.   Carry out the test as described under "Thin-layer chromatography" (vol. 1, p. 83), using a plate as prepared under the identity test A.   To a sufficient volume of disodium edetate (0.1 mol/l) VS add sodium hydroxide (~80 g/l) TS to adjust to pH 7.0, and use this solution to spray the plate uniformly until traces of moisture appear.   Dry the plate at 50°C for 30 minutes.

Prepare the following solutions immediately before use, protecting them from bright light: Dissolve 0.10 g of the test substance in sufficient methanol R to produce 10 ml; this constitutes solution A.   Dilute 2.5 ml of solution A to 10.0 ml with methanol R; this constitutes solution B.   Dissolve 5.0 mg of 4-epianhydrotetracycline hydrochloride RS in sufficient methanol R to produce 20 ml; this constitutes solution K.   Dilute 2 ml of solution K to 10 ml with methanol R; this constitutes solution C.   Dissolve 5.0 mg of 4-epitetracycline hydrochloride RS in sufficient methanol R to produce 8 ml; this constitutes solution L.   Dilute 2 ml of solution L to 10 ml with methanol R; this constitutes solution D.   Dissolve 5.0 mg of anhydrotetracycline hydrochloride RS in sufficient methanol R to produce 20 ml; this constitutes solution M.   Dilute 2 ml of solution M to 10 ml with methanol R; this constitutes solution E.   Dissolve 20 mg of chlortetracycline hydrochloride RS in sufficient methanol R to produce 20 ml; this constitutes solution N.   Dilute 2 ml of solution N to 10 ml with methanol R; this constitutes solution F.   Dissolve 10 mg of tetracycline hydrochloride RS in sufficient methanol R to produce 20 ml; this constitutes solution P.   Mix together 0.5 ml of each of the following solutions K, L, M, N and P; this constitutes solution G.

Apply separately to the plate 1 μl of each of solutions A, B, C, D, E, F, and G, and spray it very finely and uniformly with trimethylpyridine (50 g/l) TS until traces of humidity appear (about 8 ml).

As the mobile phase, use a mixture of 60 volumes of ethyl acetate R, 30 volumes of acetone R, and 6 volumes of water.   Allow the chromatogram to develop to a distance of 15 cm.   After removing the plate from the chromatographic chamber, allow it to dry in air, expose it to the vapour of ammonia

(~260 g/l) TS, and examine the chromatogram immediately in ultraviolet light (365 nm). The spot corresponding to 4-epitetracycline hydrochloride obtained with solution B is not more intense than that obtained with solution D (5% of 4-epitetracycline hydrochloride). The spots corresponding to 4-epianhydrotetracycline hydrochloride, anhydrotetracycline hydrochloride, and chlortetracycline hydrochloride obtained with solution A are not more intense than those obtained with solution C (0.5% of 4-epianhydrotetracycline hydrochloride), solution E (0.5% of anhydrotetracycline hydrochloride), and solution F (2% of chlortetracycline hydrochloride). The test is not valid unless the chromatogram obtained with solution G shows 5 clearly separated spots.

Anhydroderivatives. Dissolve about 0.2 g, accurately weighed, in sufficient hydrochloric acid (0.02 mol/l) VS to produce 50 ml. Place 10.0 ml in a separator, add 10 ml of chloroform R and 10 ml of citrate buffer, pH 5.4 TS, and shake for 2 minutes. Separate the chloroform layer and measure the absorbance at 437 nm against a solvent cell containing chloroform R; not more than 0.18 (preferably use 2-cm cells for the measurement and calculate the absorbance of a 1-cm layer).

Assay

A. Dissolve about 0.25 g, accurately weighed and previously dried at 60 °C under reduced pressure, in 5 ml of formic acid (~1080 g/l) TS and 10 ml of glacial acetic acid R1, add 10 ml of dioxan R, 5 ml of mercuric acetate/acetic acid TS, and titrate with perchloric acid (0.1 mol/l) VS as described under "Non-aqueous titration", Method A (vol. 1, p. 131). Each ml of perchloric acid (0.1 mol/l) VS is equivalent to 48.09 mg of $C_{22}H_{24}N_2O_8,HCl$.

B. Carry out the assay as described under "Microbiological assay of antibiotics" (vol. 1, p. 145), using either (a) Bacillus pumilus (NCTC 8241 or ATCC 14884) as the test organism, culture medium Cm1 with a final pH of 6.5–6.6, sterile phosphate buffer, pH 4.5 TS, an appropriate concentration of tetracycline (usually between 2 and 20 IU), and an incubation temperature of 37–39 °C, or (b) Bacillus cereus (ATCC 11778) as the test organism, culture medium Cm1 with a final pH of 5.9–6.0, sterile phosphate buffer, pH 4.5 TS, an appropriate concentration of tetracycline (usually between 0.5 and 2 IU), and an incubation temperature of 30–33 °C. The precision of the assay is such that the fiducial limits of error of the estimated potency ($P = 0.95$) are not less than 95% and not more than 105% of the estimated potency. The upper fiducial limit of error of the estimated potency ($P = 0.95$) is not less than 950 IU per mg, calculated with reference to the dried substance.

Additional Requirements for Sterile Tetracycline Hydrochloride

Undue toxicity. Carry out the test as described under "Test for undue toxicity" (vol. 1, p. 154), using 0.5 ml of a solution in sterile water R containing a quantity equivalent to 4 mg/ml.

Pyrogens.   Carry out the test as described under "Test for pyrogens" (vol. 1, p. 155) injecting, per kg of the rabbit's weight, a solution containing 5 mg of the substance to be examined in 1 ml of sterile water R.

Sterility.   Complies with the "Sterility testing of antibiotics" (vol. 1, p. 152), applying the membrane filtration test procedure.

TOLBUTAMIDUM

Tolbutamide

Molecular formula. $C_{12}H_{18}N_2O_3S$

Relative molecular mass.   270.4

Graphic formula.

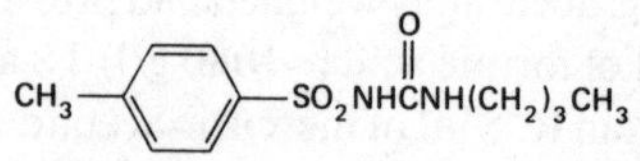

$$CH_3 \overset{}{\longrightarrow} SO_2NH\overset{\overset{\textstyle O}{\|}}{C}NH(CH_2)_3CH_3$$

Chemical name.   1-Butyl-3-(p-tolylsulfonyl)urea; N-[(butylamino)carbonyl]-4-methylbenzenesulfonamide; CAS Reg. No. 64-77-7.

Description.   A white or almost white, crystalline powder; odourless or almost odourless.

Solubility.   Practically insoluble in water; soluble in 10 parts of ethanol (~750 g/l) TS; soluble in acetone R.

Category.   Antidiabetic.

Storage.   Tolbutamide should be kept in a tightly closed container, protected from light.

Additional information.   Even in the absence of light, Tolbutamide is gradually degraded on exposure to a humid atmosphere, the decomposition being faster at higher temperatures.

REQUIREMENTS

General requirement.   Tolbutamide contains not less than 99.0% and not more than 101.0% of $C_{12}H_{18}N_2O_3S$, calculated with reference to the dried substance.

Identity tests

- Either test A alone or tests B and C may be applied.

A. Carry out the examination as described under "Spectrophotometry in the infrared region" (vol. 1, p. 40). The infrared absorption spectrum is concordant with the spectrum obtained from tolbutamide RS or with the *reference spectrum* of tolbutamide.

B. Boil 0.2 g with 8 ml of sulfuric acid (~700 g/l) TS under a reflux condenser for 30 minutes. Cool and filter. Keep the precipitate for test C. Make the filtrate strongly alkaline by adding sodium hydroxide (~300 g/l) TS, and carry out a steam distillation for 30 minutes. Collect the distillate in 30 ml of hydrochloric acid (0.1 mol/l) VS. To 2 ml of the solution containing the distillate add 0.2 g of sodium acetate R and 10 ml of sodium tetraborate (10 g/l) TS. Cool the mixture for 10 minutes in an ice-bath, add 1 ml of 4-nitroaniline TS1 and 2.7 ml of sodium nitrite (100 g/l) TS and allow to stand for 30 minutes. Add 2.5 ml of sodium hydroxide (~80 g/l) TS drop by drop; after a few minutes an intense red colour develops.

C. Wash the precipitate obtained in test B with 4 ml of water and dry at 105 °C; melting temperature, about 136 °C.

Melting range. 126–130 °C.

Heavy metals. Use 1.0 g for the preparation of the test solution as described under "Limit test for heavy metals", Procedure 3 (vol. 1, p. 118); determine the heavy metals content according to Method A (vol. 1, p. 119); not more than 20 μg/g.

Sulfated ash. Not more than 1.0 mg/g.

Loss on drying. Dry to constant weight at 105 °C; it loses not more than 5.0 mg/g.

Related substances. Carry out the test as described under "Thin-layer chromatography" (vol. 1, p. 83), using silica gel R1 as the coating substance and a mixture of 15 volumes of 2-propanol R, 3 volumes of cyclohexane R, 1 volume of ammonia (~260 g/l) TS and 1 volume of water as the mobile phase. Apply separately to the plate 5 μl of each of 2 solutions in acetone R containing (A) 10 mg of the test substance per ml and (B) 0.050 mg of 4-toluenesulfonamide R per ml. After removing the plate from the chromatographic chamber, allow it to dry in a current of warm air, heat at 110 °C for 10 minutes, spray the hot plate with sodium hypochlorite TS1 and dry in a current of cold air until a sprayed area of the plate below the line of application gives at most a very faint blue colour with 1 drop of potassium iodide/starch TS; avoid prolonged exposure to cold air. Spray the plate with potassium iodide/starch TS, allow it to stand for 5 minutes, and examine the chromatogram in daylight. Any spot obtained with solution A, other than the principal spot, is not more intense than that obtained with solution B.

Assay. Dissolve about 0.55 g, accurately weighed, in 30 ml of ethanol ($\sim$750 g/l) TS previously neutralized to phenolphthalein/ethanol TS, add 20 ml of carbon-dioxide-free water R, and titrate with carbonate-free sodium hydroxide (0.1 mol/l) VS, using phenolphthalein/ethanol TS as indicator. Repeat the operation without the substance being examined and make any necessary corrections. Each ml of carbonate-free sodium hydroxide (0.1 mol/l) VS is equivalent to 27.04 mg of $C_{12}H_{18}N_2O_3S$.

TRIMETHADIONUM

Trimethadione

Molecular formula. $C_6H_9NO_3$

Relative molecular mass. 143.1

Graphic formula.

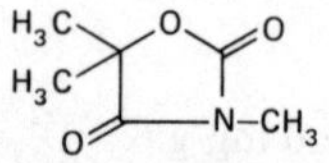

Chemical name. 3,5,5-Trimethyl-2,4-oxazolidinedione; CAS Reg. No. 127-48-0.

Description. Colourless, granular crystals; odour, slightly camphoraceous.

Solubility. Soluble in water; freely soluble in ethanol ($\sim$750 g/l) TS, ether R, and chloroform R.

Category. Anticonvulsant.

Storage. Trimethadione should be kept in a well-closed container, and stored in a cool place.

REQUIREMENTS

General requirement. Trimethadione contains not less than 98.0% and not more than 101.0% of $C_6H_9NO_3$, calculated with reference to the dried substance.

Identity tests

• Either test A alone or all 3 tests B, C, and D may be applied.

A.   Carry out the examination as described under "Spectrophotometry in the infrared region" (vol. 1, p. 40). The infrared absorption spectrum is concordant with the spectrum obtained from trimethadione RS or with the *reference spectrum* of trimethadione.

B.   To 5 ml of a 20 mg/ml solution add 2 ml of barium hydroxide (15 g/l) TS; a precipitate is immediately produced.

C.   Heat 0.5 g with 10 ml of sodium hydroxide (~80 g/l) TS on a water-bath for 30 minutes, evaporate to low bulk, cool in ice, and cautiously add hydrochloric acid (~70 g/l) TS until acid to litmus paper R. To 0.5 ml add 2 drops of ferric chloride (25 g/l) TS; a deep yellow colour is produced. Retain the remainder of the solution for test D.

D.   Extract the remainder of the solution obtained in test C 3 times with ether R, using 10 ml each time; evaporate the combined ether extracts on a water-bath for 30 minutes and scratch the inner surface of the container to induce crystallization; melting temperature, about 80 °C (α-hydroxyisobutyric acid).

Melting range.   45–47 °C, determined without previous drying.

Sulfated ash.   Not more than 1.0 mg/g.

Loss on drying.   Dry to constant weight over silica gel, desiccant, R at ambient temperature; it loses not more than 5.0 mg/g.

Assay.   Carry out the assay as described under "Gas chromatography" (vol. 1, p. 94). As an internal standard use 2-phenylethanol TS. Use the following 3 solutions (1) to 0.20 g of trimethadione RS add 5 ml of 2-phenylethanol TS and sufficient methanol R to produce 10 ml, (2) dissolve 0.20 g of the substance being examined in sufficient methanol R to produce 10 ml, and (3) to 0.20 g of the substance being examined add 5 ml of 2-phenylethanol TS and sufficient methanol R to produce 10 ml. For the procedure use a glass column 1.5 m long and 0.4 cm in internal diameter packed with an adequate quantity of an adsorbent composed of 10 g of diethylene glycol succinate R supported on 90 g of acid-washed, silanized kieselguhr R4. Maintain the column at 105 °C, use nitrogen R as the carrier gas and a flame ionization detector. Prepare chromatograms A, B, and C from solutions 1, 2 and 3, respectively. Measure the appropriate peak areas in chromatograms A, B, and C, and calculate the content of $C_6H_9NO_3$, using the data obtained from chromatograms A and C, introducing if necessary the correction resulting from chromatogram B.

TRIMETHOPRIMUM

Trimethoprim

Molecular formula. $C_{14}H_{18}N_4O_3$

Relative molecular mass. 290.3

Graphic formula.

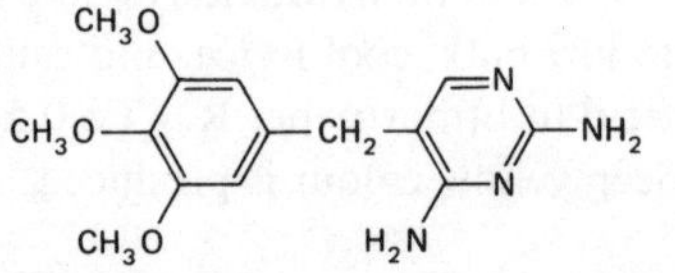

Chemical name. 2,4-Diamino-5-(3,4,5-trimethoxybenzyl)pyrimidine; 5-[(3,4,5-trimethoxyphenyl)methyl]-2,4-pyrimidinediamine; CAS Reg. No. 738-70-5.

Description. A white, crystalline powder; odourless or almost odourless.

Solubility. Sparingly soluble in water; soluble in methanol R and chloroform R; practically insoluble in ether R.

Category. Antibacterial.

Storage. Trimethoprim should be kept in a well-closed container.

REQUIREMENTS

General requirement. Trimethoprim contains not less than 98.5% and not more than 101.0% of $C_{14}H_{18}N_4O_3$, calculated with reference to the dried substance.

Identity tests

A. Carry out the examination as described under "Spectrophotometry in the infrared region" (vol. 1, p. 40). The infrared absorption spectrum is concordant with the spectrum obtained from trimethoprim RS or with the *reference spectrum* of trimethoprim.

B. Dissolve 25 mg in 5 ml of sulfuric acid (0.005 mol/l) VS, heat if necessary, and add 2 ml of a mixture of 1.6 g of potassium permanganate R dissolved in sufficient sodium hydroxide (0.1 mol/l) VS to produce 100 ml. Heat to boiling and add to the hot solution 0.4 ml of formaldehyde TS. Mix, add 1 ml of sulfuric acid (0.5 mol/l) VS, mix, and again heat to boiling. Cool to room temperature and filter. To the filtrate add 2 ml of chloroform R and shake the flask vigorously; a green fluorescence is produced in the chloroform layer when examined in ultraviolet light (365 nm).

C. Melting temperature, about 200 °C.

Sulfated ash. Not more than 1.0 mg/g.

Loss on drying. Dry to constant weight at 105 °C; it loses not more than 10 mg/g.

pH value. Shake 0.20 g with 20 ml of carbon-dioxide-free water R for 1 minute and filter; pH of the filtrate, 7.5–8.5.

Related substances

• The operations must be performed in a well-ventilated hood.

Carry out the test as described under "Thin-layer chromatography" (vol. 1, p. 83), using silica gel R2 as the coating substance and a mixture of 85 volumes of ethyl acetate R, 10 volumes of methanol R, 5 volumes of water, and 2 volumes of anhydrous formic acid R as the mobile phase; an unlined chromatographic chamber should be used and the solvent front allowed to ascend 17 cm above the line of application. Apply separately to the plate 5 μl of each of 2 solutions in a mixture of 5 volumes of chloroform R, 4.5 volumes of methanol R, and 1 volume of water containing (A) 40 mg of the test substance per ml and (B) 0.080 mg of the test substance per ml. Pour the mobile phase into the chamber and insert the plate immediately so as to avoid prior saturation of the chamber. After removing the plate from the chromatographic chamber, allow it to dry in a stream of cold air for 5 minutes, and examine the chromatogram in ultraviolet light (254 nm). Place the plate in a closed chamber containing chlorine, produced by mixing equal volumes of a 15 mg/ml solution of potassium permanganate R and hydrochloric acid (~70 g/l) TS, placed at the bottom of the chamber, and allow to stand for 20 minutes. Remove the plate from the chamber and drive off the chlorine in a current of cold air until the area below the line of application does not give any blue colour on the addition of 0.05 ml of starch/iodide TS. Spray the plate with starch/iodide TS, and examine the chromatogram in daylight. Any spot obtained with solution A, other than the principal spot, is not more intense than that obtained with solution B.

Assay. Dissolve about 0.6 g, accurately weighed, in 30 ml of glacial acetic acid R1, and titrate with perchloric acid (0.1 mol/l) VS, as described under "Non-aqueous titration", Method A (vol. 1, p. 131). Each ml of perchloric acid (0.1 mol/l) VS is equivalent to 29.03 mg of $C_{14}H_{18}N_4O_3$.

LIST OF REAGENTS, TEST SOLUTIONS, AND VOLUMETRIC SOLUTIONS

LIST OF REAGENTS, TEST SOLUTIONS, AND VOLUMETRIC SOLUTIONS

Many of the reagents, test solutions, and volumetric solutions mentioned in the *International Pharmacopoeia,* 3rd edition, volume 2, are described in volume 1, pages 167 to 211, and the exact page reference can be found by consulting the index. All other reagents, test solutions, and volumetric solutions mentioned in volume 2 are described below. As in volume 1, the reagents are denoted by the abbreviation R, the test solutions by the abbreviation TS, and the volumetric solutions, or solutions that are similarly standardized, by the abbreviation VS. Similarly named reagents differing in composition, purity etc., are distinguished by placing a numeral after the appropriate abbreviation. The designations AsTS, FeR, and FeTS refer to reagents of suitable purity for use in the limit tests for arsenic and iron. The designation Cm denotes culture media for microbiological tests. The designation RS denotes International Chemical Reference Substances.[1] The concentrations are expressed in conformity with the *Système international d'Unités* (SI) and they refer to the anhydrous substance. The reference to SRIP indicates *Specifications for reagents mentioned in the International Pharmacopoeia* (World Health Organization, Geneva, 1963). Designations used in the SRIP but now discontinued are given in square brackets. The designation *d* denotes the relative density $d\,^{20}_{20}$, i.e., measured in air at 20 °C in relation to water at 20 °C.

Acetate standard buffer TS.
Procedure. To 10 ml of acetic acid (~60 g/l) TS add 10 ml of sodium hydroxide (1 mol/l) VS and dilute with sufficient carbon-dioxide-free water R to produce 1000 ml.

Acetazolamide RS. International Chemical Reference Substance.

Acetic acid, glacial, R1. Glacial acetic acid R, that complies with the following tests:
Substances reducing dichromate. To 10 ml add 1.0 ml of potassium dichromate (0.0167 mol/l) VS and cautiously add 10 ml of sulfuric acid (~1760 g/l) TS. Cool the solution to room temperature and allow to stand for 30 minutes. While swirling the solution, dilute slowly and cautiously with 50 ml of water, cool, and add 1.5 ml of freshly prepared potassium iodide (80 g/l) TS. Titrate the liberated iodine with sodium thiosulfate (0.1 mol/l) VS, adding 3 ml of

---

[1] International Chemical Reference Substances are available from: WHO Collaborating Centre for Chemical Reference Substances, Apotekens Centrallaboratorium, Box 3045, 171 03 Solna 3, Sweden.

starch TS as the endpoint is approached.   Perform a blank titration and make any necessary corrections.   Not less than 0.60 ml of sodium thiosulfate (0.1 mol/l) VS is consumed.

Substances reducing permanganate.   Add 40 ml to 10 ml of water.   Cool to 15 °C, add 0.30 ml of potassium permanganate (0.02 mol/l) VS, and allow to stand at 15 °C for 10 minutes; the pink colour is not entirely discharged.

The present text supersedes that published in volume 1, p. 168.

Acetic anhydride/dioxan TS.
Procedure.   To 50 ml of dioxan R add 1 ml of acetic anhydride R (approximately 0.2 mol/l).

Acetyl chloride R. C_2H_3ClO.   Contains not less than 98.0% of C_2H_3ClO in both assay A and assay B (see below).
Description.   A clear, colourless or very slightly yellow liquid.
Phosphorus compounds.   Carefully treat 1 ml with 1 ml of water, add 1 ml of nitric acid (~1000 g/l) TS, boil, cool, dilute with 20 ml of water, add 10 ml of ammonium molybdate/nitric acid TS and allow to stand at about 40°C for 2 hours; no yellow precipitate is produced.
Assay.   (A) Dissolve about 1 g, accurately weighed, in 50 ml of carbonate-free sodium hydroxide (1 mol/l) VS, and titrate with sulfuric acid (0.5 mol/l) VS, using phenolphthalein/ethanol TS as indicator.   Each ml of carbonate-free sodium hydroxide (1 mol/l) VS is equivalent to 7.850 mg of C_2H_3ClO.   (B) Dilute the neutralized liquid from A to 250 ml with water, mix, and titrate 50 ml with silver nitrate (0.1 mol/l) VS, using potassium chromate (100 g/l) TS as indicator.   Each ml of silver nitrate (0.1 mol/l) VS is equivalent to 7.850 g of C_2H_3ClO.

Allopurinol RS.   International Chemical Reference Substance.

Aluminium R.   Al (SRIP, 1963, p. 29); wire, granules, or sheets.

Aluminium chloride R. $AlCl_3,6H_2O$ (SRIP, 1963, p. 30).

Aluminium chloride TS.
Procedure.   Dissolve 65.0 g of aluminium chloride R in sufficient water to produce 100 ml, add 0.5 g of charcoal R, stir for 10 minutes and filter.   While stirring, add to the filtrate sufficient sodium hydroxide (0.5 mol/l) VS to adjust the pH to 1.5.

4-Aminobenzoic acid R. $C_7H_7NO_2$.   Contains not less than 98.5% of $C_7H_7NO_2$.
Description.   White or slightly yellow crystals or a crystalline powder; odourless.
Solubility.   Soluble in 170 parts of water, in 9 parts of boiling water, in 8 parts of ethanol (~750 g/l) TS, and in 50 parts of ether R; slightly soluble in chloroform R.

Melting range.   186–189 °C.

Sulfated ash.   Not more than 1.0 mg/g.

Loss on drying.   Dry at 105 °C for 2 hours; it loses not more than 2.0 mg/g.

Assay.   Transfer to a beaker about 0.3 g, accurately weighed and previously dried at 105 °C for 2 hours, add 5 ml of hydrochloric acid (~420 g/l) TS, 50 ml of water and stir until dissolved.   Cool to about 15 °C, add about 25 g of crushed ice and slowly titrate with sodium nitrite (0.1 mol/l) VS until a glass rod dipped into the titrated solution produces an immediate blue ring when touched to starch/iodide paper R.   When the titration is complete, the endpoint is reproducible after the mixture has been allowed to stand for 1 minute.   Each ml of sodium nitrite (0.1 mol/l) VS is equivalent to 13.71 mg of $C_7H_7NO_2$.

Storage.   Store in a tightly closed container, protected from light.

2-Aminobutanol R. $C_4H_{11}NO$.

Description.   A colourless or light yellow, clear liquid.

Miscibility.   Miscible with water and methanol R.

Mass density. $\rho_{20} = 0.944–0.950$ kg/l.

Refractive index. $n_D^{20} = 1.450–1.455$.

Identification.   Dissolve 0.05 g in 4 ml of ethanol (~750 g/l) TS, add 0.5 ml of a 2.5 mg/ml solution of triketohydrindene hydrate R and warm on a water-bath; a violet colour is produced.

4-Amino-6-chloro-1,3-benzenedisulfonamide R. $C_6H_8ClN_3O_4S_2$.

Description.   A white, odourless powder.

Solubility.   Soluble in ammonia (~100 g/l) TS; practically insoluble in water and chloroform R.

Identification.   The absorption spectrum of a 5 μg/ml solution in methanol R exhibits maxima at about 223 nm, 265 nm, and 312 nm.   The absorptivity at 265 nm is about 64.0   ($E_{1cm}^{1\%} = 640$).

Sulfated ash.   Ignite 2 g; not more than 1.0 mg/g.

3-Aminopyrazole-4-carboxamide hemisulfate RS.   International Chemical Reference Substance.

Amitriptyline hydrochloride RS.   International Chemical Reference Substance.

Ammonia (~100 g/l) FeTS.

Ammonia (~100 g/l) TS that complies with the following test: Evaporate 5 ml of ammonia (~100 g/l) TS nearly to dryness on a water-bath, add 40 ml of water, 2 ml of citric acid (180 g/l) FeTS, and 2 drops of mercaptoacetic acid R; mix, make alkaline with ammonia (~100 g/l) FeTS, and dilute to 50 ml with water; no pink colour is produced.

The present text supersedes that published in volume 1, p. 168.

Ammonia (~35 g/l) TS.   Ammonia (~100 g/l) TS, diluted to contain about 35 g of NH_3 per litre (approximately 2 mol/l); d~0.985.

Ammonia (~17 g/l) TS.   Ammonia (~100 g/l) TS, diluted to contain about 17 g of NH_3 per litre (approximately 1 mol/l); d~0.992.

Ammonium chloride (100 g/l) TS.   A solution of ammonium chloride R containing about 100 g of NH_4Cl per litre.

Ammonium molybdate (45 g/l) TS.   A solution of ammonium molybdate R containing about 47 g of $(NH_4)_6Mo_7O_{24}$ per litre.

Ammonium molybdate/nitric acid TS.
Procedure.   Dissolve 50 g of ammonium sulfate R in 500 ml of nitric acid (~1000 g/l) TS using a 2000-ml conical flask or beaker. Dissolve separately in a beaker 150 g of ammonium molybdate R in 400 ml of boiling water. After cooling, pour this solution slowly, while stirring, into the acid solution and dilute with water to 1000 ml. Allow to stand for 2–3 days, and filter.
Storage.   Store in well-closed, brown glass bottles, and keep in a cool place.

Ammonium nitrate R. NH_4NO_3 (SRIP, 1963, p. 35).

Ammonium nitrate (50 g/l) TS.   A solution of ammonium nitrate R containing about 50 g of NH_4NO_3 per litre.

Ammonium oxalate (50 g/l) TS.   A solution of ammonium oxalate R containing about 50 g of $C_2H_8N_2O_4$ per litre.

Ammonium sulfamate R. $NH_4OSO_2NH_2$ (SRIP, 1963, p. 39).

Ammonium sulfamate (25 g/l) TS.   A solution of ammonium sulfamate R containing about 25 g of $NH_4OSO_2NH_2$ per litre.

Ammonium sulfamate (5 g/l) TS.   A solution of ammonium sulfamate R containing about 5 g of $NH_4OSO_2NH_2$ per litre.

Ammonium sulfate R. $(NH_4)_2SO_4$ (SRIP, 1963, p. 40).

Ampicillin RS.   International Chemical Reference Substance.

Ampicillin sodium RS.   International Chemical Reference Substance.

Ampicillin trihydrate RS.   International Chemical Reference Substance.

Amyl alcohol R. $C_5H_{12}O$ (SRIP, 1963, p. 42).

Anhydrotetracycline hydrochloride RS.   International Chemical Reference Substance.

Aniline R. C_6H_7N (SRIP, 1963, p. 43).

Aniline (25 g/l) TS. A solution of aniline R containing about 25 g of C_6H_7N per litre.

Antimony trichloride R. $SbCl_3$. Contains not less than 97.0% of $SbCl_3$.
Description. Colourless crystals.
Solubility. Very soluble in dehydrated ethanol R and in chloroform R (may form a slightly turbid solution).
Chloroform-insoluble substances. Dissolve 5.0 g in 25 ml of chloroform R, filter through a tared filtering crucible, wash the crucible with several portions of chloroform R, and dry at 105 °C; it leaves a residue of not more than 1.0 mg.
Assay. Dissolve 0.5 g, accurately weighed, in 30 ml of water containing 4.0 g of potassium sodium tartrate R, add 2 g of sodium hydrogen carbonate R, and titrate with iodine (0.1 mol/l) VS. Each ml of iodine (0.1 mol/l) VS is equivalent to 11.41 mg of $SbCl_3$.
Note: In moist air fumes may be evolved.

Antimony trichloride TS.
Procedure. Dissolve 22 g of antimony trichloride R in 100 ml of ethanol-free chloroform R, add 2.5 ml of acetyl chloride R, and allow to stand for 30 minutes.

Arsenic trioxide R1. Arsenic trioxide R that has been prepared according to either of the following methods:
1. Recrystallize arsenic trioxide R from a boiling mixture of 20 parts of hydrochloric acid (~420 g/l) TS and 5 parts of water. After cooling, collect the crystals and recrystallize them from boiling water until the mother liquor has a pH greater than 4.0. Dry the crystals to constant weight over silica gel, desiccant, R.
2. Sublime arsenic trioxide R in an appropriate apparatus.
pH Value. Heat to boiling for a few minutes 1.0 g in 20 ml of water, filter and cool; the filtrate has a pH greater than 4.0.
Chlorides. Dissolve 10 mg in sufficient water to produce 10 ml. Acidify with 1 drop of nitric acid (~1000 g/l) TS and add 2 drops of silver nitrate (0.1 mol/l) VS; the solution remains clear and colourless for not less than 2 minutes.
Sulfides. To a solution of 5.0 g in a mixture of 10 ml of sodium hydroxide (~80 g/l) TS and 15 ml of water add 2 drops of lead acetate (80 g/l) TS; the solution remains colourless.
Loss on drying. Dry to constant weight over silica gel, desiccant, R; it loses not more than 0.1 mg/g.
Sulfated ash. Not more than 0.1 mg/g.

Atropine sulfate RS. International Chemical Reference Substance.

Azo violet R. 4-(4-Nitrophenylazo)resorcinol; Magneson I; $C_{12}H_9N_3O_4$.
Description. A red powder.
Melting temperature. About 193 °C with decomposition.

Azo violet TS.

Procedure. Dissolve 0.2 g of azo violet R in a mixture of 1 volume of toluene R and 2 volumes of cyclohexane R.

Barium hydroxide R. $Ba(OH)_2,8H_2O$ (SRIP, 1963, p. 46).

Barium hydroxide (15 g/l) TS. A solution of barium hydroxide R in carbon-dioxide-free water R containing about 15 g of $Ba(OH)_2$ per litre.

Note: Barium hydroxide (15 g/l) TS must be freshly prepared.

Benzalkonium chloride TS. A mixture of alkylbenzyldimethylammonium chlorides. It contains in 1 litre not less than 470 g and not more than 530 g of alkylbenzyldimethylammonium chlorides, calculated as $C_{22}H_{40}ClN$.

Description. A clear, colourless to pale yellow, syrupy liquid; odour, aromatic.

Miscibility. Miscible with water and ethanol (~750 g/l) TS.

Assay. Dissolve 4 g, accurately weighed, in sufficient water to produce 100 ml. Transfer 25 ml to a separator, add 25 ml of chloroform R, 10 ml of sodium hydroxide (0.1 mol/l) VS, and 10 ml of freshly prepared potassium iodide (50 g/l) TS. Shake well, allow to separate, and run off the chloroform layer. Shake the aqueous solution with 3 further quantities of chloroform R, each of 10 ml, and discard the chloroform solutions. Add 40 ml of hydro-chloric acid (~420 g/l) TS, cool, and titrate with potassium iodate (0.05 mol/l) VS until the solution becomes pale brown in colour. Add 2 ml of chloroform R and continue the titration until the chloroform becomes colourless. Titrate a mixture of 20 ml of water, 6 ml of potassium iodide (80 g/l) TS, and 40 ml of hydrochloric acid (~420 g/l) TS with potassium iodate (0.05 mol/l) VS in a similar manner; the difference between the titrations represents the amount of potassium iodate (0.05 mol/l) VS required. Each ml of potassium iodate (0.05 mol/l) VS is equivalent to 35.40 mg of $C_{22}H_{40}ClN$. Determine the mass density using a pycnometer as described in "Determination of mass density and relative density" (vol. 1, p. 28) and calculate in g/l the proportion of $C_{22}H_{40}ClN$.

Note: A solution in water foams strongly when shaken.

Benzalkonium chloride TS1.

Procedure. Dilute 2 ml of benzalkonium chloride TS with sufficient water to produce 100 ml.

Benzene R. C_6H_6 (SRIP, 1963, p. 48).

Benzoic acid R. $C_7H_6O_2$. Contains not less than 99.8% of $C_7H_6O_2$.

Description. Colourless, light, feathery crystals or a white, microcrystalline powder; odour, characteristic, faint.

Solubility. Slightly soluble in water; freely soluble in ethanol (~750 g/l) TS, ether R, and chloroform R.

Methanol-insoluble substances. Dissolve 20 g in 200 ml of methanol R and digest under complete reflux for 30 minutes. Filter through a tared filtering crucible, wash thoroughly with methanol R, and dry at 105°C; it leaves a residue of not more than 1.0 mg.

Assay. Dissolve about 0.5 g, accurately weighed, in 15 ml of ethanol (~750 g/l) TS, previously neutralized to phenol red/ethanol TS, add 20 ml of water and titrate with sodium hydroxide (0.1 mol/l) VS, using phenol red/ethanol TS as indicator. Repeat the operation without the substance being examined and make any necessary correction. Each ml of sodium hydroxide (0.1 mol/l) VS is equivalent to 12.21 mg of $C_7H_6O_2$.

Benzoyl chloride R. C_7H_5ClO (SRIP, 1963, p. 50).

Benzylpenicillin potassium RS.   International Chemical Reference Substance.

Benzylpenicillin sodium RS.   International Chemical Reference Substance.

Bephenium hydroxynaphthoate RS.   International Chemical Reference Substance.

Betamethasone RS.   International Chemical Reference Substance.

Bismuth oxynitrate R.   Approximately $4BiNO_3(OH)_2,BiO(OH)$ (SRIP, 1963, p. 50).

Blue tetrazolium R. $C_{40}H_{32}Cl_2N_2O_2$.   3,3'-Dianisole-bis-[4,4'-(3,5-diphenyl) tetrazolium chloride].

Description.   Lemon-yellow crystals.

Solubility.   Slightly soluble in water; freely soluble in ethanol (~750 g/l) TS, chloroform R, and methanol R; practically insoluble in acetone R and ether R.

Molar absorptivity.   Its molar absorptivity in methanol R at 252 nm, is not less than 60 000.

Suitability test.   Prepare the following standard solution: Dissolve in ethanol (~750 g/l) TS a suitable quantity of hydrocortisone R, previously dried at 105°C for 3 hours and accurately weighed, and prepare by a step-by-step dilution a solution containing about 30 μg/ml.

Transfer 10-, 15- and 20-ml quantities of the standard solution to separate glass-stoppered 50-ml conical flasks. Add 10 ml and 5 ml, respectively, of ethanol (~750 g/l) TS to the flasks containing the 10- and 15-ml quantities of the standard solution and swirl to mix. To each of the flasks, and to a fourth flask, representing the blank, containing 20 ml of ethanol (~750 g/l) TS, add 2.0 ml of a solution prepared by dissolving 0.05 g of the blue tetrazolium R in 10 ml of ethanol (~750 g/l) TS, mix, and then add 2.0 ml of tetramethylammonium hydroxide/ethanol TS. Mix, allow the flasks to stand in the dark for 90 minutes, and determine the absorbances at 525 nm against the blank. Plot the absorbances on the abscissa and the amount of hydrocortisone on the ordinate scale of arithmetic coordinate paper, and draw the curve of best fit; the absorbance of each solution is proportional to the concentration and the absorbance of the solution containing 200 μg of hydrocortisone is not less than 0.50.

Blue tetrazolium/ethanol TS.
Procedure. Dissolve 0.5 g of blue tetrazolium R in sufficient aldehyde-free ethanol (~750 g/l) TS, warming slightly if necessary, to produce 100 ml.

Blue tetrazolium/sodium hydroxide TS.
Procedure. Immediately before use, mix 1 volume of a 2 mg/ml solution of blue tetrazolium R in water with 3 volumes of a 0.12 g/ml solution of sodium hydroxide R in methanol TS.

Bromocresol green R. $C_{21}H_{14}Br_4O_5S$ (SRIP, 1963, p. 52).

Bromocresol green/ethanol TS.
Procedure. Warm 0.1 g of bromocresol green R with 2.9 ml of sodium hydroxide (0.05 mol/l) VS and 5 ml of ethanol (~710 g/l) TS; after solution has been effected, add a sufficient quantity of ethanol (~150 g/l) TS to produce 250 ml.

Bromocresol purple R. $C_{21}H_{16}Br_2O_5S$ (SRIP, 1963, p. 52).

Bromocresol purple/ethanol TS.
Procedure. Dissolve 0.05 g of bromocresol purple R in 100 ml of ethanol (~750 g/l) TS, and filter if necessary.

Bromothymol blue/dimethylformamide TS.
Procedure. Dissolve 1.0 g of bromothymol blue R in sufficient dimethyl-formamide R to produce 100 ml.

Buffer borate, pH 8.0, TS.
Procedure. Dissolve 0.25 g of boric acid R and 0.30 g of potassium chloride R in 50 ml of carbon-dioxide-free water R, add 3.97 ml of carbonate-free sodium hydroxide (0.2 mol/l) VS, and dilute with sufficient carbon-dioxide-free water R to produce 200 ml.

Buffer borate, pH 9.0, TS.
Procedure. Dissolve 1.24 g of boric acid R in about 100 ml of water, add 8.3 ml of sodium hydroxide (1 mol/l) VS, and add sufficient water to produce 200 ml.

Buffer borate, pH 9.6, TS.
Procedure. Dissolve 0.25 g of boric acid R and 0.30 g of potassium chloride R in 50 ml of carbon-dioxide-free water R, add 36.85 ml of carbonate-free sodium hydroxide (0.2 mol/l) VS, and dilute with sufficient carbon-dioxide-free water R to produce 200 ml.

Buffer phosphate, pH 6.4, TS.
Procedure. Dissolve 1.36 g of potassium dihydrogen phosphate R in 50 ml of carbon-dioxide-free water R, add 12.60 ml of carbonate-free sodium hydroxide (0.2 mol/l) VS, and dilute with sufficient carbon-dioxide-free water R to produce 200 ml.

Buffer phosphate, pH 6.9, TS.
Procedure. Dissolve 3.40 g of potassium dihydrogen phosphate R and 3.55 g of disodium hydrogen phosphate R in sufficient carbon-dioxide-free water R to produce 1000 ml.

Buffer phthalate, pH 3.4, TS.
Procedure. Dissolve 2.04 g of potassium hydrogen phthalate R in 50 ml of carbon-dioxide-free water R, add 10.40 ml of hydrochloric acid (0.2 mol/l) VS, and dilute with sufficient carbon-dioxide-free water R to produce 200 ml.

Buffer phthalate, pH 3.5, TS.
Procedure. Dissolve 2.04 g of potassium hydrogen phthalate R in 50 ml of carbon-dioxide-free water R, add 8.40 ml of hydrochloric acid (0.2 mol/l) VS, and dilute with sufficient carbon-dioxide-free water R to produce 200 ml.

Bupivacaine hydrochloride RS.   International Chemical Reference Substance.

1-Butanol R.   [*n*-Butanol R]. $C_4H_{10}O$ (SRIP, 1963, p. 54).

tert.–**Butanol R.**   2-Methylpropan-2-ol; $(CH_3)_3COH$.
Description.   A colourless liquid or solid.
Miscibility.   Miscible with water, ethanol (~750 g/l) TS, and ether R.
Boiling range.   Not less than 95% distils between 81 and 83 °C.
Melting range.   24–26 °C.
Mass density. ρ_{20} = 0.778–0.782 kg/l.
Residue on evaporation.   Evaporate on a water-bath and dry to constant weight at 105 °C; it leaves a residue of not more than 0.05 mg/ml.

1-Butylamine R.   1-Aminobutane; $C_4H_{11}N$.
Description.   A colourless to pale yellow inflammable liquid.
Miscibility.   Miscible with water, ethanol (~750 g/l) TS, and ether R.
Boiling range.   Not less than 95% distils between 76 and 78 °C.
Mass density. ρ_{20} = about 0.740 kg/l.
Water.   Determine as described under "Determination of water by the Karl Fischer method" (vol. 1, p. 135), using about 5 ml of the liquid; not more than 10 mg/ml.
Acid impurities.   To 50 ml add 5 drops of azo violet TS, and titrate quickly with sodium methoxide (0.1 mol/l) VS to a deep blue endpoint, taking precautions to prevent absorption of atmospheric carbon dioxide, e.g., by use of an atmosphere of nitrogen; not more than 1.0 ml of sodium methoxide (0.1 mol/l) VS is required for neutralization.

Cadmium acetate R. $(CH_3CO_2)_2Cd,2H_2O$. Contains not less than 98.0% of $(CH_3CO_2)Cd,2H_2O$.
Description. Colourless crystals.
Solubility. Soluble in water.
Assay. Dissolve 1 g, accurately weighed, in 50 ml of water, add 25 ml of ammonia (~260 g/l) TS, and titrate with disodium edetate (0.1 mol/l) VS, using methylthymol blue mixture R as indicator, until the blue solution becomes colourless or grey. Each ml of disodium edetate (0.1 mol/l) VS is equivalent to 26.65 mg of $(CH_3CO_2)_2Cd,2H_2O$.

Caffeine RS. International Chemical Reference Substance.

Calcium hydroxide R. $Ca(OH)_2$ (SRIP, 1963, p. 59).

Calcium hydroxide TS.
Procedure. Prepare a saturated solution of calcium hydroxide R.
Note: Calcium hydroxide TS must be freshly prepared.

Carbomer R. Carbomer suitable for thin-layer chromatography. A high relative molecular mass cross-linked polymer of acrylic acid; it contains a large proportion (56–68%) of carboxylic acid (-COOH) groups after drying at 80 °C for 1 hour.
pH value. The pH of a 10 g/l suspension is about 3.
Viscosity. Whilst stirring continuously, prepare a suspension containing 2.5 g in 500 ml of water. Maintain at 25 ± 0.2 °C for 30 minutes, then add 0.2 ml of phenolphthalein/ethanol TS, 1 ml of bromothymol blue/ethanol TS and, whilst stirring, neutralize using a mixture of equal volumes of sodium hydroxide (~400 g/l) TS and water until a uniform blue colour is obtained (check the pH which must be 7.3–7.8). The dynamic viscosity of the neutralized preparation is 30–40 Pa · s (300–400 poise).

Cellulose R1. Microcrystalline cellulose suitable for thin-layer chromatography.
Description. A fine, white homogeneous powder.
Particle size. Less than 30 μm.
Note: A suspension of about 25 g of cellulose R1 in 90 ml of water is used in the preparation of the coating for thin-layer chromatographic plates.

Cellulose R2. Cellulose suitable for thin-layer chromatography.
Description. A fine, white homogeneous powder.
Particle size. Less than 30 μm.
Note: A suspension of about 15 of cellulose R2 in 100 ml of water is used in the preparation of the coating for thin-layer chromatographic plates.

Cellulose R3. Cellulose suitable for thin-layer chromatography.
Description. A fine, white homogeneous powder.
Composition. Cellulose (particle size less than 30 μm) containing a fluorescent indicator having an optimal intensity at 254 nm.

Note: A suspension of about 25 g of cellulose R3 in 100 ml of water is used in the preparation of the coating for thin-layer chromatographic plates.

Ceric ammonium sulfate R. Ammonium cerium(IV) sulfate dihydrate, $Ce(SO_4)_2,2(NH_4)_2SO_4,2H_2O$. Contains not less than 95.0% of $Ce(SO_4)_2,2(NH_4)_2SO_4,2H_2O$.
Description. Yellow crystals or an orange-yellow, crystalline powder.
Solubility. Slowly soluble in water; insoluble in ethanol ($\sim$750 g/l) TS.
Assay. Dissolve about 1 g, accurately weighed, in 50 ml of sulfuric acid ($\sim$100 g/l) TS, add 0.1 ml of a 10 mg/ml solution of osmium tetroxide R, and titrate with sodium arsenite (0.05 mol/l) VS, using *o*-phenanthroline TS as indicator. Each ml of sodium arsenite (0.05 mol/l) VS is equivalent to 63.26 mg of $Ce(SO_4)_2,2(NH_4)_2SO_4,2H_2O$.

Ceric ammonium sulfate/nitric acid TS.
Procedure. Dissolve 5 g of ceric ammonium sulfate R in sufficient nitric acid ($\sim$130 g/l) TS to produce 100 ml.

Ceric ammonium sulfate (0.1 mol/l) VS.
Procedure. Dissolve 65.0 g of ceric ammonium sulfate R in a mixture of 500 ml of water and 30 ml of sulfuric acid ($\sim$1760 g/l) TS. Allow to cool and dilute to 1000 ml with water.
Method of standardization. Ascertain the exact concentration of the 0.1 mol/l solution in the following manner: Accurately weigh about 0.2 g of arsenic trioxide R1 and dissolve by gently heating in 15 ml of sodium hydroxide (0.2 mol/l) VS. Add to the clear solution 50 ml of sulfuric acid ($\sim$100 g/l) TS, 0.15 ml of a 2.5 mg/ml solution of osmium tetroxide R in sulfuric acid ($\sim$100 g/l) TS, and 0.1 ml of *o*-phenanthroline TS. Titrate the solution with the ceric ammonium sulfate solution until the red colour disappears. Titrate slowly as the endpoint is approached.

Chloramphenicol RS. International Chemical Reference Substance.

Chloroform, ethanol-free, R.
Procedure. Shake 20 ml of chloroform R gently but thoroughly with 20 ml of water for 3 minutes, draw off the chloroform layer, and wash twice more with 20-ml quantities of water. Finally filter the chloroform through a dry filter-paper, shake it well with 5 g of powdered anhydrous sodium sulfate R for 5 minutes, allow the mixture to stand for 2 hours, and decant or filter the clear chloroform.

5-Chloro-2-methylaminobenzophenone RS. International Chemical Reference Substance.

2-Chloro-4-nitroaniline R. $C_6H_5ClN_2O_2$.
Description. A yellow to brown, crystalline powder.
Solubility. Slightly soluble in water; soluble in ethanol ($\sim$750 g/l) TS.

Melting range.   106–108 °C.

Sulfated ash.   Not more than 0.5 mg/g.

2-(4-Chloro-3-sulfamoyl)benzoic acid RS.   International Chemical Reference Substance.

Chlorphenamine hydrogen maleate RS.   International Chemical Reference Substance.

Chlorpromazine hydrochloride RS.   International Chemical Reference Substance.

Chlortalidone RS.   International Chemical Reference Substance.

Chlortetracycline hydrochloride RS.   International Chemical Reference Substance.

Chromic acid TS.
Procedure.   Dissolve 84 g of chromium trioxide R in 700 ml of water and add slowly while stirring 400 ml of sulfuric acid (~1760 g/l) TS.

Chromium trioxide R. CrO_3 (SRIP, 1963, p. 68).

Cinchonidine R. $C_{19}H_{22}N_2O$.
Description.   A white, crystalline powder.
Solubility.   Soluble in ethanol (~750 g/l) TS.
Melting temperature.   About 207 °C.
Specific optical rotation.   Use a 50 mg/ml solution in ethanol (~750 g/l) TS; $[\alpha]_D^{20\,°C} = -105$ to $-110\,°$.

Citrate buffer, pH 5.4, TS.
Procedure.   Dissolve 2.101 g of citric acid R in water, add 20 ml of sodium hydroxide (1 mol/l) VS, and dilute with sufficient water to produce 100 ml. Mix 76.5 ml of this solution with 23.5 ml of sodium hydroxide (0.1 mol/l) VS.

Citric acid, copper-free, R.   Citric acid R, that complies with the following additional test: Dissolve 0.50 g in 20 ml of water, make alkaline with ammonia (~100 g/l) TS, dilute to 50 ml with water, and add 1 ml of sodium diethyldithiocarbamate (0.8 g/l) TS; no yellow colour is produced.

Citric acid (20 g/l) TS.   A solution of citric acid R containing about 20 g of $C_6H_8O_7$ per litre.

Cloxacillin sodium RS.   International Chemical Reference Substance.

Cobaltous chloride TS.
Procedure.   Dissolve 6.5 g of cobaltous chloride R in a sufficient quantity of a mixture of 2.5 ml of hydrochloric acid (~250 g/l) TS and 97.5 ml of water to produce 100 ml.

Colbatous thiocyanate TS.
Procedure. Dissolve 6.8 g of cobaltous chloride R and 4.3 g of ammonium thiocyanate R in sufficient water to produce 100 ml.

Codeine R. $C_{18}H_{21}NO_3,H_2O$.
Description. Colourless crystals or a white, crystalline powder; odourless.
Solubility. Slightly soluble in water; freely soluble in ethanol (~750 g/l) TS and ether R.
Melting temperature. About 156 °C.
Specific optical rotation. Use a 20 mg/ml solution in ethanol (~750 g/l) TS; $[\alpha]_D^{20\,°C} = -142$ to -146 °.

Colecalciferol RS. International Chemical Reference Substance.

Copper(II) acetate R. $C_4H_6CuO_4,H_2O$. Contains not less than 98.0% of $C_4H_6CuO_4,H_2O$.
Description. Blue-green crystals or powder; odour, resembling that of acetic acid.
Solubility. Soluble in water.
Assay. Dissolve 0.8 g, accurately weighed, in 50 ml of water, add 2 ml of acetic acid (~300 g/l) TS and 3 g of potassium iodide R, and titrate the liberated iodine with sodium thiosulfate (0.1 mol/l) VS, using starch TS as indicator, until only a faint blue colour remains; add 2 g of potassium thiocyanate R and continue the titration until the blue colour disappears. Each ml of sodium thiosulfate (0.1 mol/l) VS is equivalent to 19.97 mg of $C_4H_6CuO_4,H_2O$.

Copper edetate TS.
Procedure. To 2 ml of a 20 mg/ml solution of copper(II) acetate R, add 2 ml of disodium edetate (0.1 mol/l) VS, and dilute to 50 ml with water.

Copper(II) sulfate (80 g/l) TS. A solution of copper(II) sulfate R containing about 80 g of $CuSO_4$ per litre (approximately 0.5 mol/l).

Copper(II) sulfate/ammonia TS.
Procedure. Dissolve 50 g of copper(II) sulfate R in 1000 ml of ammonia (~35 g/l) TS.

Copper(II) sulfate/pyridine TS.
Procedure. Dissolve 4 g of copper(II) sulfate R in 90 ml of water and add 30 ml of pyridine R.
Note: Copper(II) sulfate/pyridine TS must be freshly prepared.

o-Cresol R. 2-Methylphenol; C_7H_8O.
Description. Colourless to pale brownish-yellow crystals or liquid; odour, resembling that of phenol.
Miscibility. Miscible with ethanol (~750 g/l) TS, ether R, and chloroform R; miscible with about 50 parts of water.

Mass density. ρ_{20} = about 1.05 kg/l.

Refractive index. n_D^{20} = 1.540–1.550.

Boiling temperature. About 190 °C.

Freezing temperature. Not below 30.5 °C.

Residue on evaporation. Evaporate on a water-bath and dry to constant weight at 105 °C; it leaves a residue of not more than 1.0 mg/ml.

Storage. Store in a tightly closed container, protected from light and oxygen.

Note: On exposure to light and air *o*-cresol R darkens in colour.

Cyanide/oxalate/thiosulfate TS.

Procedure. To 2.0 ml of ammonia (~100 g/l) TS, add in the following order: 1.5 ml of ammonium oxalate (50 g/l) TS, 15 ml of potassium cyanide (50 g/l) TS, 45 ml of sodium acetate (60 g/l) TS, 120 ml of sodium thiosulfate (320 g/l) TS, 75 ml of sodium acetate (60 g/l) TS, and 35 ml of hydrochloric acid (1 mol/l) VS.

Note: Cyanide/oxalate/thiosulfate TS must be prepared immediately before use.

Cyanoethylmethyl silicone gum R.

A suitable grade to be used in gas-liquid chromatography.

Cyanogen bromide TS.

Caution. Very toxic; avoid inhalation of vapours.

Procedure. Add drop by drop, while cooling, potassium cyanide (100 g/l) TS to bromine TS1 until the colour disappears.

Note: Cyanogen bromide TS must be prepared immediately before use.

Cyclohexane R1.

Cyclohexane R showing a fluorescence that is not more intense than that of a solution of 2 μg/ml of quinine R in sulfuric acid (0.05 mol/l) VS when measured at 460 nm using a 1-cm layer and an excitation beam at 365 nm.

Dapsone RS.

International Chemical Reference Substance.

Dexamethasone RS.

International Chemical Reference Substance.

Dexamethasone acetate RS.

International Chemical Reference Substance.

Diammonium hydrogen phosphate R

[ammonium phosphate R]. $(NH_4)_2HPO_4$ (SRIP, 1963, p. 38).

Diammonium hydrogen phosphate (100 g/l) TS.

A solution of diammonium hydrogen phosphate R containing about 100 g of $(NH_4)_2HPO_4$ per litre.

Diazepam RS.

International Chemical Reference Substance.

Diazobenzenesulfonic acid TS.

Procedure. To 0.9 g of sulfanilic acid R add 10 ml of hydrochloric acid (~250 g/l) TS and sufficient water to produce 100 ml. To 3 ml of this solution add 5 ml of sodium nitrite (3 g/l) TS, cool in ice for 5 minutes, add a further 20 ml of sodium nitrite (3 g/l) TS, and again cool in ice; dilute with water to 100 ml, keeping the solution cold.

Note: Diazobenzenesulfonic acid TS must be freshly prepared and should not be used until at least 15 minutes after its preparation.

Diazomethane TS.

Caution. Diazomethane is explosive in the gaseous state and its explosive decomposition is easily initiated by rough surfaces. Do not use apparatus with ground-glass joints or boiling stones of any kind. Diazomethane is highly toxic and all operations should be conducted under a well-ventilated hood.

Procedure. Prepare a solution of 0.4 g of potassium hydroxide R in 10 ml of ethanol (~750 g/l) TS and add it to a solution of 2.14 g of N-methyl-N-nitrosotoluene-4-sulfonamide R in 30 ml of ether R while cooling in ice. If a precipitate forms, add just sufficient ethanol (~750 g/l) TS to dissolve it. After 5 minutes, gently distil the ethereal diazomethane solution from a water-bath. Diazomethane TS contains about 10 g of CH_2N_2 per litre.

Alternative procedures. Other procedures for the evolution of diazomethane, using other starting materials, may also be employed, provided the resulting solution has the required concentration of CH_2N_2.

Diazoxide RS. International Chemical Reference Substance.

Dibutyl ether R. Di-n-butyl ether, $C_8H_{18}O$.

Caution. Dibutyl ether R tends to form explosive peroxides, especially when anhydrous.

Description. A colourless liquid.

Miscibility. Practically immiscible with water; miscible with ethanol (~750 g/l) TS and ether R.

Boiling range. 140–143 °C.

Mass density. $\rho_{20} = 0.769$ kg/l.

Refractive index. $n_D^{20} = 1.344$.

Dibutyl phthalate R. Di-n-butyl phthalate, $C_{16}H_{22}O_4$.

Description. A clear, colourless or faintly coloured liquid.

Miscibility. Very slightly miscible with water; miscible with ethanol (~750 g/l) TS and ether R.

Mass density. $\rho_{20} = 1.043$–1.048 kg/l.

Refractive index. $n_D^{20} = 1.492$–1.495.

Sulfated ash. Not more than 0.2 mg/ml.

Dichloroethane R. 1,2-Dichloroethane, $C_2H_4Cl_2$ (SRIP, 1963, p. 76).

2,6-Dichloroquinone chlorimide R. $C_6H_2Cl_3NO$ (SRIP, 1963, p. 77).

2,6-Dichloroquinone chlorimide/ethanol TS.
Procedure.   Dissolve 0.5 g of 2,6-dichloroquinone chlorimide R in sufficient
ethanol (~750 g/l) TS to produce 100 ml.

Dicoumarol RS.   International Chemical Reference Substance.

Diethoxytetrahydrofuran R. $C_8H_{16}O_3$.   Mixture of the cis and trans isomers.
Description.   Colourless or slightly yellow, clear liquid.
Miscibility.   Practically immiscible with water; miscible with ethanol
(~750 g/l) TS and ether R.
Mass density. ρ_{20} = about 0.975 kg/l.
Refractive index. n_D^{20} = 1.418.

Diethoxytetrahydrofuran/acetic acid TS.
Procedure.   Mix 1 ml of diethoxytetrahydrofuran R with sufficient glacial
acetic acid R to produce 100 ml.

Diethylamine R. $C_4H_{11}N$.   Contains not less than 99.5% of $C_4H_{11}N$.
Description.   A clear, colourless liquid.
Mass density. ρ_{20} = 0.702–0.704 kg/l.
Refractive index. n_D^{20} = 1.384–1.386.
Assay.   Add about 3 g, accurately weighed, to 50 ml of sulfuric acid (0.5 mol/l)
VS and titrate the excess acid with sodium hydroxide (1 mol/l) VS, using
methyl red/ethanol TS as indicator.   Each ml of sulfuric acid (0.5 mol/l) VS is
equivalent to 73.14 mg of $C_4H_{11}N$.

Diethylcarbamazine dihydrogen citrate RS.   International Chemical Reference
Substance.

Diethylene glycol succinate R.   A suitable grade to be used in gas-liquid
chromatography.

Digitonin R. $C_{55}H_{90}O_{29}$ (SRIP, 1963, p. 78).

Digitonin TS.
Procedure.   Dissolve 0.10 g of digitonin R in sufficient ethanol (~710 g/l) TS
to produce 10 ml.
Note: Digitonin TS must be freshly prepared.

Digitoxin RS.   International Chemical Reference Substance.

Digoxin RS.   International Chemical Reference Substance.

Dimethylamine R. C_2H_7N.
Description.   A low-boiling liquid, 7 °C; odour, characteristic.
Solubility.   Soluble in water, ethanol (~750 g/l) TS, and ether R.

Dimethylamine/ethanol TS. A solution of dimethylamine R in ethanol (~750 g/l) TS containing about 330 g/l of C_2H_7N.

Assay. Dilute 2 ml to 10 ml with ethanol (~750 g/l) TS. Transfer 2 ml to a flask containing 50.0 ml of sulfuric acid (0.05 mol/l) VS and mix. Titrate the excess acid with sodium hydroxide (0.1 mol/l) VS, using methyl red/ethanol TS as indicator. Each ml of sulfuric acid (0.05 mol/l) VS is equivalent to 4.508 mg of C_2H_7N.

4-Dimethylaminobenzaldehyde R [dimethylaminobenzaldehyde R]. $C_9H_{11}NO$ (SRIP, 1963, p. 78).

4-Dimethylaminobenzaldehyde TS1.
Procedure. Dissolve 0.125 g of 4-dimethylaminobenzaldehyde R in a cooled mixture of 65 ml of sulfuric acid (~1760 g/l) TS and 35 ml of water and add 0.2 ml of ferric chloride (25 g/l) TS.
Note: 4-Dimethylaminobenzaldehyde TS1 must be freshly prepared.

4-Dimethylaminobenzaldehyde TS2.
Procedure. Dissolve 0.80 g of 4-dimethylaminobenzaldehyde R in a cooled mixture of 80 g of ethanol (~750 g/l) TS and 20 g of sulfuric acid (~1760 g/l) TS.

4-Dimethylaminobenzaldehyde TS3.
Procedure. Dissolve 0.5 g of 4-dimethylaminobenzaldehyde R in 50 ml of ethanol (~750 g/l) TS, add 1 ml of hydrochloric acid (~420 g/l) TS, and dilute with sufficient ethanol (~750 g/l) TS to produce 100 ml.

4-Dimethylaminobenzaldehyde TS4.
Procedure. Dissolve 2 g of 4-dimethylaminobenzaldehyde R in a mixture of 5 ml of hydrochloric acid (~420 g/l) TS and 95 ml of glacial acetic acid R.

4-Dimethylaminocinnamaldehyde R. $C_{11}H_{13}NO$.
Description. Orange crystals, or a crystalline powder; odour, characteristic.
Solubility. Practically insoluble in water; freely soluble in hydrochloric acid (~70 g/l) TS; sparingly soluble in ethanol (~750 g/l) TS and ether R.

4-Dimethylaminocinnamaldehyde TS1.
Procedure. Dissolve 2 g of 4-dimethylaminocinnamaldehyde R in a mixture of 100 ml of hydrochloric acid (5 mol/l) VS and 100 ml of ethanol (~750 g/l) TS.
Storage. Store the solution at a temperature of about 0 °C.

4-Dimethylaminocinnamaldehyde TS2.
Procedure. Dilute 20 ml of 4-dimethylaminocinnamaldehyde TS1 with sufficient ethanol (~750 g/l) TS to produce 100 ml.
Note: 4-Dimethylaminocinnamaldehyde TS2 must be freshly prepared.

Dinitrobenzene R. $C_6H_4N_2O_4$ (SRIP, 1963, p. 79).

Dinitrobenzene/ethanol TS.
Procedure. Dissolve 1 g of dinitrobenzene R in sufficient ethanol (~750 g/l) TS to produce 100 ml.

Dinonyl phthalate R. $C_{26}H_{42}O_4$.
Description. A colourless to pale yellow, viscous liquid.
Mass density. $\rho_{20} = 0.97$–0.98 kg/l.
Refractive index. $n_D^{20} = 1.482$–1.489.
Water. Determine as described under "Determination of water by the Karl Fischer method" (vol. 1, p. 135), using about 2 ml of the liquid; not more than 1.0 mg/ml.
Acidity. Shake 5.0 g with 25 ml of water for 1 minute. Allow to stand, filter the aqueous layer and add to it 5 drops of phenolphthalein/ethanol TS; not more than 0.3 ml of carbonate-free sodium hydroxide (0.1 mol/l) VS is required for the neutralization (0.5 mg/g expressed as phthalic acid).

Diphenylamine R. $C_{12}H_{11}N$ (SRIP, 1963, p. 81).

Disodium chromotropate R [chromotropic acid sodium salt R].
 $C_{10}H_6Na_2O_8S_2,2H_2O$.
Description. A yellow to light-brown powder.
Solubility. Freely soluble in water; insoluble in ethanol (~750 g/l) TS.
Identification. To 0.5 ml of a 2 mg/ml solution add 10 ml of water and 1 drop of ferric chloride (25 g/l) TS; a green colour is produced.
Sensitivity. Dissolve 5 mg in 10 ml of a mixture of 9 ml of sulfuric acid (~1760 g/l) TS and 4 ml of water. Separately dilute 0.5 ml of formaldehyde TS with water to make 1000 ml. Transfer to each of two separate test-tubes 5 ml of the disodium chromotropate solution, to one add 0.2 ml of the formaldehyde solution, and heat both tubes in a water-bath for 30 minutes; a violet colour is produced in the tube containing the formaldehyde solution.

Disodium chromotropate (10 g/l) TS. A solution of disodium chromotropate R containing about 9.5 g of $C_{10}H_6Na_2O_8S_2$ per litre.

Disodium edetate (50 g/l) TS. A solution of disodium edetate R containing about 50 g of $C_{10}H_{14}N_2Na_2O_8$ per litre.

Disodium edetate (0.1 mol/l) VS. Disodium edetate R, dissolved in water to contain 33.62 g of $C_{10}H_{14}N_2Na_2O_8$ in 1000 ml.
Method of standardization. Ascertain the exact concentration of the solution following an appropriate method, e.g., as described under disodium edetate (0.05 mol/l) VS in volume 1, p. 179.

Disodium hydrogen phosphate R [sodium phosphate R]. $Na_2HPO_4,12H_2O$ (SRIP, 1963, p. 192).

Disodium hydrogen phosphate (40 g/l) TS. A solution of disodium hydrogen phosphate R containing about 40 g of Na_2HPO_4 per litre.

Dithizone R. $C_{13}H_{12}N_4S$ (SRIP, 1963, p. 83).

4-Epianhydrotetracycline hydrochloride RS. International Chemical Reference Substance.

Epinephrine hydrogen tartrate R. Epinephrine hydrogen tartrate R as described in the monograph in volume 2, p. 110, which complies with the following test for the absence of levarterenol:
Levarterenol. Carry out descending paper chromatography (vol. 1, p. 84). Mix 4 volumes of 1-butanol R, 1 volume of glacial acetic acid R, and 5 volumes of water, shake and allow the two layers to separate. Use the lower layer as the stationary phase and the upper layer as the mobile phase. Apply to the paper 20 μl of a solution containing 50 mg/ml of epinephrine hydrogen tartrate R, develop for 5 hours, dry the paper, and spray with a freshly prepared 4.4 mg/ml solution of potassium ferricyanide R dissolved in buffer borate, pH 8.0, TS or another buffer having the same pH may be used; only 1 spot appears, which is pink.

4-Epitetracycline hydrochloride RS. International Chemical Reference Substance.

Ergometrine hydrogen maleate RS. International Chemical Reference Substance.

Ergotamine tartrate RS. International Chemical Reference Substance.

Estrone RS. International Chemical Reference Substance.

Ethambutol hydrochloride RS. International Chemical Reference Substance.

Ethanol, neutralized, TS.
Procedure. To a suitable quantity of ethanol (~750 g/l) TS add 0.5 ml of phenolphthalein/ethanol TS and just sufficient carbonate-free sodium hydroxide (0.02 mol/l) VS or (0.1 mol/l) VS to produce a faint pink colour.
Note: Prepare neutralized ethanol TS just prior to use.

Ethanol (~750 g/l), aldehyde-free TS [ethanol, aldehyde-free, (95 per cent.) R]. (SRIP, 1963, p. 84).

Ethanol (~675 g/l) TS. A solution of about 842 ml of ethanol (~750 g/l) TS diluted with water to 1000 ml.

Ethanol (~600 g/l) TS. A solution of about 735 ml of ethanol (~750 g/l) TS diluted with water to 1000 ml.

Ethinylestradiol RS. International Chemical Reference Substance.

Ethosuximide RS. International Chemical Reference Substance.

Ethylenediamine R. $C_2H_8N_2$.

Description.   A colourless to pale yellow, clear liquid; odour, ammonia-like.

Miscibility.   Miscible with water and ethanol (~750 g/l) TS; slightly miscible with ether R.

Boiling temperature.   About 116 °C.

Mass density. ρ_{20} = about 0.898 kg/l.

Storage.   Store in a tightly closed container, protected from air and acidic vapours.

Ethyl iodide R. C_2H_5I (SRIP, 1963, p. 87).

Ethylmethylketone R. C_4H_8O.

Description.   A clear, colourless, mobile liquid; odour, characteristic.

Miscibility.   Miscible with water, ethanol (~750 g/l) TS, ether R, and chloroform R.

Boiling range.   79–80 °C.

Mass density. ρ_{20} = about 0.805 kg/l.

Ferric ammonium sulfate TS1.

Procedure.   Dissolve 0.2 g of ferric ammonium sulfate R in 50 ml of water, add 6 ml of nitric acid (~1000 g/l) TS and sufficient water to produce 100 ml.

Ferric ammonium sulfate TS2.

Procedure.   Dissolve 8.3 g of ferric ammonium sulfate R in sufficient sulfuric acid (0.25 mol/l) VS to produce 1000 ml.

Firebrick, pink, R.   A suitable grade for use in gas chromatography with an average particle size of about 180–250 μm.

Fluphenazine decanoate RS.   International Chemical Reference Substance.

Fluphenazine enantate RS.   International Chemical Reference Substance.

Fluphenazine hydrochloride RS.   International Chemical Reference Substance.

Folic acid RS.   International Chemical Reference Substance.

Formaldehyde TS [formaldehyde R].   (SRIP, 1963, p. 91).

Formaldehyde/sulfuric acid TS.

Procedure.   To 10 ml of sulfuric acid (~1760 g/l) TS add 0.2 ml of formaldehyde TS.

Shelf-life.   Use within 1 month after preparation.

Formamide R. CH_3NO (SRIP, 1963, p. 92).

Formic acid, anhydrous, R. CH_2O_2, $d \sim 1.22$. Contains not less than 98.0% of CH_2O_2.

Description. A colourless liquid; odour, pungent.

Miscibility. Miscible with water and ethanol ($\sim$750 g/l) TS.

Chlorides. Dilute 1 ml to 15 ml with water and proceed as described under "Limit test for chlorides" (vol. 1, p. 116). Anhydrous formic acid R contains not more than 0.50 mg/g.

Sulfates. Dilute 0.5 ml to 15 ml with water and proceed as described under "Limit test for sulfates" (vol. 1, p. 116). Anhydrous formic acid R contains not more than 1.5 mg/g.

Residue on evaporation. Evaporate on a water-bath and dry to constant weight at 105 °C; leaves not more than 0.5 mg/g of residue.

Assay. To a tared flask containing about 10 ml of water, quickly add about 1 ml of the test liquid, and weigh. Dilute with 50 ml of water, and titrate with carbonate-free sodium hydroxide (1 mol/l) VS, using phenolphthalein/ethanol TS as indicator. Each ml of carbonate-free sodium hydroxide (1 mol/l) VS is equivalent to 46.03 mg of CH_2O_2.

Fuchsin, basic, R [magenta, basic R]. A mixture of rosaniline hydrochloride, $(H_2NC_6H_4)_2C{:}C_6H_3(CH_3){:}NH_2^+Cl^-$, and pararosaniline hydrochloride, $(H_2NC_6H_4)_2C{:}C_6H_4{:}NH_2^+Cl^-$.

Description. Crystals or crystalline fragments, with a glossy, greenish-bronze lustre.

Solubility. Soluble in water, ethanol ($\sim$750 g/l) TS, and amyl alcohol R.

Loss on drying. Dry to constant weight at 105 °C; it loses not more than 0.10 g/g.

Sulfated ash. Ignite 1 g with 0.5 ml of sulfuric acid ($\sim$1760 g/l) TS; not more than 3.0 mg/g.

Fuchsin TS.

Procedure. Pour carefully 40 ml of sulfuric acid ($\sim$1760 g/l) TS into 60 ml of water. Allow to cool and add 100 ml of a 1 g/l solution of basic fuchsin R. Dilute with water to 200 ml and allow to stand. An orange-yellow colour develops. Immediately before use dilute the solution with an equal volume of glacial acetic acid R.

Furosemide RS. International Chemical Reference Substance.

Griseofulvin RS. International Chemical Reference Substance.

Haloperidol RS. International Chemical Reference Substance.

Hexane R. *n*-Hexane, C_6H_{14}.

Description. A colourless, mobile, highly inflammable liquid.

Boiling range. Distils completely over a range of 1 °C between 67.5 and 69.5 °C.

Mass density. $\rho_{20} = 0.658$–0.659 kg/l

Refractive index. $n_D^{20} = 1.374$–1.375.

Hydrazine hydrate R. N_2H_4,H_2O. Contains not less than 98.0% of N_2H_4,H_2O.

Description. A clear, colourless liquid.

Miscibility. Miscible with water.

Residue on evaporation. Evaporate to dryness on a water-bath; it leaves a residue of not more than 5.0 mg/g.

Assay. Dilute 1 g to 200 ml with water. Neutralize 20 ml of this solution with hydrochloric acid (~420 g/l) TS and add 10 ml in excess. Add 5 ml of potassium cyanide (100 g/l) TS, titrate with potassium iodate (0.05 mol/l) VS until the brown colour which first forms becomes pale, add starch TS, and continue the titration until the blue colour disappears. Each ml of potassium iodate (0.05 mol/l) VS is equivalent to 2.503 mg of N_2H_4,H_2O.

Hydrochloric acid (~250 g/l) FeTS. Hydrochloric acid (~250 g/l) TS that complies with the following additional test: Evaporate 5 ml nearly to dryness on a water-bath, add 40 ml of water, 2 ml of citric acid (180 g/l) FeTS, and 2 drops of mercaptoacetic acid R; mix, make alkaline with ammonia (~100 g/l) FeTS, and dilute to 50 ml with water; no pink colour is produced.

Hydrochloric acid, brominated, AsTS.

Procedure. To 100 ml of hydrochloric acid (~250 g/l) AsTS add 1 ml of bromine AsTS.

Hydrochloric acid (5 mol/l) VS. Hydrochloric acid (~250 g/l) TS, diluted with water to contain 182.35 g of HCl in 1000 ml.

Method of standardization. Ascertain the exact concentration of the solution following the method described under hydrochloric acid (1 mol/l) VS, volume 1, p. 184.

Hydrochloric acid (0.2 mol/l) VS. Hydrochloric acid (~250 g/l) TS, diluted with water to contain 7.293 g of HCl in 1000 ml.

Method of standardization. Ascertain the exact concentration of the solution following the method described under hydrochloric acid (1 mol/l) VS, volume 1, p. 184.

Hydrochloric acid (0.02 mol/l) VS. Hydrochloric acid (~250 g/l) TS, diluted with water to contain 0.7293 g of HCl in 1000 ml.

Method of standardization. Ascertain the exact concentration of the solution following the method described under hydrochloric acid (1 mol/l) VS, volume 1, p. 184.

Hydrochloric acid (0.001 mol/l) VS. Hydrochloric acid (~250 g/l) TS, diluted with water to contain 36.47 mg of HCl in 1000 ml.

Method of standardization. Ascertain the exact concentration of the solution following the method described under hydrochloric acid (1 mol/l) VS, volume 1, p. 184.

Hydrochlorothiazide RS. International Chemical Reference Substance.

Hydrocortisone R. $C_{21}H_{30}O_5$. Use Hydrocortisone as described in the monograph in volume 2, p. 149.

Hydrocortisone RS. International Chemical Reference Substance.

Hydrocortisone acetate RS. International Chemical Reference Substance.

Hydrogen peroxide (~330 g/l) TS [hydrogen peroxide (30 per cent.) R]. (SRIP, 1963, p. 97).

Hydroxyethylcellulose R. Contains not less than 20 % of $C_2H_5O_2$, calculated with reference to the dried substance.
Description. A white or yellowish, flaky, heterogeneous mass; odourless.
Solubility. Practically insoluble in ethanol (~750 g/l) TS; after soaking for several hours in water, freely soluble in water.
Colour of solution. Transfer 2 g to a 200-ml glass-stoppered, conical flask, add 200 ml of carbon-dioxide-free water R, shake, and allow to stand for 30 minutes. Repeat this operation until the substance has dissolved and filter through sintered glass. Observe 5 ml of the filtrate; it is colourless (keep the filtrate for the acidity or alkalinity test).
Loss on drying. To 1.0 g add 25 ml of water, stir, and allow to stand. Repeat this operation until dissolved. Evaporate on a water-bath and dry to constant weight at 110 °C; it loses not more than 0.10 g/g. (Keep the dried substance for the assay).
Acidity or alkalinity. To 10 ml of the filtrate obtained from the test for colour of solution, add 2 drops of bromothymol blue/ethanol TS; a yellow colour is produced. Add 0.5 ml of potassium hydroxide (0.01 mol/l) VS; a green or blue solution is produced.
Assay. Place into a boiling flask as described under "Determination of methoxyl" (vol. 1, p. 136), 0.5 ml of acetic anhydride R, 0.05–0.10 g of phenol R, 0.20 g of red phosphorus R, and 5.0 ml of hydriodic acid (~970 g/l) TS; connect the flask to the condenser, pass a slow, uniform stream of carbon dioxide R through the solution, and heat for 60 minutes. Cool for 10 minutes and add 0.035 g, accurately weighed, of the dried substance obtained in the test for loss on drying. Proceed with this mixture as described under "Determination of methoxyl". For the calculation, take an average of 3 determinations. Each ml of sodium thiosulfate (0.1 mol/l) VS is equivalent to 1.018 mg of $C_2H_5O_2$.

Hydroxyethylcellulose TS.
Procedure. Place 50 ml of water in a 100 ml beaker and add 2.0 g of hydroxyethylcellulose R. After 15 hours, stir the solution for 1 minute and centrifuge for 15 minutes. Using a pipette, separate 20 ml of the supernatant liquid.
Note: Hydroxyethylcellulose TS must be freshly prepared.

Hydroxylamine hydrochloride R. NH_2OH,HCl (SRIP, 1963, p. 99).

(–)-3-(4-Hydroxy-3-methoxyphenyl)-2-methylalanine RS.   International Chemical Reference Substance.

Ibuprofen RS.   International Chemical Reference Substance.

Imidazole R.   Glyoxaline, $C_3H_4N_2$.   Contains not less than 99.0% of $C_3H_4N_2$.
Description.   A white, crystalline powder.
Solubility.   Soluble in water and ethanol (~750 g/l) TS.
Melting range.   89–93 °C.
Sulfated ash.   Not more than 0.5 mg/g.
Assay.   Dissolve 0.3 g in 50 ml of water and titrate with sulfuric acid (0.05 mol/l) VS, using bromocresol green/ethanol TS as indicator.   Each ml of sulfuric acid (0.05 mol/l) VS is equivalent to 6.808 mg of $C_3H_4N_2$.

Imidazole, recrystallized, R.
Procedure.   Dissolve 25 g of imidazole R in 100 ml of hot toluene R and cool in an ice-bath, while stirring.   Filter off the crystals with suction using filter-paper Whatman No. 54 or No. 541.   Repeat the crystallization and filtration, sucking as dry as possible.   Slurry wash the resulting crystals with about 50 ml of ether R and filter.   Repeat this process and then wash the crystals on the filter with ether R and suck as dry as possible.   Transfer to a shallow dish and dry at room temperature under reduced pressure (not exceeding 0.6 kPa or about 5 mm of mercury) over silica gel, desiccant, R.
Storage.   Store in a tightly closed container.

Imidazole/mercuric chloride TS.
Procedure.   Dissolve 8.25 g of recrystallized imidazole R in 60 ml of water and add 10 ml of hydrochloric acid (5 mol/l) VS.   Under continuous stirring add, drop by drop, 10 ml of mercuric chloride (2.7 g/l) TS.   If a cloudy solution results, discard and prepare a further solution by adding the mercuric chloride solution more slowly.   Adjust the pH to 6.80 ± 0.05 with hydrochloric acid (5 mol/l) VS (about 4 ml is required) and add sufficient water to produce 100 ml.

Indometacin RS.   International Chemical Reference Substance.

Iodine/ethanol TS.
Procedure.   Dissolve 10 g of iodine R in sufficient ethanol (~750 g/l) TS to produce 1000 ml.

Isoniazid RS.   International Chemical Reference Substance.

Kieselguhr R1.   Kieselguhr G.
Description.   A greyish-white powder, of an average particle size between 10 and 40 μm, containing per kg about 150 g of calcium sulfate, hemihydrate.

Kieselguhr R2. Kieselguhr GF254.

Description. A greyish-white powder, of an average particle size between 10 and 40 μm, containing per kg about 150 g of calcium sulfate, hemihydrate and an adequate amount (usually about 15 g/kg) of a fluorescent indicator having a maximum absorption at 254 nm.

Kieselguhr R3.

Description. A greyish-white powder, of an average particle size between 170 and 200 μm.

Kieselguhr R4.

Description. A greyish-white powder, of an average particle size between 70 and 150 μm.

Kieselguhr R5. Kieselguhr H.

Description. A fine, greyish-white powder; the grey colour becomes more pronounced on triturating the powder with water. The average particle size is between 10 and 40 μm.

Levarterenol hydrogen tartrate R. $C_8H_{11}NO_3,C_4H_6O_6,H_2O$. Contains not more than 99% of $C_8H_{11}NO_3,C_4H_6O_6$, calculated with reference to the anhydrous substance.

Description. A white, or almost white, crystalline powder; odourless.

Solubility. Soluble in water; slightly soluble in ethanol ($\sim$750 g/l) TS; practically insoluble in ether R.

Specific optical rotation. Use a 50 mg/ml solution; $[\alpha]_D^{20\,°C} = -10$ to $-13°C$.

Water. Determine as described under "Determination of water by the Karl Fischer Method", Method A (vol. 1, p. 135), using about 0.5 g of the substance; not less than 45 mg/g and not more than 58 mg/g.

Assay. Dissolve about 0.4 g, accurately weighed, in glacial acetic acid R, and titrate with perchloric acid (0.1 mol/l) VS as described under "Non-aqueous titration", Method A (vol. 1, p. 131). Each ml of perchloric acid (0.1 ml/l) VS is equivalent to 31.93 mg of $C_8H_{11}NO_3,C_4H_6O_6$.

Levodopa RS. International Chemical Reference Substance.

Lidocaine RS. International Chemical Reference Substance.

Lindane RS. International Chemical Reference Substance.

Lithium R. Li.

Description. A soft metal whose freshly cut surface is silvery-grey, tarnishing rapidly in air.

Solubility. Reacts violently with water, yielding hydrogen and a solution of lithium hydroxide; soluble in methanol R, yielding hydrogen and a solution of lithium methoxide; practically insoluble in ether R.

Lithium methoxide (0.1 mol/l) VS.

Procedure. Dissolve 0.694 g of lithium R and add sufficient toluene R to produce 1000 ml.

Method of standardization. Ascertain the exact concentration of the 0.1 mol/l solution in the following manner: Dissolve about 0.15 g, accurately weighed, of benzoic acid R in 25 ml of dimethylformamide R and titrate with the lithium methoxide solution to a red endpoint, using quinaldine red/methanol TS as indicator, as described under "Non-aqueous titration", Method B (vol. 1, p. 132). Each 12.21 mg of benzoic acid is equivalent to 1 ml of lithium methoxide (0.1 mol/l) VS. Lithium methoxide solutions must be standardized immediately before use.

Litmus R.   (SRIP, 1963, p. 108).

Litmus TS.

Procedure. Boil 10 g of litmus R with 40 ml of ethanol (~710 g/l) TS for 1 hour and pour away the clear liquid; repeat this operation twice with 30 ml of ethanol (~710 g/l) TS. Digest the washed litmus with 100 ml of water and filter.

Litmus paper R.   (SRIP, 1963, p. 109).

Macrogol 20M R.   Polyethylene glycol 20 000. A suitable grade to be used in gas-liquid chromatography.

Magnesium sulfate (50 g/l) TS.   A solution of magnesium sulfate R containing about 50 g of $MgSO_4$ per litre.

Mercuric chloride R. $HgCl_2$ (SRIP, 1963, p. 113).

Mercuric chloride (65 g/l) TS.   A solution of mercuric chloride R containing about 65 g of $HgCl_2$ per litre (approximately 0.25 mol/l).

Mercuric chloride (2.7 g/l) TS.   A solution of mercuric chloride R containing about 2.7 g of $HgCl_2$ per litre.

Mercury R.   Hg (SRIP, 1963, p. 115).

Methyldopa RS.   International Chemical Reference Substance.

Methylisobutylketone R.   Isopropylacetone, $C_6H_{12}O$. (SRIP, 1963, p. 119).

N-Methyl-N-nitrosotoluene-4-sulfonamide R. $C_8H_{10}N_2O_3S$.

Description. A yellow, crystalline powder.

Solubility. Insoluble in water; soluble in ethanol (~750 g/l) TS and ether R.

Melting temperature. About 60 °C.

Methyl orange/acetone TS.   A saturated solution of methyl orange R in acetone R.

N-Methylpiperazine R. $C_5H_{12}N_2$.
Mass density. $\rho_{20} = 0.902$ kg/l.
Refractive index. $n_D^{20} = 1.466$.

Methyl silicone gum R. A suitable grade to be used in gas-liquid chromatography.

Methyltestosterone RS. International Chemical Reference Substance.

Methylthioninium chloride (1 g/l) TS. A solution of methylthioninium chloride R containing about 1 g of $C_{16}H_{18}ClN_3S$ per litre.

Methylthymol blue R. Tetrasodium [$3H$-2,1-benzoxathiol-3-ylidenebis[(6-hydroxy-5-isopropyl-2-methyl-m-phenylene)methylenenitrilo]]tetraacetic acid S,S-dioxide; $C_{37}H_{44}N_2Na_4O_{13}S$.
Description. A brownish-black powder.
Solubility. Freely soluble in water; very slightly soluble in ethanol ($\sim$750 g/l) TS.

Methylthymol blue mixture R.
Procedure. Mix 1 part of methylthymol blue R with 100 parts of potassium nitrate R.

Metronidazole RS. International Chemical Reference Substance.

1-Naphthol R. $C_{10}H_8O$.
Description. Colourless crystals or a white, crystalline powder; odour, characteristic.
Solubility. Soluble in 5 parts of ethanol ($\sim$750 g/l) TS (may form a slightly opalescent, colourless or almost colourless solution).
Melting range. 93–96 °C.
Sulfated ash. Not more than 0.5 mg/g.

1-Naphthol TS1.
Procedure. Dissolve 0.10 g of 1-naphthol R in 3 ml of sodium hydroxide ($\sim$150 g/l) TS and dilute with sufficient water to produce 100 ml.
Note: 1-Naphthol TS1 must be prepared immediately before use.

1-Naphtholbenzein R. $C_{27}H_{20}O_3$.
Description. A reddish-brown powder.
Solubility. Practically insoluble in water; soluble in ethanol ($\sim$750 g/l) TS, benzene R, ether R, and glacial acetic acid R.

1-Naphtholbenzein/acetic acid TS.
Procedure. Dissolve 0.2 g of 1-naphtholbenzein R in sufficient glacial acetic acid R to produce 100 ml.

N-(1-Naphthyl)ethylenediamine hydrochloride R. $C_{12}H_{14}N_2$,2HCl (SRIP, 1963, p. 124).

N-(1-Naphthyl)ethylenediamine hydrochloride (5 g/l) TS. A solution of *N*-(1-naphthyl)ethylenediamine hydrochloride R containing about 5 g of $C_{12}H_{14}N_2,2HCl$ per litre.

N-(1-Naphthyl)ethylenediamine hydrochloride (1 g/l) TS. A solution of *N*-(1-naphthyl)ethylenediamine hydrochloride R containing about 1 g of $C_{12}H_{14}N_2,2HCl$ per litre.

N-(1-Naphthyl)ethylenediamine hydrochloride/ethanol TS.
Procedure. Dissolve 5 g of *N*-(1-naphthyl)ethylenediamine hydrochloride R in sufficient ethanol (~750 g/l) TS to produce 1000 ml.

Nicotinamide RS. International Chemical Reference Substance.

Nicotinic acid RS. International Chemical Reference Substance.

Nitric acid, fuming, R. HNO_3 (SRIP, 1963, p. 126); *d* ~1.5.

4-Nitroaniline R [*p*-nitroaniline R]. $C_6H_6N_2O_2$ (SRIP, 1963, p. 127).

4-Nitroaniline TS1.
Procedure. Dissolve 5 g of 4-nitroaniline R in sufficient hydrochloric acid (1 mol/l) VS to produce 1000 ml.

4-Nitroaniline TS2.
Procedure. Dissolve 0.4 g of 4-nitroaniline R in 60 ml of hydrochloric acid (1 mol/l) VS, cool to 15 °C, and add sufficient sodium nitrite (100 g/l) TS until 1 drop of the mixture turns starch/iodine paper R blue.
Note: 4-Nitroaniline TS2 must be freshly prepared.

4-Nitrobenzoyl chloride R [*p*-nitrobenzoyl chloride R]. $C_7H_4ClNO_3$ (SRIP, 1963, p. 128).

Nitrogen, oxygen-free, R. Nitrogen R which has been freed from oxygen by passing it through alkaline pyrogallol TS.

1-Nitroso-2-naphthol-3,6-disodium disulfonate R [1-nitroso-2-naphthol-3,6-disodium sulfonate R]. $C_{10}H_5NNa_2O_8S_2$ (SRIP, 1963, p. 129).

1-Nitroso-2-naphthol-3,6-disodium disulfonate (2 g/l) TS. A solution of 1-nitroso-2-naphthol-3,6-disodium disulfonate R containing about 2 g of $C_{10}H_5NNa_2O_8S_2$ per litre.

Norethisterone RS. International Chemical Reference Substance.

Norethisterone acetate RS. International Chemical Reference Substance.

Opalescence standard TS1.
Procedure. Dilute 15 ml of opalescence stock standard TS with sufficient water to produce 1000 ml.
Shelf-life. Use within 24 hours after preparation.

Opalescence standard TS2.

Procedure. Dilute 5.0 ml of opalescence standard TS1 with sufficient water to produce 100 ml. Mix well and shake before use.

Note: Opalescence standard TS2 must be freshly prepared.

Opalescence stock standard TS.

Procedure. Dissolve 1.0 g of hydrazine sulfate R in sufficient water to produce 100 ml and allow to stand for 4–6 hours. To 25.0 ml of this solution add a solution of 2.5 g of methenamine R dissolved in 25.0 ml of water, mix well, and allow to stand for 24 hours.

Storage. Store in a glass container free from surface defects.

Shelf-life. Use within 2 months after preparation.

Osmium tetroxide R. OsO_4.

Caution. The fumes are corrosive to the eyes, the mucous membranes, and the skin.

Description. Yellow, needle-shaped crystals or a yellow, crystalline mass; hygroscopic; light sensitive; odour, pungent.

Solubility. Soluble in water, ethanol (~750 g/l) TS, and ether R.

Oxytetracycline hydrochloride RS. International Chemical Reference Substance.

Papaverine hydrochloride RS. International Chemical Reference Substance.

Perchloric acid (0.05 mol/l) VS.

Procedure. To 900 ml of glacial acetic acid R1 at about 25°C, add 4.2 ml of perchloric acid (~1170 g/l) TS, mix, add 15 ml of acetic anhydride R, and mix again. Cool to room temperature, add sufficient glacial acetic acid R1 to produce 1000 ml, and allow to stand for 24 hours.

Water and method of standardization. Determine the content of water and ascertain the exact concentration of the solution following the method described under perchloric acid (0.1 mol/l) VS, volume 1, p. 194.

Petroleum, light, R1.

Description. A colourless, very volatile, highly inflammable liquid.

Boiling range. 40–60 °C.

Mass density. $\rho_{20} = 0.630-0.650$ kg/l.

2-Phenoxyethanol R. $C_8H_{10}O_2$.

Description. A clear, colourless, oily liquid; odour, faintly aromatic.

Miscibility. Slightly miscible with water; freely miscible with ethanol (~750 g/l) TS and ether R.

Mass density. ρ_{20} = about 1.1 kg/l.

Refractive index. n_D^{20} = about 1.537.

Freezing point. Not below 12.0 °C.

Phenoxymethylpenicillin RS. International Chemical Reference Substance.

Phenoxymethylpenicillin calcium RS. International Chemical Reference Substance.

Phenoxymethylpenicillin potassium RS. International Chemical Reference Substance.

2-Phenylethanol R. $C_8H_{10}O$. A suitable grade to be used in gas-liquid chromatography.

2-Phenylethanol TS.
Procedure. Dissolve 1 g of 2-phenylethanol R in sufficient methanol R to produce 50 ml.

Phenylhydrazine R. $C_6H_8N_2$ (SRIP, 1963, p. 140).

Phenylhydrazine hydrochloride R. $C_6H_8N_2$,HCl (SRIP, 1963, p. 140).

Phenylhydrazine/sulfuric acid TS.
Procedure. Dissolve 65 mg of phenylhydrazine hydrochloride R, previously recrystallized from ethanol (~710 g/l) TS, in a sufficient quantity of a mixture of 170 ml of sulfuric acid (~1760 g/l) TS and 80 ml of water to produce 100 ml.
Note: Phenylhydrazine/sulfuric acid TS must be freshly prepared.

Phenytoin RS. International Chemical Reference Substance.

Phosphate/citrate buffer pH 4.5, TS.
Procedure. Dissolve 2.15 g of disodium hydrogen phosphate R in 30 ml of water and adjust the pH of the solution to 4.5 with citric acid (20 g/l) TS.

Phosphomolybdic acid R. H_3PO_4,$12MoO_3$,$24H_2O$ (SRIP, 1963, p. 141).

Phosphorus, red R.
Description. A dark red powder.
Solubility. Insoluble in water and dilute acids.
Soluble matter. Heat 2.0 g with 30 ml of acetic acid (~300 g/l) TS on a water-bath for 15 minutes, cool, dilute to 50 ml, filter, evaporate 25 ml of the filtrate on a water-bath and dry at 110 °C for 2 hours; the residue weighs not more than 50 mg.
Yellow phosphorus. Shake 5.0 g with 20 ml of carbon disulfide R in a glass-stoppered cylinder, filter, and immerse in the filtrate a strip of filter-paper, 10 cm by 0.5 cm, previously immersed in copper(II) sulfate (80 g/l) TS, and allow to dry in the air; no stain is produced.
Loss on drying. Dry to constant weight over sulfuric acid (~1760 g/l) TS; it loses not more than 10 mg/g.

Platinic chloride R. H_2PtCl_6,$6H_2O$ (SRIP, 1963, p. 144).

Platinic chloride (60 g/l) TS. A solution of platinic chloride R containing about 63 g of H_2PtCl_6 per litre.

Potassio-cupric tartrate TS.

Procedure. Dissolve 7 g of copper(II) sulfate R in sufficient water to produce 100 ml. Separately dissolve 35 g of potassium sodium tartrate R and 10 g of sodium hydroxide R in 100 ml of water. Shortly before use, mix together equal volumes of both solutions.

Potassio-mercuric iodide TS.

Procedure. Dissolve 1.355 g of mercuric chloride R in 60 ml of water; separately dissolve 5 g of potassium iodide R in 20 ml of water; mix the two solutions and dilute to 100 ml with water.

Potassio-mercuric iodide, alkaline, TS.

Procedure. Dissolve 3.5 g of potassium iodide R and 1.25 g of mercuric chloride R in 80 ml of water, add while stirring a cold saturated solution of mercuric chloride R in water until a slight red precipitate remains. Then add 12 g of sodium hydroxide R and mix to dissolve, add a little more of the saturated solution of mercuric chloride R and sufficient water to produce 100 ml; allow to stand for 24 hours and decant the clear liquid.

Potassium bromate R. $KBrO_3$ (SRIP, 1963, p. 147).

Potassium bromate (50 g/l) TS. A solution of potassium bromate R containing about 50 g of $KBrO_3$ per litre.

Potassium bromate (0.0167 mol/l) VS. Potassium bromate R, dissolved in water to contain 2.784 g of $KBrO_3$ in 1000 ml.

Potassium bromide (0.119 g/l) TS. A solution of potassium bromide R containing about 0.1190 g of KBr per litre.

Potassium chromate R. K_2CrO_4 (SRIP, 1963, p. 152).

Potassium chromate (100 g/l) TS. A solution of potassium chromate R containing about 97 g of K_2CrO_4 per litre (approximately 0.5 mol/l).

Potassium cyanide R. KCN (SRIP, 1963, p. 153).

Potassium cyanide (100 g/l) TS. A solution of potassium cyanide R containing about 100 g of KCN per litre.

Potassium cyanide (50 g/l) TS. A solution of potassium cyanide R containing about 50 g of KCN per litre.

Potassium dichromate (100 g/l) TS. A solution of potassium dichromate R containing about 98 g of $K_2Cr_2O_7$ per litre (approximately 0.4 mol/l).

Potassium ferricyanide (50 g/l) TS.

Procedure. Wash about 5 g of crystalline potassium ferricyanide R with a little water and dissolve the washed crystals in sufficient water to produce 100 ml.

Note: Potassium ferricyanide (50 g/l) TS must be freshly prepared.

Potassium ferrocyanide R. K$_4$Fe(CN)$_6$,3H$_2$O (SRIP, 1963, p. 156).

Potassium ferrocyanide (45 g/l) TS. A solution of potassium ferrocyanide R containing about 50 g of K$_4$Fe(CN)$_6$ per litre.

Potassium hydroxide/ethanol TS2.
Procedure. Dissolve 112 g of potassium hydroxide R in sufficient ethanol (~710 g/l) TS to produce 1000 ml (approximately 2 mol/l).

Potassium hydroxide/methanol TS.
Procedure. Dissolve 30 g of potassium hydroxide R in sufficient methanol R to produce 1000 ml.

Potassium hydroxide (0.01 mol/l) VS. Potassium hydroxide R, dissolved in water to contain 0.5610 g of KOH in 1000 ml.
Method of standardization. Ascertain the exact concentration of the solution following the method described under potassium hydroxide (1 mol/l) VS, volume 1, p. 199.

Potassium hydroxide/ethanol (1 mol/l) VS.
Potassium hydroxide R, dissolved in ethanol (~710 g/l) TS to contain 56.10 g of KOH in 1000 ml.
Method of standardization. Ascertain the exact concentration of the solution following the method described under potassium hydroxide/ethanol (0.5 mol/l) VS, volume 1, p. 200.

Potassium iodate R. KIO$_3$ (SRIP, 1963, p. 160).

Potassium iodate (0.05 mol/l) VS. Potassium iodate R, dissolved in water to contain 10.70 g of KIO$_3$ in 1000 ml.
Method of standardization. Ascertain the exact concentration of the 0.05 mol/l solution in the following manner. Place 10.0 ml of the potassium iodate solution in a glass-stoppered flask, dilute with 200 ml of water, add 2 g of potassium iodide R, and 25 ml of sulfuric acid (~100 g/l) TS. Allow the solution to stand for 10 minutes and titrate the liberated iodine with sodium thiosulfate (0.1 mol/l) VS, adding 3 ml of starch TS as the endpoint is approached. Correct for a blank determined on the same quantities of the same reagents.

Potassium iodate (0.01 mol/l) VS. Potassium iodate R, dissolved in water to contain 2.140 g of KIO$_3$ in 1000 ml.
Method of standardization. Ascertain the exact concentration of the solution following the method described under potassium iodate (0.05 mol/l) VS.

Potassium iodide (400 g/l) TS. A solution of potassium iodide R containing about 400 g of KI per litre.

Potassium iodide (300 g/l) TS. A solution of potassium iodide R containing about 300 g of KI per litre.

Potassium iodide (60 g/l) TS. A solution of potassium iodide R containing about 60 g of KI per litre.

Potassium iodide/starch TS1.
Procedure. Dissolve 10 g of potassium iodide R in 95 ml of water and add to it 5 ml of starch TS.
Note: Potassium iodide/starch TS1 must be freshly prepared.

Potassium iodobismuthate TS1.
Procedure. Dissolve 100 g of tartaric acid R in 400 ml of water and add 8.5 g of bismuth oxynitrate R. Shake the solution for 1 hour, add 200 ml of potassium iodide (400 g/l) TS, and mix. Allow to stand for 24 hours and filter.

Potassium iodobismuthate TS2.
Procedure. Dissolve 100 g of tartaric acid R in 500 ml of water and add 50 ml of potassium iodobismuthate TS1.

Potassium iodoplatinate TS.
Procedure. Dissolve 2.5 g of platinic chloride R in 50 ml of water, add 45 ml of a 0.1 g/ml solution of potassium iodide R, and dilute to 100 ml with water.
Storage. Store in amber glass containers.

Potassium periodate R. KIO_4 (SRIP, 1963, p. 164).

Potassium periodate TS.
Procedure. To 2.8 g of potassium periodate R add 200 ml of water followed by 20 ml of sulfuric acid (~1760 g/l) TS added drop by drop while shaking to effect solution; cool and add sufficient water to produce 1000 ml.

Potassium permanganate (0.002 mol/l) VS. Potassium permanganate R, dissolved in water to contain 0.3161 g of $KMnO_4$ in 1000 ml.
Method of standardization. Ascertain the exact concentration of the solution following the method described under potassium permanganate (0.02 mol/l) VS, volume 1, p. 201.

Potassium sodium tartrate R [sodium potassium tartrate R]. $C_4H_4KNaO_6,4H_2O$ (SRIP, 1963, p. 193).

Potassium thiocyanate R. KCNS. Contains not less than 99.0% of KCNS, calculated with reference to the dried substance.
Description. Colourless crystals.
Solubility. Soluble in 0.5 part of water and in 15 parts of dehydrated ethanol R.
Alkalinity. A 0.1 g/ml solution in carbon-dioxide-free water R is not alkaline to bromothymol blue/ethanol TS.

Ammonia. Boil 1.0 g with 5 ml of sodium hydroxide (~80 g/l) TS; no ammonia is evolved.

Chlorides. Dissolve 1.0 g in a solution of 1 g of ammonium nitrate R in 30 ml of hydrogen peroxide (~60 g/l) TS containing not more than 1 μg/g of chlorides, add 1 g of sodium hydroxide R, and warm gently; when the vigorous reaction subsides add a further 30 ml of hydrogen peroxide (~60 g/l) TS and boil for 2 minutes. Cool, add 5 ml of nitric acid (~1000 g/l) TS and 1 ml of silver nitrate (40 g/l) TS; any opalescence produced is not greater than that produced by treating 1 ml of hydrochloric acid (0.01 mol/1) VS in the same manner.

Sulfates. Dissolve 0.50 g in 20 ml of water and proceed as described under "Limit test for sulfates" (vol. 1, p. 116); not more than 1.0 mg/g.

Other sulfur compounds. Dissolve 1.0 g in 50 ml of water, add 2 ml of hydrochloric acid (~70 g/l) TS, and titrate with iodine (0.1 mol/l) VS; not more than 0.5 ml of iodine (0.1 mol/l) VS is required.

Loss on drying. Dry to constant weight at 105 °C; it loses not more than 20 mg/g.

Assay. Dissolve about 0.4 g, accurately weighed, in 50 ml of water, add 5 ml of nitric acid (~1000 g/l) TS, 50 ml of silver nitrate (0.1 mol/l) VS, and 5 ml of ferric ammonium sulfate (45 g/l) TS, and titrate the excess of silver nitrate with ammonium thiocyanate (0.1 mol/l) VS. Each ml of silver nitrate (0.1 mol/l) VS is equivalent to 9.718 mg of KCNS.

Note: Potassium thiocyanate R is deliquescent.

Prednisolone RS. International Chemical Reference Substance.

Primaquine diphosphate RS. International Chemical Reference Substance.

Procaine hydrochloride RS. International Chemical Reference Substance.

Progesterone RS. International Chemical Reference Substance.

1-Propanol R. *n*-Propanol; propan-1-ol, C_3H_8O.
Description. A clear, colourless liquid.
Miscibility. Miscible with water and ethanol (~750 g/l) TS.
Boiling range. Not less than 95% distils between 95 and 98 °C.
Mass density. ρ_{20} = about 0.803 kg/l.
Residue on evaporation. Evaporate on a water-bath and dry to constant weight at 105 °C; it leaves a residue of not more than 0.1 mg/g.

2-Propanol R [*iso*-propanol R]; isopropyl alcohol; C_3H_8O (SRIP, 1963, p. 167).

Propranolol hydrochloride RS. International Chemical Reference Subtance.

Propylene glycol R. $C_3H_8O_2$ (SRIP, 1963, p. 168).

Pyridostigmine bromide RS. International Chemical Reference Substance.

Pyrogallol R. Pyrogallic acid; 1,2,3-trihydroxybenzene, $C_6H_6O_3$ (SRIP, 1963, p. 170).

Pyrogallol, alkaline, TS.
Procedure. Dissolve 0.5 g of pyrogallol R in 2 ml of water. Dissolve separately 12 g of potassium hydroxide R in 8 ml of water. Immediately before use mix the two solutions.

Quinaldine red R. 2-(*p*-Dimethylaminostyryl)quinoline ethiodide; $C_{21}H_{23}IN_2$.
Description. A dark blue-black powder.
Solubility. Sparingly soluble in water; freely soluble in ethanol (~750 g/l) TS.
Melting temperature. About 260 °C with decomposition.

Quinaldine red/ethanol TS.
Procedure. Dissolve 0.1 g of quinaldine red R in 100 ml of ethanol (~750 g/l) TS.

Quinaldine red/methanol TS.
Procedure. Dissolve 1.0 g of quinaldine red R in sufficient methanol R to produce 100 ml.

Quinine R. $C_{20}H_{24}N_2O_2$.
Description. A white, microcrystalline powder; odourless.
Solubility. Very slightly soluble in water; slightly soluble in boiling water; very soluble in ethanol (~750 g/l) TS; soluble in ether R and benzene R.
Melting temperature. About 175 °C.
Identification. Very dilute solutions containing sulfuric acid (~100 g/l) TS show a blue fluorescence. Acid solutions are levorotatory. Dissolve about 5 mg in a mixture of 5 ml of water and 0.3 ml of hydrochloric acid (~70 g/l) TS. Mix the solution with 0.2 ml of bromine TS1 and add 1 ml of ammonia (~35 g/l) TS; an emerald green colour is produced.

Reserpine RS. International Chemical Reference Substance.

Riboflavin RS. International Chemical Reference Substance.

Salicylic acid R. $C_7H_6O_3$. Salicylic acid as described in the monograph in volume 2, p. 28.

Selenious acid R. H_2SeO_3. Contains not less than 93% of H_2SeO_3.
Description. Colourless or white crystals.
Solubility. Soluble in water and ethanol (~750 g/l) TS.
Assay. Transfer about 0.1 g, accurately weighed, to a glass-stoppered flask, and dissolve in 50 ml of water. Add 10 ml of potassium iodide (300 g/l) TS and 5 ml of hydrochloric acid (~420 g/l) TS, mix, insert the stopper into the flask, and allow to stand for 10 minutes. Dilute with 50 ml of water, add 3 ml of starch TS, and titrate with sodium thiosulfate (0.1 mol/l) VS until the colour is

no longer diminished, then titrate with iodine (0.1 mol/l) VS to a blue colour. Subtract the volume of iodine (0.1 mol/l) VS from the volume of sodium thiosulfate (0.1 mol/l) VS equivalent to selenious acid. Each ml of sodium thiosulfate (0.1 mol/l) VS is equivalent to 3.225 mg of H_2SeO_3.

Note: Selenious acid R effloresces in dry air and is hygroscopic in moist air.

Selenious acid/sulfuric acid TS.
Procedure. Dissolve 10 mg of selenious acid R in 2 ml of sulfuric acid (~1760 g/l) TS.

Silica gel R1. Silica gel G.
Description. A white, homogeneous powder.
Composition. A mixture of silica gel (particle size 10–40 μm) and calcium sulfate, hemihydrate (about 130 g/kg).

Silica gel R2. Silica gel HF(UV254).
Description. A white, homogeneous powder.
Composition. Silica gel (particle size 10–40 μm) containing a fluorescent indicator having an optimal intensity at 254 nm (about 15 g/kg).

Silica gel R3. Silica gel H.
Description. A white, homogeneous powder.
Particle size. 10–40 μm.

Silica gel R4. Silica gel GF (UV 254).
Description. A white, homogeneous powder.
Composition. A mixture of silica gel (particle size 10–40 μm) and calcium sulfate, hemihydrate (about 130 g/kg) containing a fluorescent indicator having an optimal intensity at 254 nm (about 15 g/kg).

Silica gel R5. Silica gel 60.
Description. A white, homogeneous powder.
Average pore size. 6 nm.

Silver oxide R. Ag_2O.
Description. A brownish-black, heavy powder; odourless.
Solubility. Practically insoluble in water; freely soluble in nitric acid (~130 g/l) TS and ammonia (~260 g/l) TS.
Substances insoluble in nitric acid. Dissolve 5 g in a mixture of 5 ml of nitric acid (~1000 g/l) TS and 10 ml of water, dilute to about 65 ml with water, and filter any undissolved residue on a tared filtering crucible (retain the filtrate for the test for substances not precipitated by hydrochloric acid). Wash the crucible with water until the last washing shows no opalescence with 1 drop of hydrochloric acid (~250 g/l) TS, and dry to constant weight at 105 °C; not more than 0.2 mg/g.

Substances not precipitated by hydrochloric acid. Dilute the filtrate obtained in the test for substances insoluble in nitric acid to 250 ml with water, heat to boiling, and add dropwise sufficient hydrochloric acid ($\sim$250 g/l) TS to precipitate all of the silver (about 5 ml), avoiding any great excess. Cool, dilute to 300 ml with water, and allow to stand overnight. Filter, evaporate 200 ml of the filtrate to dryness in a suitable tared porcelain dish, and ignite; not more than 0.5 mg/g.

Alkalinity. Heat 2 g with 40 ml of water on a water-bath for 15 minutes, cool, and dilute to 50 ml with water. Filter, discarding the first 10 ml of the filtrate. To 25 ml of the subsequent filtrate add 2 drops of phenolphthalein/ethanol TS, and titrate with hydrochloric acid (0.02 mol/l) VS to the disappearance of any pink colour; not more than 0.20 ml is required.

Sodium R. Na (SRIP, 1963, p. 175).

Sodium acetate R. $C_2H_3NaO_2,3H_2O$. Contains not less than 99.0% of $C_2H_3NaO_2,3H_2O$.

The present text supersedes that published in volume 1, p. 202.

Description. Colourless crystals.

Solubility. Very soluble in water; sparingly soluble in ethanol ($\sim$750 g/l) TS.

Clarity and colour of solution. A 0.1 g/ml solution is clear and colourless.

pH value. pH of a 50 mg/ml solution, 7.5–9.2.

Iron. Use 8 g; the solution complies with the "Limit test for iron" (vol. 1, p. 121); not more than 5.0 μg/g.

Heavy metals. Use 1.0 g for the preparation of the test solution as described in "Limit test for heavy metals", Procedure 1 (vol. 1, p. 118); determine the heavy metals content according to Method A; not more than 10 μg/g.

Substances reducing permanganate. Dissolve 1 g in 100 ml of boiling water, add 2 ml of sulfuric acid ($\sim$100 g/l) TS and 0.05 ml of potassium permanganate (0.02 mol/l) VS, and boil for 5 minutes; the pink colour does not entirely disappear.

Assay. Dissolve about 0.4 g, accurately weighed, in 100 ml of glacial acetic acid R and 5 ml of acetic anhydride R. After 5 minutes add 10 drops of 1-naphtholbenzein/acetic acid TS, and titrate to a green endpoint with perchloric acid (0.1 mol/l) VS as described under "Non-aqueous titration", Method A (vol. 1, p. 131). Each ml of perchloric acid (0.1 mol/l) VS is equivalent to 13.61 mg of $C_2H_3NaO_2,3H_2O$.

Sodium acetate (60 g/l) TS. A solution of sodium acetate R containing about 60 g of $C_2H_3NaO_2$ per litre.

Sodium acetate (50 g/l) TS. A solution of sodium acetate R containing about 50 g of $C_2H_3NaO_2$ per litre.

Sodium arsenite (0.1 mol/l) VS.

Procedure. Dissolve 5 g of arsenic trioxide R in a mixture of 20 ml of sodium hydroxide (~80 g/l) TS and 20 ml of water, dilute to 400 ml with water and add hydrochloric acid (~70 g/l) TS until the solution is neutral to litmus paper R. Dissolve 2 g of sodium hydrogen carbonate R in the prepared solution and dilute to 500 ml with water.

Method of standardization. Ascertain the exact concentration of the solution following the method described under sodium arsenite (0.05 mol/l) VS.

Storage. Add 1 drop of mercury R for the preservation of the solution.

Sodium arsenite (0.05 mol/l) VS.

Procedure. Dissolve 5 g of arsenic trioxide R in a mixture of 20 ml of sodium hydroxide (~80 g/l) TS and 20 ml of water, dilute to 400 ml with water, and add hydrochloric acid (~70 g/l) TS until the solution is neutral to litmus paper R. Dissolve 4 g of sodium hydrogen carbonate R in the prepared solution and dilute to 1000 ml with water.

Method of standardization. Ascertain the exact concentration of the 0.05 mol/l solution in the following manner: Dilute 25 ml with 50 ml of water, add 5 g of sodium hydrogen carbonate R, and titrate with iodine (0.1 mol/l) VS, using starch TS as indicator.

Storage. Add 1 drop of mercury R for the preservation of the solution.

Sodium carbonate, anhydrous, FeR. Anhydrous sodium carbonate R that complies with the following additional test: Dissolve 4.0 g in 25 ml of water, add 8 ml of hydrochloric acid (~250 g/l) FeTS, and proceed with the "Limit test for iron" (vol. 1, p. 121), using 2 ml of iron standard FeTS; not more than 10 μg/g.

Sodium carbonate (200 g/l) TS. A solution of sodium carbonate R containing 200 g of Na_2CO_3 per litre.

Sodium carbonate (75 g/l) TS. A solution of sodium carbonate R containing about 75 g of Na_2CO_3 per litre.

Sodium carbonate (10 g/l) TS. A solution of sodium carbonate R containing about 10.6 g of Na_2CO_3 per litre (approximately 0.1 mol/l).

Sodium chloride, pyrogen-free, R. Sodium chloride R which complies with the following additional test:

Pyrogens. Carry out the test as described under "Test for pyrogens" (vol. 1, p. 155) injecting, per kg of the rabbit's weight, a solution containing 9 mg in 10 ml of sterile water R.

Sodium diethyldithiocarbamate R. $C_5H_{10}NNaS_2,3H_2O$ (SRIP, 1963, p. 183).

Sodium diethyldithiocarbamate (0.8 g/l) TS. A solution of sodium diethyldithiocarbamate R containing about 0.8 g of $C_5H_{10}NNaS_2$ per litre.

Sodium dihydrogen phosphate R [sodium biphosphate]; sodium phosphate, monobasic; NaH$_2$PO$_4$,H$_2$O (SRIP, 1963, p. 178).

Sodium dihydrogen phosphate (45 g/l) TS. A solution of sodium dihydrogen phosphate R containing about 47 g of NaH$_2$PO$_4$ per litre.

Sodium hydrogen carbonate R [sodium bicarbonate]; NaHCO$_3$ (SRIP, 1963, p. 177).

Sodium hydrogen carbonate (40 g/l) TS. A solution of sodium hydrogen carbonate R containing about 42 g of NaHCO$_3$ per litre (approximately 0.5 mol/l).

Sodium hydroxide (~150 g/l) TS. A solution of sodium hydroxide R containing about 150 g of NaOH per litre.

Sodium hydroxide (10 g/l) TS. A solution of sodium hydroxide R containing about 10 g of NaOH per litre (approximately 0.25 mol/l).

Sodium hydroxide/methanol TS.
Procedure. Dissolve 40 g of sodium hydroxide R in sufficient methanol R to produce 1000 ml.

Sodium hydroxide (0.5 mol/l) VS. Sodium hydroxide R, dissolved in water to contain 20.00 g of NaOH in 1000 ml.
Method of standardization. Ascertain the exact concentration of the solution following the method described under sodium hydroxide (1 mol/l) VS, volume 1, p. 204.

Sodium hydroxide (0.02 mol/l) VS. Sodium hydroxide R, dissolved in water to contain 0.8001 g of NaOH in 1000 ml.
Method of standardization. Ascertain the exact concentration of the solution following the method described under sodium hydroxide (1 mol/l) VS, volume 1, p. 204.

Sodium hydroxide (0.001 mol/l) VS. Sodium hydroxide R, dissolved in water to contain 40.01 mg of NaOH in 1000 ml.
Method of standardization. Ascertain the exact concentration of the solution following the method described under sodium hydroxide (1 mol/l) VS, volume 1, p. 204.

Sodium hypochlorite (~40 g/l) TS.
Description. A pale, greenish yellow, clear liquid; odour, resembling that of chlorine.
Assay. Introduce 3 ml into a glass-stoppered flask, weigh accurately, and add 50 ml of water. Add 2 g of potassium iodide R and 10 ml of acetic acid (~300 g/l) TS, and titrate the liberated iodine with sodium thiosulfate

(0.1 mol/l) VS, adding 3 ml of starch TS as the endpoint is approached. Each ml of sodium thiosulfate (0.1 mol/l) VS is equivalent to 3.723 mg of NaOCl.

Storage. Sodium hypochlorite (~40 g/l) TS must be kept in a light-resistant container at a temperature not exceeding 25 °C.

Sodium hypochlorite TS1.

Procedure. Dilute 10 ml of sodium hypochlorite (~40 g/l) TS to 100 ml with water (contains approximately 0.5% of chlorine).

Sodium metabisulfite R. $Na_2O_5S_2$ (SRIP, 1963, p. 187).

Sodium metaperiodate R. Sodium periodate $NaIO_4$. Contains not less than 98.0% of $NaIO_4$.

Description. White crystals or a white, crystalline powder.

Solubility. Soluble in water.

Assay. Dissolve 0.5 g in 100 ml of water. Add 3 g of sodium hydrogen carbonate R and 3 g of potassium iodide R, and titrate the liberated iodine with sodium arsenite (0.05 mol/l) VS. Each ml of sodium arsenite (0.05 mol/l) VS is equivalent to 10.69 mg of $NaIO_4$.

Sodium methoxide (0.1 mol/l) VS.

Procedure. Cool in ice-water 150 ml of dehydrated methanol R and add in small portions 2.5 g of freshly cut sodium R. When the metal has dissolved, add sufficient toluene R to produce 1000 ml.

Method of standardization. Ascertain the exact concentration of the 0.1 mol/l solution in the following manner: Titrate 0.10 g of benzoic acid R, accurately weighed, as described under "Non-aqueous titration", Method B (vol. 1, p. 132). Each 12.21 mg of $C_7H_6O_6$ is equivalent to 1 ml of sodium methoxide (0.1 mol/l) VS.

Note: Sodium methoxide (0.1 mol/l) VS must be standardized immediately before use.

Sodium molybdotungstophosphate TS.

Procedure. Boil under a reflux condenser for 2 hours 350 ml of water with 50 g of sodium tungstate R, 12 g of phosphomolybdic acid R, and 25 ml of phosphoric acid (~1440 g/l) TS; cool and add sufficient water to produce 500 ml.

Sodium 1,2-naphthoquinone-4-sulfonate R. $C_{10}H_5NaO_5S$.

Description. A yellow or orange, crystalline powder.

Solubility. Soluble in water; insoluble in ethanol (~750 g/l) TS.

Sodium 1,2-naphthoquinone-4-sulfonate (5 g/l) TS. A solution of sodium 1,2-naphthoquinone-4-sulfonate R containing about 5 g of $C_{10}H_5NaO_5S$ per litre.

Sodium nitrite (100 g/l) TS. A solution of sodium nitrite R containing about 100 g of $NaNO_2$ per litre.

Sodium nitrite (3 g/l) TS. A solution of sodium nitrite R containing about 3 g of $NaNO_2$ per litre.
Note: Sodium nitrite (3 g/l) TS must be freshly prepared.

Sodium nitrite (1 g/l) TS. A solution of sodium nitrite R containing about 1 g of $NaNO_2$ per litre.
Note: Sodium nitrite (1 g/l) TS must be freshly prepared.

Sodium nitroprusside R. $Na_2Fe(NO)(CN)_5,2H_2O$ (SRIP, 1963, p. 190).

Sodium nitroprusside (45 g/l) TS. A solution of sodium nitroprusside R containing about 45 g of $Na_2Fe(NO)(CN)_5$ per litre.
Note: Sodium nitroprusside (45 g/l) TS must be freshly prepared.

Sodium tetraborate (10 g/l) TS. A solution of sodium tetraborate R containing about 10 g of $Na_2B_4O_7$ per litre.

Sodium thiosulfate (320 g/l) TS. A solution of sodium thiosulfate R containing about 320 g of $Na_2S_2O_3$ per litre.

Sodium thiosulfate (0.1 mol/l) VS. *Add the following text to volume 1, p. 207: Method of standardization* (alternative procedure). Ascertain the exact concentration of the 0.1 mol/l solution in the following manner: To about 40 ml of water in a glass-stoppered conical flask, add 10.0 ml of potassium bromate (0.0167 mol/l) VS, 1 g of potassium iodide R, and 3 ml of sulfuric acid ($\sim$1760 g/l) TS. Allow the solution to stand for 5 minutes, and titrate the liberated iodine with the sodium thiosulfate solution, adding 3 ml of starch TS as the endpoint is approached. Perform a blank determination on the same quantities of the reagents and make any necessary corrections.

Sodium thiosulfate (0.02 mol/l) VS. Sodium thiosulfate R, dissolved in water to contain 3.164 g of $Na_2S_2O_3$ in 1000 ml.
Method of standardization. Ascertain the exact concentration of the solution following the method described under sodium thiosulfate (0.1 mol/l) VS.

Sodium tungstate R. $Na_2O_4W,2H_2O$ (SRIP, 1963, p. 197).

Sorbitol R. $C_6H_{14}O_6$. Contains not less than 97.0% of $C_6H_{14}O_6$.
Description. White granules or powder or a white, crystalline mass.
Solubility. Very soluble in water; sparingly soluble in ethanol ($\sim$750 g/l) TS; practically insoluble in ether R and chloroform R.
Assay. Dissolve about 0.2 g, previously dried and accurately weighed, in sufficient water to produce 100 ml. Transfer 10.0 ml to an iodine flask, add 50.0 ml of potassium periodate TS, and heat for 15 minutes on a water-bath.

Cool, add 2.5 g of potassium iodide R, stopper tightly, and shake well. Allow to stand for 5 minutes protected from light and titrate with sodium thiosulfate (0.1 mol/l) VS, using 3 ml of starch TS as an indicator. Perform a blank titration and make any necessary corrections. Each ml of sodium thiosulfate (0.1 mol/l) VS is equivalent to 1.822 mg of $C_6H_{14}O_6$.

Storage. Store in a tightly closed container.

Starch iodide TS.

Procedure. Dissolve 0.75 g of potassium iodide R in 5 ml of water and 2 g of zinc chloride R in 10 ml of water, mix the two solutions, and add 100 ml of water. Heat the solution to boiling and add, with constant stirring, a suspension of 5 g of corn or potato starch R in 35 ml of water. Boil for 2 minutes and cool.

Storage. Store in a well-closed container and keep in a cool place.

Strychnine sulfate R. $C_{42}H_{44}N_4O_4,H_2SO_4,5H_2O$ (SRIP, 1963, p. 200).

Sulfamethoxazole RS.   International Chemical Reference Substance.

Sulfamethoxypyridazine RS.   International Chemical Reference Substance.

Sulfamic acid R. H_3NO_3S.

Description. Colourless or white crystals.

Solubility. Soluble in water; slightly soluble in ethanol (~750 g/l) TS.

Sulfamic acid (50 g/l) TS.   A solution of sulfamic acid R containing about 50 g of H_3NO_3S per litre.

Note: Sulfamic acid (50 g/l) TS must be freshly prepared.

Sulfanilamide RS.   International Chemical Reference Substance.

Sulfanilic acid R. $C_6H_7NO_3S$ (SRIP, 1963, p. 201).

Sulfuric acid (~700 g/l) TS.

Procedure. Slowly add sulfuric acid (~1760 g/l) TS to an equal weight of water while gently stirring and cool; d~1.40.

Sulfuric acid (~635 g/l) TS.   Sulfuric acid (~1760 g/l) TS, diluted with water to contain about 635 g of H_2SO_4 per litre; d~1.36.

Sulfuric acid (~570 g/l) TS.

Procedure. Slowly add 3 volumes of sulfuric acid (~1760 g/l) TS to 7 volumes of water while gently stirring and cool; d~1.33.

Sulfuric acid (~50 g/l) TS.

Procedure. To 50 ml of sulfuric acid (~100 g/l) TS add about 50 ml of water and mix.

Sulfuric acid/ethanol TS.

Procedure. Cool separately 10 ml of ethanol (~750 g/l) TS and 90 ml of sulfuric acid (~1760 g/l) TS to about −5 °C. Carefully add the acid to the ethanol, keeping the solution as cool as possible, and mix gently.

Sulfuric acid (0.25 mol/l) VS. Sulfuric acid (~1760 g/l) TS, diluted with water to contain 24.52 g of H_2SO_4 in 1000 ml.

Method of standardization. Ascertain the exact concentration of the solution following the method decribed under sulfuric acid (0.5 mol/l) VS, volume 1, p. 209.

Sulfuric acid (0.1 mol/l) VS. Sulfuric acid (~1760 g/l) TS, diluted with water to contain 9.808 g of H_2SO_4 in 1000 ml.

Method of standardization. Ascertain the exact concentration of the solution following the method described under sulfuric acid (0.5 mol/l) VS, volume 1, p. 209.

Sulfurous acid TS [sulfurous acid R]. (SRIP, 1963, p. 204).

Tartaric acid R. $C_4H_6O_6$ (SRIP, 1963, p. 205).

Tartaric acid (10 g/l) TS. A solution of tartaric acid R containing about 10 g of $C_4H_6O_6$ per litre.

Tartaric acid (5 g/l) TS. A solution of tartaric acid R containing about 5 g of $C_4H_6O_6$ per litre.

Testosterone propionate RS. International Chemical Reference Substance.

Tetrabutylammonium hydroxide (0.1 mol/l) VS.

Procedure. Dissolve 40 g of tetrabutylammonium iodide R in 90 ml of dehydrated ethanol R, add 20 g of finely powdered, purified silver oxide R, and shake vigorously for 1 hour. Centrifuge a small volume of the mixture and test the supernatant liquid for iodides. If a positive reaction is obtained, add an additional 2 g of silver oxide R and shake for a further 30 minutes. Repeat this procedure until the liquid is free from iodides, filter the mixture through a fine sintered glass filter, and rinse the reaction vessel and the filter with 3 quantities of dry benzene R, each of 50 ml. Add the washings to the filtrate and dilute to 1000 ml with dry benzene R. Pass dry carbon-dioxide-free nitrogen R through the solution for 5 minutes.

Method of standardization. Titrate 10 ml of dimethylformamide R with the tetrabutylammonium hydroxide solution, using 3 drops of thymol blue/methanol TS as indicator, until a pure blue colour is obtained. Immediately add about 0.06 g of benzoic acid R, accurately weighed, stir to effect solution, and titrate with the tetrabutylammonium hydroxide solution until the full blue colour of the indicator is again obtained. The solution must be protected from atmospheric carbon dioxide throughout the titration. From the volume of the titrant used in the second titration ascertain the exact concentration of the 0.1 mol/l solution. Each 12.21 mg of benzoic acid is equivalent to 1 ml of tetrabutylammonium hydroxide (0.1 mol/l) VS.

Note: Tetrabutylammonium hydroxide (0.1 mol/l) VS must be standardized immediately before use.

Tetrabutylammonium iodide R. $C_{16}H_{36}IN$. Contains not less than 98.0% of $C_{16}H_{36}IN$.

Description. White or slightly cream-coloured crystals or a crystalline powder.

Solubility. Soluble in ethanol (~750 g/l) TS.

Sulfated ash. Not more than 0.2 mg/g.

Assay. Dissolve about 1.2 g, accurately weighed, in 30 ml of water. Add 50 ml of silver nitrate (0.1 mol/l) VS and 5 ml of nitric acid (~130 g/l) TS. Titrate the excess of silver nitrate with ammonium thiocyanate (0.1 mol/l) VS, using ferric ammonium sulfate (45 g/l) TS as indicator. Each ml of silver nitrate (0.1 mol/l) VS is equivalent to 36.94 mg of $C_{16}H_{36}IN$.

Tetrachloroethane R. 1,1,2,2-Tetrachloroethane, $C_2H_2Cl_4$.

Description. A clear, colourless liquid.

Miscibility. Miscible with 400 parts of water; miscible with ethanol (~750 g/l) TS and ether R.

Boiling range. Not less than 95% distils between 142 and 147 °C.

Refractive index. $n_D^{20} = 1.493–1.495$.

Mass density. $\rho_{20} = 1.590–1.595$ kg/l.

Tetracycline hydrochloride RS. International Chemical Reference Substance.

n-Tetradecane R. $C_{14}H_{30}$.

Description. A clear and colourless liquid.

Miscibility. Miscible with ethanol (~750 g/l) TS.

Mass density. $\rho_{20} =$ about 0.76 kg/l.

Refractive index. $n_D^{20} = 1.428–1.429$.

Tetramethylammonium hydroxide (~100 g/l) TS. Contains about 100 g/l of $(CH_3)_4NOH$ in water.

Description. A clear and colourless liquid; odour, strong, ammonia-like.

Residue on evaporation. Evaporate 5 ml on a water-bath and dry at 105 °C for 1 hour; it leaves a residue of not more than 1.0 mg (0.2 mg/g).

Ammonia and other amines. Weigh accurately a quantity of the solution, equivalent to about 0.3 g of $(CH_3)_4NOH$, in a low-form weighing bottle tared with 5 ml of water. Add a slight excess of hydrochloric acid (1 mol/l) VS (about 4 ml), evaporate to dryness on a water-bath, and dry at 105 °C for 2 hours. The weight of the residue obtained, multiplied by 0.8317, represents the quantity in mg of $(CH_3)_4NOH$ corresponding to within $\pm 0.2\%$ of that found in the assay.

Assay. Weigh accurately a glass-stoppered flask containing about 15 ml of water. Add a quantity of the solution equivalent to about 0.2 g of $(CH_3)_4NOH$, and weigh again. Add methyl red/ethanol TS and titrate with hydrochloric acid (0.1 mol/l) VS. Each ml of hydrochloric acid (0.1 mol/l) VS is equivalent to 9.115 mg of $(CH_3)_4NOH$.

Storage. Store in a tightly closed container.

Tetramethylammonium hydroxide/ethanol TS.

Procedure. Dilute 10 ml of tetramethylammonium hydroxide ($\sim$100 g/l) TS with sufficient ethanol ($\sim$750 g/l) TS to produce 100 ml.

4,4'-Thiodianiline RS. International Chemical Reference Substance.

Note: 4,4'-Thiodianiline RS decomposes on storage, especially on exposure to the air. If a slight decomposition is suspected, the substance can be purified by treatment of a solution in methanol R with activated charcoal.

Thiourea R. CH_4N_2S (SRIP, 1963, p. 207).

Thiourea (0.1 g/l) TS. A solution of thiourea R containing 0.1 g of CH_4N_2S per litre.

Thymol R. $C_{10}H_{14}O$.

Description. Colourless, often large crystals, or a white, crystalline powder; odour, aromatic, resembling that of thyme.

Solubility. Soluble in about 1000 parts of water, in 1 part of ethanol ($\sim$750 g/l) TS, in 1 part of chloroform R, and in 1.5 parts of ether R.

Melting range. Between 48 and 51 °C; when the melted substance is cooled, it remains liquid at a considerably lower temperature.

Residue on volatilization. Volatilize 2 g on a water-bath and dry to constant weight at 105 °C; it leaves a residue of not more than 0.5 mg/g.

Storage. Store in tightly closed containers, protected from light.

Thymol TS1.

Procedure. Dissolve 0.225 g of thymol R in sufficient carbon tetrachloride R to produce 100 ml.

Thymol TS2.

Procedure. Dilute 10 ml of thymol TS1 to 100 ml with carbon tetrachloride R.

Thymol TS3.

Procedure. Dilute 10 ml of thymol TS1 to 150 ml with carbon tetrachloride R.

Thymol blue R. Thymolsulfonphthalein, $C_{27}H_{30}O_5S$ (SRIP, 1963, p. 207).

Thymol blue/dimethylformamide TS.
Procedure. Dissolve 0.3 g of thymol blue R in sufficient dimethylformamide R to produce 100 ml.

Thymol blue/ethanol TS.
Procedure. Dissolve 0.1 g of thymol blue R in sufficient ethanol (~750 g/l) TS to produce 100 ml; filter if necessary.

Thymol blue/methanol TS.
Procedure. Dissolve 0.3 g of thymol blue R in sufficient methanol R to produce 100 ml.

Thymolphthalein/dimethylformamide TS.
Procedure. Dissolve 0.1 g of thymolphthalein R in sufficient dimethylformamide R to produce 100 ml.

Titanium dioxide R. TiO_2.
Description. A white powder; odourless.
Solubility. Practically insoluble in water; slowly soluble, when heated, in sulfuric acid (~1760 g/l) TS.

Titanium dioxide/sulfuric acid TS.
Procedure. To 0.1 g of titanium dioxide R add 100 ml of sulfuric acid (~1760 g/l) TS. Heat cautiously with occasional stirring until a clear solution is effected and fumes are evolved; cool.
Storage. Store in glass-stoppered bottles.

Tolbutamide RS. International Chemical Reference Substance.

4-Toluenesulfonamide R. $C_7H_9NO_2S$.
Melting range. 135–137 °C.

4-Toluenesulfonic acid R. $C_7H_8O_3S,H_2O$. Contains not less than 98.0% of $C_7H_8O_3S$.
Description. Colourless crystals or a white, crystalline powder.
Solubility. Soluble in water, ethanol (~750 g/l) TS and ether R.
Melting range. 100–105 °C.
Sulfated ash. Not more than 1.0 mg/g.
Assay. Dissolve 0.8 g, accurately weighed, in 50 ml of water and titrate with sodium hydroxide (0.1 mol/l) VS, using phenolphthalein/ethanol TS as indicator. Each ml of sodium hydroxide (0.1 mol/l) VS is equivalent to 19.02 mg of $C_7H_8O_3S,H_2O$.

4-Toluenesulfonic acid/ethanol TS.
Procedure. Dissolve 20 g of 4-toluenesulfonic acid R in sufficient ethanol (~750 g/l) TS to produce 100 ml.

Tosylchloramide sodium R. $C_7H_7ClNNaO_2S,3H_2O$. Contains not less than 98.0% of $C_7H_7ClNNaO_2S,3H_2O$.

Description. White crystals or a white, crystalline powder; odour, resembling that of chlorine.

Solubility. Soluble in 7 parts of water and in 2 parts of boiling water; soluble in ethanol (~750 g/l) TS; insoluble in chloroform R and ether R.

Sodium chloride. Treat 1.0 g with 15 ml of dehydrated ethanol R without the aid of heat, and filter; it leaves a residue of not more than 15 mg.

Assay. Dissolve 0.4 g, accurately weighed, in 50 ml of water, placed in a glass-stoppered vessel. Add 10 ml of potassium iodide (80 g/l) TS and 5 ml of sulfuric acid (~100 g/l) TS. Allow to stand for 10 minutes and titrate the liberated iodine with sodium thiosulfate (0.1 mol/l) VS. Each ml of sodium thiosulfate (0.1 mol/l) VS is equivalent to 14.08 mg of $C_7H_7ClNNaO_2S,3H_2O$.

Note: Tosylchloramide sodium R is efflorescent.

Tosylchloramide sodium (15 g/l) TS. A solution of tosylchloramide sodium R containing about 16 g of $C_7H_7ClNNaO_2S$ per litre.

Trichloroacetic acid R. $C_2HCl_3O_2$. (SRIP, 1963, p. 209).

Trichloroethylene R. C_2HCl_3.

Description. A colourless or pale blue, clear, mobile liquid; odour, characteristic, resembling that of chloroform.

Miscibility. Almost immiscible with water; miscible with dehydrated ethanol R, ether R, and chloroform R.

Trichlorotrifluoroethane R. 1,1,2-Trichloro-1,2,2-trifluoroethane. $C_2Cl_3F_3$.

Description. A colourless, volatile liquid.

Miscibility. Immiscible with water; miscible with acetone R and ether R.

Trichlorotrifluoroethane TS.

Procedure. Mix 0.05 μl of trichlorotrifluoroethane R with 1.0 ml of dichloromethane R (other suitable solvents can be used).

Triketohydrindene hydrate R. Ninhydrin, $C_9H_4O_3,H_2O$ (SRIP, 1963, p. 210).

Triketohydrindene/cadmium TS.

Procedure. Dissolve 0.050 g of cadmium acetate R in a mixture of 5 ml of water and 1 ml of glacial acetic acid R and add sufficient ethylmethylketone R to produce 50 ml. Dissolve 20 mg of triketohydrindene hydrate R in 10 ml of this solution.

Note: Prepare immediately before use.

Trimethadione RS. International Chemical Reference Substance.

Trimethoprim RS. International Chemical Reference Substance.

Trimethylpyridine R. $C_8H_{11}N$. 2,4,6-Trimethylpyridine; sym. collidine.
Description. Liquid; odour, aromatic.
Miscibility. More miscible with cold water than with hot water; miscible with ethanol (~750 g/l) TS; ether R, and methanol R.
Relative density. $d_4^{20} = 0.914$.
Refractive index. $n_D^{20} = 1.498$.

Trimethylpyridine (50 g/l) TS. A solution of trimethylpyridine R containing about 50 g of $C_8H_{11}N$ per litre.

Trinitrophenol R. $C_6H_3N_3O_7$ (SRIP, 1963, p. 211).

Trinitrophenol (7 g/l) TS. A solution of trinitrophenol R containing 7 g of $C_6H_3N_3O_7$ per litre.

Trinitrophenol, alkaline, TS.
Procedure. Mix 20 ml of a 10 mg/ml solution of trinitrophenol R with 10 ml of a 50 mg/ml solution of sodium hydroxide R, dilute with water to 100 ml, and mix.
Note: After preparation alkaline trinitrophenol TS should be used for only 48 hours.

Tyrosine R. $C_9H_{11}NO_3$ (SRIP, 1963, p. 212).

Urea R. CH_4N_2O (SRIP, 1963, p. 214).

Vanillin R. $C_8H_8O_3$ (SRIP, 1963, p. 214).

Vanillin (10 g/l) TS. A solution of vanillin R containing about 10 g of $C_8H_8O_3$ per litre.

Water, ammonia-free, R. Water that complies with the following additional test: to 50 ml add 2 ml of alkaline potassio-mercuric iodide TS; no colour is produced.

Water, carbon-dioxide-free and ammonia-free, R. Ammonia-free water R that has been treated as described under carbon-dioxide-free water R, volume 1, p. 211.

Water, sterile, R. Sterile water that complies with the following additional test:
Pyrogens. Carry out the test as described under "Test for pyrogens" (vol. 1, p. 155) injecting, per kg of the rabbit's weight, 10 ml of water that has been rendered isotonic by the addition of pyrogen-free sodium chloride R.

Xylene R. C_8H_{10} (SRIP, 1963, p. 215).

Zinc chloride R. $ZnCl_2$ (SRIP, 1963, p. 217).

Zinc standard (20 μg/ml Zn) TS.

Procedure. To 4.398 g of zinc sulfate R add 1 ml of acetic acid (~300 g/l) TS and dilute with sufficient water to produce 1000 ml. Dilute 1 ml of this solution to 100 ml with water.

Zinc sulfate R. $ZnSO_4,7H_2O$. Contains not less than 99.0% and not more than 105.0% of $ZnSO_4,7H_2O$.

Description. Colourless crystals or a white, crystalline powder; odourless; efflorescent.

Solubility. Very soluble in water; practically insoluble in ethanol (~750 g/l) TS.

Clarity and colour of solution. A 0.05 g/ml solution is clear and colourless.

Chlorides. Dissolve 0.7 g in a mixture of 2 ml of nitric acid (~130 g/l) TS and 30 ml of water, and proceed as described under "Limit test for chlorides" (vol. 1, p. 116); not more than 0.35 mg/g.

Iron. Use 0.4 g; the solution complies with the "Limit test for iron" (vol. 1, p. 121); not more than 0.10 mg/g.

pH value. pH of a 0.05 g/ml solution, 4.4–5.6.

Assay. Dissolve about 0.2 g, accurately weighed, in 5 ml of acetic acid (~60 g/l) TS, and proceed with the titration as described under "Complexometric titrations" (vol. 1, p. 129). Each ml of disodium edetate (0.05 mol/l) VS is equivalent to 14.38 mg of $ZnSO_4,7H_2O$.

Storage. Store at a temperature below 35 °C, in a tightly closed container.

Zirconyl nitrate R. Contains not less than 43.5% and not more than 45.5% of ZrO_2.

Description. A white powder.

Solubility. Soluble in water giving a solution that is clear or not more than faintly turbid.

Assay. Dissolve about 0.1 g, accurately weighed, in 5 ml of sulfuric acid (~1760 g/l) TS and add carefully 50 ml of water. Add, with stirring, 5 ml of hydrogen peroxide (~330 g/l) TS and 350 ml of diammonium hydrogen phosphate (100 g/l) TS. Add 40 ml of sulfuric acid (~1760 g/l) TS and keep the mixture at a temperature of 40–50 °C for 2 hours. Filter and wash with not more than 200 ml of cold ammonium nitrate (50 g/l) TS until the washings no longer give the reaction A for orthophosphates described under "General identification tests" (vol. 1, p. 114). Dry and ignite to constant weight. Each g of residue is equivalent to 0.4647 g of ZrO_2.

Zirconyl nitrate TS.

Procedure. Dissolve 0.1 g of zirconyl nitrate R in a mixture of 60 ml of hydrochloric acid (~420 g/l) TS and 40 ml of water.

INDEX

INDEX

For the convenience of users of volume 2, the reagents, test solutions, and volumetric solutions described in volume 1 are also listed in this index. The numbers printed in bold type, preceding the page numbers, indicate the volume in which the indexed item is to be found.

T